PROGRESS IN CLINICAL AND BIOLOGICAL RESEARCH

Series Editors
Nathan Back
George J. Brewer

Vincent P. Eijsvoogel
Robert Grover
Kurt Hirschhorn

Seymour S. Kety
Sidney Udenfriend
Jonathan W. Uhr

RECENT TITLES

ANIMAL MODELS OF
INHERITED METABOLIC DISEASES

ANIMAL MODELS OF INHERITED METABOLIC DISEASES

Proceedings of the International Symposium
on Animal Models of Inherited Metabolic Disease
Held in Bethesda, Maryland
October 19–20, 1981

Editors

Robert J. Desnick, Ph.D., M.D.
Chief, Division of Medical Genetics
Mount Sinai School of Medicine
New York, New York

Donald F. Patterson, D.V.M., D. Sc.
Chief, Section of Medical Genetics
School of Veterinary Medicine
University of Pennsylvania
Philadelphia, Pennsylvania

Dante G. Scarpelli, M.D., Ph.D.
Chairman, Department of Pathology
Northwestern University Medical School
Chicago, Illinois

ALAN R. LISS, INC. • NEW YORK

Address all Inquiries to the Publisher
Alan R. Liss, Inc., 150 Fifth Avenue, New York, NY 10011

Copyright © 1982 Alan R. Liss, Inc.

Printed in the United States of America.

Library of Congress Cataloging in Publication Data

Main entry under title:

Animal models of inherited metabolic diseases.

(Progress in clinical and biological research;
v. 94)

Based on the papers presented at the symposium held in Oct. 1981, at the National Institutes of Health, sponsored by the Registry of Comparative Pathology of the Armed Forces Institute of Pathology, and by the Universities Associated for Research and Education in Pathology, Inc.

Includes index and bibliographies.

1. Metabolism, Inborn errors of--Animal models--Congresses.   I. Desnick, Robert J.   II. Patterson, Donald F.   III. Scarpelli, Dante G., 1927-
IV. Registry of Comparative Pathology.
V. Universities Associated for Research and Education in Pathology.   VI. Series.   [DNLM: 1. Disease models, Animal.   2. Models, Genetic--Congresses.
3. Metabolism, Inborn errors--Congresses.   W1
PR668E v.94 / WD 205 A598 1981]
RC627.8.A54   616.3'907   82-8961
ISBN 0-8451-0094-7   AACR2

Contents

Contributors

Robert J. Adams, D.V.M. [449]
Assistant Professor, Division of Comparative Medicine, The Johns Hopkins University School of Medicine, 601 North Wolfe Street, Baltimore, MD 21205

David M. Alessi, B.S. [165]
Department of Pathology, Michigan State University, East Lansing, MI 48824

Thaddeus Anderson, V.M.D. [435]
School of Veterinary Medicine, The University of Pennsylvania, 39th and Pine Streets H1, Philadelphia, PA 19104

W. French Anderson, M.D., Ph.D. [11]
Chief, Laboratory of Molecular Hematology, National Heart, Lung, and Blood Institute, Department of Health and Human Services, National Institutes of Health, Bethesda, MD 20205

A.M. Appel, Ph.D. [213]
Research Assistant Professor of Medicine, Department of Pediatrics, The Children's Hospital of Buffalo, State University of New York, 219 Bryant Street, Buffalo, NY 14222

G.D. Aurbach, M.D. [353]
National Institute of Arthritis, Diabetes, and Digestive and Kidney Diseases, Department of Health and Human Services, National Institutes of Health, Bethesda, MD 20205

Henry J. Baker, D.V.M. [203,213]
Professor and Chairman, Department of Comparative Medicine, The University of Alabama at Birmingham, University Station, Birmingham, AL 35294

Kurt Bernirschke, Ph.D., M.D. [1]
Professor of Pathology and Reproductive Medicine, University of California; Director of Research, Zoological Society of San Diego, San Diego, CA 92112

Fred G. Biddle, Ph.D. [309]
Assistant Professor, Departments of Medical Biochemistry and Pediatrics, University of Calgary, Faculty of Medicine, Calgary, Alberta T2N 1N4 Canada

The boldface number in brackets following each contributor's name indicates the opening page number of that author's article.

Kenneth C. Bovee, D.V.M., M.Med.Sc. [435]
Corinne R. and Henry Bower Professor of Medicine, Chairman, Department of Clinical Studies, School of Veterinary Medicine, University of Pennsylvania, 3800 Spruce Street, Philadelphia, PA 19104

Kenneth S. Brown, M.D. [245,251]
Laboratory of Development Biology and Anomalies, National Institute of Dental Research, Department of Health and Human Sciences, National Institutes of Health, Bethesda, MD 20205

Scott Brown, V.M.D. [435]
School of Veterinary Medicine, University of Pennsylvania, 39th and Pine Streets H1, Philadelphia, PA 19104

Leslie P. Bullock, D.V.M. [369]
Associate Professor, Comparative Medicine, Senior Research Associate, Medicine, The Milton S. Hershey Medical Center, The Pennsylvania State University, Hershey, PA 17033

Linda C. Cork, D.V.M., Ph.D. [449]
Assistant Professor, Division of Comparative Medicine and Department of Pathology, The Johns Hopkins University School of Medicine, 514 Pathology, 601 North Wolfe Street, Baltimore, MD 21205

James G. Cunningham, D.V.M. [165]
Associate Professor, Department of Physiology, Michigan State University, East Lansing, MI 48824

Albert W. Dade, D.V.M., Ph.D. [165]
Professor, Department of Pathology, Tuskegee Institute, Tuskegee, AL 36088

Beverly A. Dale, Ph.D. [251]
Research Associate Professor, Departments of Medicine and Periodontics, The University of Washington, Seattle, WA 98195

Glyn Dawson, Ph.D. [165]
Associate Professor of Pediatrics and Biochemistry, Department of Biochemistry, University of Chicago, Chicago, IL 60637

Robert J. Desnick, Ph.D., M.D. [xv,27,177]
Arthur J. and Nellie Z. Cohen Professor of Pediatrics and Genetics, Chief, Division of Medical Genetics, Mount Sinai School of Medicine, 100th Street and Fifth Avenue, New York, NY 10029

W. Jean Dodds, D.V.M. [117]
Research Director of Laboratories for Veterinary Science, Division of Laboratories and Research, New York State Department of Health, Empire State Plaza, Albany, NY 12201

Jan M. Friedman, M.D., Ph.D. [459]
Assistant Professor of Obstetrics and Gynecology and Pediatrics, Head, Division of Clinical Genetics, University of Texas Health Science Center, 5323 Harry Hines Boulevard, Dallas, TX 75235

Lauretta W. Gerrity, D.V.M. [459]
Research Fellow, Division of Clinical Genetics, Department of Obstetrics and Gynecology, University of Texas Health Science Center, 5323 Harry Hines Boulevard, Dallas, TX 75235

M.H. Goldschmidt, B.VMS., M.Sc. [435]
Assistant Professor, Department of Pathology, School of Veterinary

Medicine, University of Pennsylvania, 39th and Pine Streets H1, Philadelphia, PA 19174

John W. Griffin, M.D. [449]
Associate Professor, Department of Neurology, The Johns Hopkins University School of Medicine, 601 North Wolfe Street, Baltimore, MD 21205

Jean-Louis Guenet, D.V.M., D.Sc. [265]
Institut Pasteur de Paris, 75724 Paris, France

Leslie C. Harne, [245,251]
Laboratory of Development Biology and Anomalies, National Institute of Dental Research, Department of Health and Human Services, National Institutes of Health, Bethesda, MD 20205

Mark E. Haskins, V.M.D., Ph.D. [27,93,177]
Assistant Professor, Sections of Pathology and Medical Genetics, School of Veterinary Medicine and Genetics Center, The University of Pennsylvania, 39th and Pine Streets H1, Philadelphia, PA 19104

Gerald A. Hegreberg D.V.M., Ph.D. [229]
Associate Professor, Department of Veterinary Microbiology and Pathology, Washington State University, Pullman, WA 99164

Karen A. Holbrook, Ph.D. [251]
Research Associate Professor, Departments of Biological Structure and Medicine, The University of Washington, Seattle, WA 98195

Peter F. Jezyk, V.M.D., Ph.D. [93,177]
Associate Professor of Medicine, Section of Medical Genetics, School of Veterinary Medicine and Genetics Center, The University of Pennsylvania, 39th and Pine Streets H1, Philadelphia, PA 19104

Robert D. Jolly, V.M.D., D.Sc. [145]
Reader, Department of Veterinary Pathology, Faculty of Veterinary Science, Massey University, Palmerston North, New Zealand

Margaret Z. Jones, M.D. [5,165]
Professor, Department of Pathology, Michigan State University, East Lansing, MI 48824

T.C. Jones, D.V.M. [5]
Professor, Department of Comparative Medicine, Harvard Medical School, New England Regional Primate Research Center, Southborough, MA 01772

Roger A. Laine, Ph.D. [165]
Associate Professor, Department of Biochemistry, University of Kentucky, Lexington, KY 40536

Trevor Lukey, M.Sc. [309]
Departments of Medical Biochemistry and Pediatrics, University of Calgary, Faculty of Medicine, Calgary, Alberta T2N 1N4 Canada

Nancy S. Magnuson, Ph.D. [271]
Assistant Professor, Department of Veterinary Microbiology and Pathology, Washington State University, Pullman, WA 99164

Pierre Maroteaux, M.D. [265]
Hôpital Necker – Enfants Malades, Institut Pasteur de Paris, 75724 Paris, France

James Martinell, Ph.D. [11]
Laboratory of Molecular Hematology, National Heart, Lung, and Blood

Institute, Department of Health and Human Services, National Institutes of Health, Bethesda, MD 20205

Margaret M. McGovern, Ph.D. [27,177]
Division of Medical Genetics, Mount Sinai School of Medicine, 100th Street and Fifth Avenue, New York, NY 10029

George Migaki, D.V.M. [473]
Chief Pathologist, Registry of Comparative Pathology, Armed Forces Institute of Pathology, Washington, D.C. 20306

Ulreh V. Mostosky, D.V.M. [165]
Professor, Department of Small Animal Surgery and Medicine, Michigan State University, East Lansing, MI 48824

William G. Nash, Ph.D. [67]
Section of Genetics, Laboratory of Viral Carcinogenesis, National Cancer Institute, Frederick, MD 21701

Stephen J. O'Brien, Ph.D. [67]
Section of Genetics, Laboratory of Viral Carcinogenesis, National Cancer Institute, Frederick, MD 21701

Donald F. Patterson, D.V.M., D.Sc. [xv,93,177,505]
Professor of Veterinary Medicine and Genetics, Chief, Section of Medical Genetics, School of Veterinary Medicine, University of Pennsylvania, 39th and Pine Streets H1, Philadelphia, PA 19104

Lance E. Perryman, D.V.M., Ph.D. [271]
Associate Professor, Department of Veterinary Microbiology and Pathology, Washington State University, Pullman, WA 99164

Raymond A. Popp, Ph.D. [11]
Oak Ridge National Laboratory, Oak Ridge, TN 37830

Michel Potier, Ph.D. [221]
Associate Professor, Hospital St. Justine, University of Montreal, C.P. 6128 Succursale A, Montreal, Quebec H3C 3J7 Canada

Donald L. Price, M.D. [449]
Professor of Neurology and Pathology, Division of Neuropathology, Departments of Pathology and Neurology, The Johns Hopkins University School of Medicine, 601 North Wolfe Street, Baltimore, MD 21205

Mario C. Rattazzi, M.D. [203,213]
Professor, The Children's Hospital of Buffalo, Department of Pediatrics, State University of New York, 219 Bryant Street, Buffalo, NY 14222

Roger H. Reeves, B.S. [67]
Section of Genetics, Laboratory of Viral Carcinogenesis, National Cancer Institute, Frederick, MD 21701

John C. Roder, Ph.D. [315]
Assistant Professor, Department of Microbiology and Immunology, Queens University, Kingston, Ontario K7L 3N6 Canada

Dante G. Scarpelli, M.D., Ph.D. [xv]
Magerstadt Professor and Chairman, Department of Pathology, Northwestern University Medical School, Chicago, IL 60611

Edward H. Schuchman, B.S. [27]
Division of Medical Genetics, Mount Sinai School of Medicine, 100th Street and Fifth Avenue, New York, NY 10029

Stanton Segal, M.D. [435]
Professor of Pediatrics, Children's Hospital of Pennsylvania, Philadelphia, PA 19104

Jules R. Selden, V.M.D. [381]
Research Associate, Section of Cell Surface Immunogenetics, Sloan-Kettering Institute for Cancer Research, 1275 York Avenue, New York, NY 10021

Harvey S. Singer, M.D. [203]
Associate Professor of Neurology, The Johns Hopkins Hospital, Baltimore, MD 21205

Joseph E. Smith, D.V.M., Ph.D. [421]
Professor, Department of Pathology, College of Veterinary Medicine, Kansas State University, Veterinary Medical Center, Manhattan, KS 66506

Floyd F. Snyder, Ph.D. [309]
Assistant Professor, Departments of Medical Biochemistry and Pediatrics, The University of Calgary, Faculty of Medicine, Calgary, Alberta T2N 1N4 Canada

Marcia J. Sparling, B.Sc. [309]
Departments of Medical Biochemistry and Pediatrics, The University of Calgary, Calgary, Alberta T2N 1N4 Canada

Ritta Stanescu, M.D. [265]
Hôpital Necker – Enfants Malades, Institut Pasteur de Paris, 75724 Paris, France

Viktor Stanescu, M.D. [265]
Hôpital Necker – Enfants Malades, Institut Pasteur de Paris, 75724 Paris, France

Deborah T. Vine, M.D. [177]
Division of Medical Genetics, Mount Sinai School of Medicine, 100th Street and Fifth Avenue, New York, NY 10029

Joseph R. Vorro, Ph.D. [165]
Associate Professor, Department of Anatomy, Michigan State University, East Lansing, MI 48824

Steven U. Walkley, D.V.M., Ph.D. [203]
Assistant Professor, Department of Neuroscience, Albert Einstein College of Medicine, Bronx, NY 10461

Ada L.M. Watson, B.A. [327]
Immunogenetics Laboratory Supervisor, Division of Immunogenetics, Sidney Farber Cancer Institute, 44 Binney Street, Boston, MA 02115

Harold L. Watson, M.S. [203]
Research Assistant, Department of Comparative Medicine, The University of Alabama at Birmingham, University Station, Birmingham, AL 35294

J. Barry Whitney III, Ph.D. [11,133]
Assistant Professor, Department of Cell and Molecular Biology, Medical College of Georgia, Augusta, GA 30912

Christine S.F Williams, D.V.M. [165]
Associate Professor, Department of Pathology, Michigan State University, East Lansing, MI 48824

Cheryl A. Winkler, M.S. [67]
Section of Genetics, Laboratory of Viral Carcinogenesis, National Cancer Institute, Frederick, MD 21701

Robert W. Wissler, Ph.D., M.D. [xv]
Professor, Department of Pathology, The University of Chicago, Chicago, IL 60637

George L. Wolff, Ph.D. [463]
National Center for Toxicological Research, Food and Drug Administration, Jefferson, AR 72079

James E. Womack, Ph.D. [221]
Associate Professor, Department of Veterinary Pathology, Texas A&M University, College Station, TX 77843

Philip A. Wood, D.V.M., M.S. [203]
Fellow, Department of Comparative Medicine, The University of Alabama at Birmingham, University Station, Birmingham, AL 35294

Denise L.S. Yan, B.S. [221]
Department of Veterinary Pathology, Texas A&M University, College Station, TX 77843

Edmond J. Yunis, M.D. [327]
Chief, Division of Immunogenetics, Professor of Pathology, Sidney Farber Cancer Institute, Harvard Medical School, 44 Binney Street, Boston, MA 02115

Preface

In October 1981, veterinarians, physicians and scientists from several continents convened at the National Institutes of Health to discuss their most recent studies on animal models of human disease. This symposium—"Animal Models of Inherited Metabolic Disease"—was sponsored by the Registry of Comparative Pathology of the Armed Forces Institute of Pathology, and by the Universities Associated for Research and Education in Pathology, Inc. The chapters in this book are based on the papers presented at the symposium.

The symposium was supported in part by a grant (RR 00301) from the Division of Research Resources, National Institutes of Health. In addition, we acknowledge the generous support of the Charles River Breeding Laboratories, Inc. and Hazelton Research Animals, Inc.

We hope that the scientific information recorded in this volume will not only provide a resource for veterinarians and physicians, but will stimulate efforts to identify and characterize new animal models of human disease. It is anticipated that the study of animal models will provide further insights into the molecular pathology of their human counterparts, and based on this information, the design and evaluation of new therapeutic strategies. Such studies should ultimately lead to better health care and effective treatment for the many patients and families who suffer from these unfortunate "experiments of nature".

R.J. Desnick, Ph.D., M.D.
D.F. Patterson, D.V.M., D.Sc.
D.G. Scarpelli, M.D., Ph.D.

INTRODUCTION AND ACKNOWLEDGEMENTS

Robert W. Wissler, Ph.D., M.D.

Department of Pathology
The University of Chicago
Chicago, Illinois 60637

It is my privilege to introduce and welcome you to this symposium and to what we believe will be a very lively and thought provoking monograph. The monograph is designed to provide the biochemical scientific community with new information and innovative possibilities for developing new animal models of genetic disease.

The Scientific Advisory Committee of the Registry, which I chaired at that time, developed the concepts for this symposium. It was recognized that there was a great unfulfilled need for "recognition and preservation of genetic disorders which otherwise might be lost." It was the hope that many of the mutations which now go unrecognized would be observed and preserved if it became clearer to veterinarians and pathologists what some of the needs are. It also seemed to us at that time that the types of clues of linkage of genetic models to hair coat, odor, age at death, enzyme and electrophoretic parameters, etc., needed to be more widely recognized and utilized if astute observation and follow-up were to help in the identification and preservation of new and valuable mutations which might otherwise be inadvertently discarded.

This was planned as a companion for the "Workshop on Needs for New Animal Models of Human Disease" which was held here in 1980 under the leadership of Dr. Donald Hackel. The resulting publication in the American Journal of Pathology and widespread distribution, along with much of the excellent discussion that occurred, has been widely recognized as an important contribution to comparative pathology and to the experimental pathology of human disease of the future.

The grant which supports the Registry of Comparative Pathology is from the Animal Resources Branch, Division of Research Resources, National Institutes of Health. I do want to acknowledge and highlight this support because it has been seminal in the many pioneering efforts that this Registry has successfully undertaken. Dr. Dante Scarpelli and I have been the principal links of this Registry to the Board of Directors of Universities Associated for Research and Education in Pathology which has, from the Registry's inception, been its main sponsor and has, over and above our grant-related relationship, recognized the value of comparative pathology and provided a constant source of intellectual support and interest which needs to be emphasized as we open this symposium. Also providing valuable support and use of its facilities is the Armed Forces Institute of Pathology where the Registry is located.

The committee that set about to develop this program included not only the Scientific Advisory Committee of the Registry, chaired by Dr. Dante Scarpelli and consisting of Drs. C.C. Capen, D.B. Hackel, T.C. Jones, R.M. Lewis, and G. Majno along with staff (Drs. G. Migaki and S.R. Jones), but also three valuable special consultants, Drs. D.F. Patterson, R.J. Desnick, and G.A. Hegreberg. They have developed a program which we feel provides an excellent reflection of the ultramodern contributions being made in the areas of genetic modeling for the understanding of human diseases. We believe that the contributors they have chosen and the time provided for free-flowing discussion should lead to new concepts and plans for recognizing and preserving badly needed genetic models of disease.

Finally, I want to recognize several hidden heroes and heroines of this planning process and of the valuable volume which it has yielded.

First and foremost, there is Dr. George Migaki, the Chief Pathologist for the Registry of Comparative Pathology. As is true with almost everything the Registry does, Dr. Migaki has played a key role in planning, implementing and preparing these proceedings for publication. In this he has been assisted, not only by the Scientific Advisory

Committee to the Registry and the special consultants mentioned above, but also by Merryanna Swartz, his able Research Assistant, and Charmaine Goetz, the most capable Senior Secretary of the Registry. We also want to acknowledge with gratitude the financial assistance of the Charles River Breeding Laboratories and Hazleton Research Animals, Inc.

We have had extraordinary help from Dr. John Holman of the Animal Resources Branch in developing the arrangements for this meeting in Building 31 at the National Institutes of Health. We appreciate the skillful work of John Bowers and his co-workers in recording and transcribing the discussions so these could be corrected for publication while the participants are in attendance.

A special dividend of this symposium and its publication will be an exemplary "Compendium of Inherited Metabolic Diseases in Animals," worked up by Dr. Migaki and his staff with special assistance from Charlotte Kenton of the National Library of Medicine. Included are many models and references gleaned from the brand new "Bibliography of Naturally Occurring Animal Models of Human Disease" (and its companion volume on Induced Animal Models) edited by Drs. Gerald Hegreberg and Charles Leathers, Washington State University School of Veterinary Medicine in Pullman. It was also valuable, as Dr. Migaki points out in his introduction to the compendium and its bibliography, to be able to utilize the rather recent two volume work on "Spontaneous Animal Models of Human Disease" published by Academic Press and compiled by Drs. E.J. Andrews, B.C. Ward, and N.H. Altman. Of course, he utilized our favorite source, i.e., the Registry's own handbook: Animal Models of Human Disease, which has now developed into a valuable resource with ten fascicles and 232 models, many of which are of special relevance to this monograph.

Thus begins what Dr. Scarpelli and I believe will be a most successful symposium which, if we all do our part, should bring together the best thinking of ways to increase the yield of Animal Models of Inherited Metabolic Diseases which will be identified, preserved and utilized in the next ten years.

Animal Models of Inherited Metabolic Diseases, pages 1-3
© 1982 Alan R. Liss, Inc., 150 Fifth Avenue, New York, NY 10011

INTRODUCTORY REMARKS
SYMPOSIUM ON ANIMAL MODELS OF INHERITED METABOLIC DISEASES

Kurt Benirschke, M.D.

Professor of Pathology and Reproductive Medicine
University of California, San Diego
La Jolla, California
and
Director of Research
San Diego Zoo
San Diego, California

It is ironic that while we hold a conference on the
usefulness and methods of identification of "animal models
of inherited metabolic disease" there are a number of bills
being considered on the Hill that would severely limit the
use of animals in research, if not eliminate it altogether.
We are incredulous of these activities because of our
knowledge that insights gained from such models have materially aided us in a better understanding of human disease
and thereby helping to combat it or, at times, even eliminate its curses. Clearly, we owe a deep gratitude to
animals that have given us this insight and must persevere
in their proper and humane employment for biomedical
research purposes. As one person who has upheld the notion
of "one medicine," convinced of the conservation employed
in genetic structure and biological mechanisms, I have recently benefited from the reverse situation, the use of a
well-understood human genetic error in gaining insight into
a disease of lemurs. In pectus excavatum, the dominant
mode of inheritance and relative innocuous nature of this
human condition was mirrored when a similar if not identical condition was discovered in the black and white ruffed
lemur, Lemur variegatus (Benirschke, 1980). Thus, biological knowledge in man was able to contribute materially
in breeding programs designed to rescue a very severely
endangered species. My recent exposure to endangered
species allows me to state unequivocally that "one medicine"

is indeed a viable and most necessary concept for the future. And it is with this in mind that I would like to introduce the first session of this symposium.

By-and-large, most inborn errors of metabolism have been considered to be the result of homozygosity of autosomal genes carried in the heterozygous state by apparently normal individuals. Employing specially designed testing schemes it is at times possible to identify these heterozygous carriers. In general, this is the case only once the metabolic abnormality is fully understood through intense study of affected individuals. When the disease is uncommon or when it is lethal at early ages it may be difficult to obtain this knowledge from the study of afflicted patients. In such circumstances then, the availability of appropriate models may be of invaluable help. In other cases, the ability to modulate the disease by experimental therapy in animal models is of utmost benefit to affected patients. This concept has now been expanded by recent studies of hemoglobinopathies to add the important role of noncoding sequences (introns) and flanking regions with assumed regulatory roles. This necessitates a rethinking of these previous notions of inherited disease and forms a basis for this conference. In a broader sense, the comparison of genetic defects in animals with those that are similar or identical in humans also gives valuable evolutionary insights and is indeed crossfertilizing. And it is with these thoughts that knowledge gained from the genetics of experimental animals helps to understand and combat human disease that this symposium was conceived. After years of cataloguing animal models for human disease and making the knowledge of the past available to a wider circle of scientists through the Registry of Comparative Pathology it was felt necessary to bring into clearer focus the broader common aspects of inborn errors, namely the genetic basis, the means of detection, and the common biological parameters. How can we learn to better understand the nucleic acid anomalies that we subsume to be the basis of the mutation? Are there better means to detect new animal models than their random discovery by accident? It is time we redirect our thinking of the future of animal models. It is probably wasteful to hope that the right model for such a disease as cystic fibrosis will just happen along. Instead, it may be more judicious to rapidly inbreed potential heterozygotes and more rapidly screen for abnormalities, a process that has led to so much progress in the understanding of the genetics of mice. To enhance this process of discovery we chose to bring together representatives of different disciplines to bring their most modern views and knowledge to this conference. We will open then our first portion of the symposium with a consideration of the genetic basis of disease and hear from Dr. Nienhuis on "Gene Structure, Organization, and Expression."

Benirschke K (1980). Pectus excavatum in ruffed lemurs (Lemur (Varecia) variegatus). In XXII International Symposium Erkrank. Zootiere, Berlin: Akademic-Verlag, pp 169-172.

Animal Models of Inherited Metabolic Diseases, pages 5-7
© **1982 Alan R. Liss, Inc., 150 Fifth Avenue, New York, NY 10011**

ANIMAL MODELS OF INHERITED METABOLIC DISEASE - AN OVERVIEW

T.C. Jones, D.V.M.

Harvard Medical School

New England Regional Primate Research Center
Southborough, Massachusetts

This publication is part of a continuing program of communication among scientists interested in research on disease problems in man and other animals. Among the barriers to effective use of animal models in the study of human disease problems are the dfficulties of communication between investigators of differing disciplines and objectives. Other publications on this theme resulting from the sponsorship of the Registry of Comparative Pathology at the Armed Forces Institute of Pathology are listed in the references to follow.

The papers in this volume, along with the comments and questions raised by the participants, stimulates one to reflect upon the contributions to the understanding and control of infectious diseases of man and animals made by investigators and health workers in the past two centuries. Revolutionary changes in combating disease started slowly in the eighteenth century with such pioneers as Edward Jenner; continued in the nineteenth century by scientists symbolized by Louis Pasteur, and built upon by a small but dedicated cadre in the twentieth century. Almost all of the plagues of the early 1900's which took their toll in death and suffering from man and animals are now either eradicated or under control in the United States. Animal models played a significant part in leading to the understanding of infectious diseases and made their control possible. Most of the resources now available for the study of inherited diseases would probably not exist were it not for the great triumphs over infectious diseases in the late nineteenth and twentieth centuries.

It is interesting to note the increased number of inherited animal models of disease in which a defective enzyme has been identified and found to be chemically identical to the affected enzyme in the human disease. The deficient enzyme invariable points toward a defective gene. Chemically identical single defective enzymes, for example, have been identified in human patients and other species with gangliosidoses. A further example: all but one of the specific inherited defects in blood coagulation recognized in human patients have now been identified in at least one animal species. In the reports that follow, more examples will be added to the close parallels of metabolic disease in man and other animals.

Does the repeated occurrence of mutations in several species at the same or comparable part of the genome indicate a point of increased vulnerability? Or is this simply a result of the manner in which the abnormal human and animal phenotypes are distinguished from the rest of the population? Is it also possible that past emphasis placed on certain lines of research has led to identification of some model systems and not others? The number of animal models of metabolic disease which have been identified and studied has reached a point at which more scientific and philosophical questions may be answered. This symposium has provided a broader basis for the consideration of the value and future use of specific animal models.

In the papers which follow in this volume, one will find examples of the perceptive study of animal and human disease in concert, with comparisons giving new insights into the nature of the animal as well as the human disease. The unity and the diversity in nature become increasingly evident from studies such as described in these pages.

Listed below are publications sponsored by the Registry of Comparative Pathology which deal with comparative aspects of disease in humans and animals:

Comparative Pathology Bulletin, Registry of Comparative Pathology, Armed Forces Institute of Pathology, Washington, published quarterly since 1969.

"Comparative Morphology of Hematopoietic Neoplasms," National Cancer Institute Monograph 32, National Institutes of Health, Bethesda, 1969.

Animal Models of Human Disease, American Journal of Pathology, a description of an animal model published in each issue since January 1972.

"Handbook: Animal Models of Human Disease," Registry of Comparative Pathology, Armed Forces Institute of Pathology, Washington, yearly fascicles since 1972.

"Hemoglobin: Comparative Molecular Biology Models for the Study of Disease," Annals of the New York Academy of Sciences, Volume 241, 1974.

"The Pathology of Fishes," The University of Wisconsin Press, Madison, 1975.

"Animals as Monitors of Environmental Pollutants," National Academy of Sciences, Washington, 1979.

"Comparative Pathology of Zoo Animals," Smithsonian Institution Press, Washington, 1980.

Needs for New Animal Models of Human Disease, American Journal of Pathology, December 1980 Supplement.

SECTION I.
GENETIC BASIS OF DISEASE

Animal Models of Inherited Metabolic Diseases, pages 11–26
© **1982 Alan R. Liss, Inc., 150 Fifth Avenue, New York, NY 10011**

MOUSE MODELS OF HUMAN THALASSEMIA

W. French Anderson, James Martinell,
J. Barry Whitney, III,* and Raymond A. Popp**
Laboratory of Molecular Hematology
National Heart, Lung, and Blood Institute
National Institutes of Health
Bethesda, Maryland 20205

The group of diseases called the thalassemias is the largest single-gene health problem in the world according the World Health Organization. The thalassemias are lethal hereditary anemias in which the infants cannot make their own blood. Patients with homozygous α-thalassemia, in which there is an inability to make the α-globin chains, are normally stillborn, suffering the condition called hydrops fetalis. Patients homozygous for β-thalassemia, in which there is an inability to make the β-globin chains, must be transfused every 3 to 4 weeks starting at approximately 6 months of age for the rest of their lives. With modern care, these patients now can live into their twenties. This latter condition is called Cooley's anemia, named after Dr. Thomas Cooley, who first described the disease in 1925. The details of the clinical syndromes are described in hematology textbooks.

---

* Present address: Department of Cell and Molecular
  Biology, Medical College of Georgia,
  Augusta, Georgia 30912

** Address: Oak Ridge National Laboratory
  Oak Ridge, Tennessee 37830

Thanks to the methodological advances resulting from recombinant DNA technology, the molecular organization of the globin gene loci are known for a number of animals (human, several primates, sheep, goat, rabbit, mouse, and chicken). The human globin loci are shown in Figure 1. The α-like globin genes are on human chromosome 16 and the β-like genes on chromosome 11. In each case the transcription of globin mRNA is from left to right (as drawn), and the order of activation of the genes during development is also from left to right. Thus, the left hand genes, zeta and epsilon, are expressed during embryologic; development then the alpha and gamma genes are activated during the fetal period, and finally the adult delta and beta globin genes are switched on after birth. The hemoglobins found during each developmental period are listed on the figure.

The mouse globin loci have a similar organization. The mouse equivalent of the human zeta gene is x; the mouse equivalents of the epsilon gene are y and z. There does not appear to be in the mouse a gene which is exactly equivalent to the human fetal globin gene. Therefore, the human/mouse equivalents are:

$$
\begin{array}{lll}
\underline{\text{Human}} & & \underline{\text{Mouse}} \\
\text{Gower 1 } (\zeta_2\varepsilon_2) & \longrightarrow \text{EI} & (x_2y_2) \\[4pt]
\text{Gower 2 } (\alpha_2\varepsilon_2) & \longrightarrow \begin{cases} \text{EII} & (\alpha_2y_2) \\ \text{EIII} & (\alpha_2z_2) \end{cases} \\[8pt]
\text{A } (\alpha_2\beta_2) & \text{Adult} & (\alpha_2\beta_2)
\end{array}
$$

Mice have a number of globin gene alleles at both the α and the β loci. There are, in addition, two α- and two β-globin genes so that each strain of mouse can have one or two types of α- and one or two types of β-globin. Consequently, the planning and interpretation of experiments involving the mouse globin genes is rather complex. To simplify the discussion below, I will omit all genetic information except that which is required. The references provide complete information.

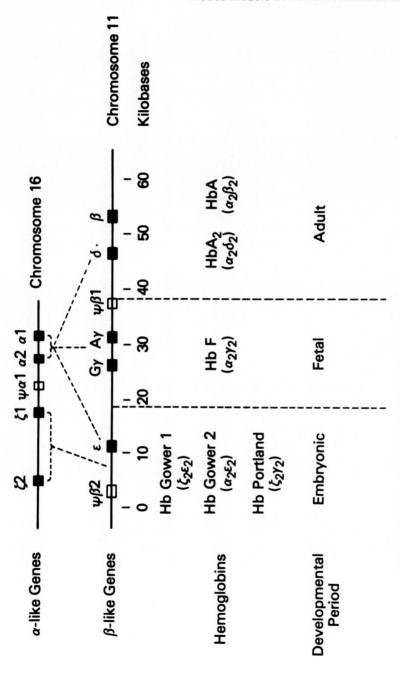

Figure 1. Organization of the human globin genes.

MOUSE MODELS

Three stocks of mice, two from the Oak Ridge National Laboratory and one from the Jackson Laboratory, have an abnormality in their ability to synthesize α-globin chains.

Oak Ridge Mice: A large scale mutagenic project aimed at finding abnormalities at the globin loci in mice was carried out at the Oak Ridge National Laboratory in 1973 (Russell et al., 1976). 8621 progeny of irradiated males or females were examined for hemoglobin abnormalities; five were positive. Of these five, 3 were found to have sustained a loss of α-globin synthesis from the irradiated parent (the other two were: a tandem duplication involving the part of mouse chromosome 7 carrying the β-globin locus, and a double non-dysjunction involving chromosome 7). Of the three α-thalassemia type mutants, one was sterile. Therefore, two mouse mutants have been propagated and are called 27HB and 352HB (after the original "number" 27 female and number 352 male who were the F1 offspring of two different irradiated males; HB stands for hemoglobin). The 27HB and 352HB mutations have been placed onto a number of genetic backgrounds.

Jackson Laboratory Mouse: Dr. Barry Whitney screened approximately 500 progeny of mice, which had been subjected to chemical mutagenesis for other reasons, for globin chain abnormalities (Whitney and Russell, 1980). He found no structural chain mutations, but he did find one mouse who was unable to make α-globin chains from one of his two chromosomes. This mouse was the offspring of a male which had been injected with the mutagen triethylene-melamine. He named the globin mutation in this mouse, Hba^{th-J}. This mutation, also, has been put on a number of genetic backgrounds.

Phenotypic Characteristics

Since the thalassemia mutation is lethal in the homozygous state (see below), all studies have been done on heterozygotes. The three thalassemic mutations appear similar. Each produces a microcytic, hypochromic anemia. They have elevated reticulocytes and red blood cell

TABLE 1. Hematologic Values for Progeny of 27HB Mice

α/β ratio	Retic. (%)	Hct (%)	Hb (g/dl)	RBC (x10^6/mm^3)	MCV (μm^3)	Hb/cell (g x 10^{-12})
Normal	3.9	47.5	15.6	10.5	45.2	14.9
Abnormal	6.6	44.6	14.7	12.4	36.3	11.9
Level of significance.	<0.001	<0.002	<0.05	<0.001	<0.001	<0.001

For experimental details see Popp and Enlow, 1977.

number, and have reduced hematocrit, hemoglobin level, mean cell volume, and hemoglobin concentration (Popp and Enlow, 1977) as shown in Table I. The erythrocyte half-life is reduced from a value of 12.7 days for normal cells to 10.3 days for thalassemic red blood cells injected into normal mice (Popp et al., 1978). Blood smears reveal microcytosis, anisocytosis and erythrocyte inclusion bodies (Popp and Enlow, 1977). Scanning electron micros-copy demonstrates the irregular size and shape of many of the thalassemic erythrocytes (Popp et al., 1979) as shown in Figure 2. All these properties are similar to those seen in hemoglobin H disease (heterozygous α-thalassemia) in humans.

The fundamental characteristic of α-thalassemia is a reduction in the α/β globin chain ratio. All three mouse stocks have a similar reduction (Martinell et al., 1981). Analysis of α- and β-globin polypeptide synthesis was carried out as follows. Reticulocyte-rich blood from either a thalassemic mouse (TH) or a normal sibling (NS) was incubated with radioactive leucine. The globin chains were separated by carboxymethyl-cellulose chromatography. The total dpm under each peak was determined and is shown in Table 2 along with the α/β globin chain ratios.

Table 2.   α/β Ratios of Globin Chains Labeled in Intact Reticulocytes.

Mouse	Total dpm α	Total dpm β	α/β	Normalized α/β
352HB NS	196,000	178,000	1.10	1.00
352HB TH	221,000	263,000	0.84	0.76
27HB NS	210,000	208,000	1.01	1.00
27HB TH	350,000	395,000	0.89	0.88

Similar results have been obtained for the Hba[th-J] mutant. The α/β globin ratio is reduced approximately 20% in all studies that have been done. An α/β ratio of 0.5 would be expected in heterozygous α-thalassemia where one-half of the α-globin genes have been deleted. Thus,

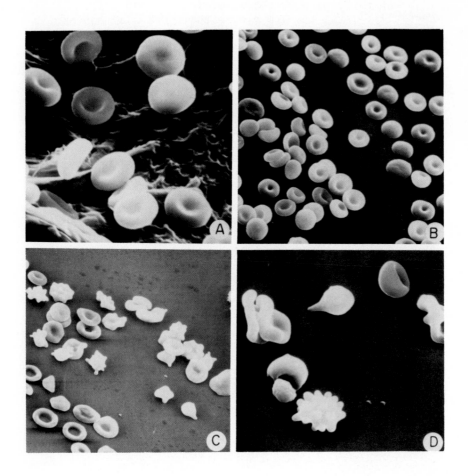

Figure 2. Scanning electron micrographs of erythrocytes.
(A) Normal, 5000x; (B) Normal, 2100x; (C) 352HB, 2000x; (D)
352HB, 5000x.

thalassemic mouse erythroid cells appear to compensate partially for the non-expressing α-globin genes. It has been recognized for many years that the bone marrow cells of human patients with thalassemia also compensate partially; i.e., the α/β globin chain ratio is not as abnormal in nucleated erythroid precursors as it is in enucleated peripheral blood erythrocytes.

Peptide analysis has demonstrated the total absence of α-globin chains derived from the mutant chromosome in heterozygous α-thalassemic mice (Popp et al., 1979). In other words, only the α-globin chains from the normal parent are expressed in heterozygous thalassemic red cells. By an appropriate selection of parentage, it is possible to identify which α-globin chains come from the chromosome inherited from each parent.

Just as in human thalassemia, the globin mRNA levels exactly reflect the globin polypeptide ratio (Martinell et al., 1981). Extensive liquid hybridization studies were carried out in order to obtain accurate α/β globin mRNA ratios. α- and β-globin cDNA probes were labeled with different isotopes so that double-label hybridization could measure α and β globin mRNA simultaneously in the same experiment. The mean value of a number of experiments revealed the following data:

Table 3.

Mouse	Normalized α/β globin mRNA
Normal	1.00
352HB	0.81
27HB	0.78
Hb^{th-J}	0.75

Thus, the α/β globin mRNA ratio for all three mouse mutants is around 0.8.

In human α-thalassemia, hemoglobin H (β4) is found in the circulating erythrocytes. This tetramer results from the lack of sufficient α-globin chains to complex with all the β-globin that is synthesized. In Figure 3 evidence is presented that a "Hb H" molecule is found in the peripheral blood of the α-thalassemic mice (Anderson, 1980). In like manner, human fetuses have excess fetal globin (gamma) chains, and consequently have γ4 tetramers (Hb Bart's) in their erythrocytes. Even though the mouse does not have a true fetal globin, a related tetramer to Hb Bart's, namely y4, can be identified (see Figure 4) (Popp et al., 1980a). The exact equivalent in humans would be an epsilon-4 which has not yet been identified. This finding of y4, together with the ratios of E1 and EII observed in fetal thalassemic mouse blood, strongly suggests that the x gene is also non-functional in these mutants. Therefore, there appear to be no functional α-like globin genes (embryonic or adult) in the chromosome containing the thalassemic mutation.

Genotype

Using recombinant DNA techniques, it is possible to determine whether or not a given gene is present in the genome of an organism. By choosing the appropriate strains of mice for study, and by using specific α-globin gene probes, it can be shown by Southern blot analysis that the two adult α-globin genes are deleted from the mutant chromo some (Whitney et al., 1981). The x gene is also assumed to-be deleted. Figure 5 illustrates a Southern blot analysis. The figure legend describes the results.

Deletion of the two adult α-globin genes in humans is a common cause of α-thalassemia. Thus, the mouse mutants appear to be true models of the human disease.

USES OF THE MOUSE MUTANTS

It is now possible to microinject globin (and other) genes into the nucleus of adult or embryonic cells (Anderson et al., 1980; Gordon et al., 1980; Wagner et al., 1981). Therefore, it might be possible to develop the techniques for curing a genetic disease by injecting a normal α-globin gene into the fertilized thalassemic mouse egg. If the α-globin gene expressed itself, the α/β globin imbalance might be corrected. Such an experiment is probably doomed to failure, however, because the homozygous thalassemic embryo appears to die at around 5 to 5-1/2

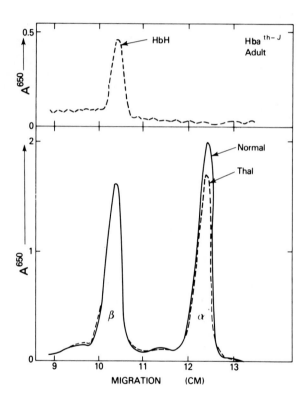

<u>Figure 3.</u> Urea polyacrylamide gel patterns of peripheral-blood globin chains from normal and Hba^{th-J} mice.

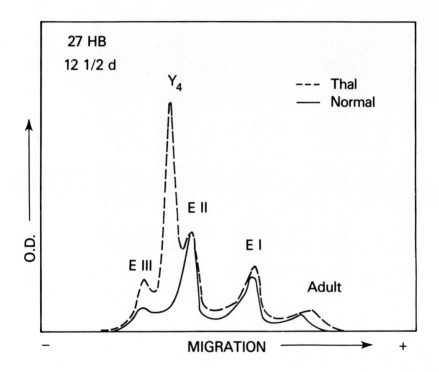

<u>Figure 4.</u> Cellulose acetate electrophoretic profiles of hemoglobins from normal and thalassemic (27HB) embryonic mice.

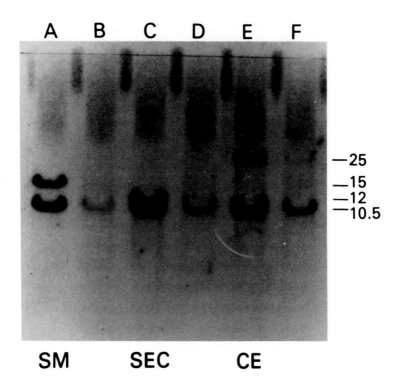

Figure 5. Southern blot analysis of the α-globin genomic
DNA fragments of normal and thalassemic mice. Southern
blots (30 μg per lane) of Eco RI fragments were hybridized
with a radiolabeled 3 kb fragment which contains a cloned
gene for α-globin. DNA from normal mice was in lanes A
(strain SM/J), C (strain SEC/1Re), and E (strain CE/J).
DNA in lanes B, D, and F came from mice that carried one
normal CE/J chromosome and, respectively, the mutated
chromosome Hba^{th-J}, 352HB, or 27HB. Sizes are shown in
kb. A 12 kb band would be expected if the α-globin genes
were present from the thalassemic chromosome. No 12 kb
band can be seen even after long periods of exposure.

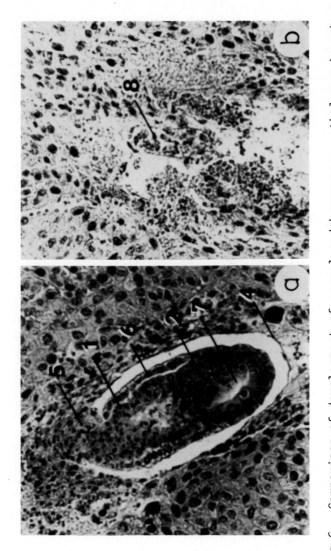

Figure 6. Comparison of development of normal and homozygous α-thalassemic embryos. a. Late egg cylinder stage of normal embryo; 6.5 days x 150. b. Necrotic remains of a presumed α-thalassemic homozygote; 6.5 days x 150. Extraembryonic ectoderm (1), embryonic ectoderm (2), trophectoderm (4), ectoplacental cone (5), visceral yolk sac (6), amnionic cavity (7) degenerate blastocyst (8).

days, and this is several days before the globin genes are activated (Popp et al., 1980b). Figure 6 shows two 6-1/2 day embryos; the one on the left is normal, while the one on the right is degenerated and is presumed to have arisen from a homozygous α-thalassemic zygote. The trophectoderm appears to degenerate in these latter implants, and thus rapidly produce the death of the embryo. Since all three mutants demonstrate this same property, it is likely that the deletion which removes the α-globin genes also removes a linked "development" gene. It might be possible by "walking" down the normal mouse chromosome from the α-globin genes to locate this developmental gene. If it were possible to locate and isolate this putative gene, it could be cloned and studied. Furthermore, it might be possible to cure homozygous α-thalassemic mice by coinjection of the developmental gene along with a normal α-globin gene.

CONCLUSION

In conclusion, three mouse mutants have been shown to be models of the human disease α-thalassemia. However, since an additional gene(s) is affected, these mutants represent a particularly severe condition in which death occurs in the homozygous embryo, even before globin genes are activated. A search is underway to locate the putative developmental gene which is thought to be linked to the α-globin gene.

REFERENCES

Anderson WF (1980). Regulation of globin gene expression at the molecular level. Ann NY Acad Sci 344:262.

Anderson WF, Killos L, Sanders-Haigh L, Kretschmer PJ, Diacumakos EG (1980). Replication and expression of thymidine kinase and human globin genes microinjected into mouse fibroblasts. Proc Natl Acad Sci USA 77:5399.

Gordon JW, Scangos GA, Plotkin DJ, Barbosa JA, Ruddle FH (1980). Genetic transformation of mouse embryos by microinjection of purified DNA. Proc Natl Acad Sci USA 77:7380.

Martinell J, Whitney JB III, Popp RA, Russell LB, Anderson WF (1981). Three mouse models of human thalassemia. Proc Natl Acad Sci USA 78:5056.

Popp RA, Bradshaw BS, Skow LC (1980b). Effects of alpha thalassemia on mouse development. Differentiation 17:205.

Popp RA, Enlow MK (1977). Radiation-induced α-thalassemia in mice. Am J Vet Res 38:569.

Popp RA, Francis MC, Bradshaw BS (1978). Erythrocyte life span in alpha thalassemic mice. Birth Defects: Original Article Series, XIV:181.

Popp RA, Skow LC, Whitney JB III (1980a). Expression of embryonic hemoglobin genes in α-thalassemic mice and in β-duplication mice. Ann NY Acad Sci 344:280.

Popp RA, Stratton LP, Hawley DK, Effron K (1979). Hemoglobin of mice with radiation-induced mutations at the hemoglobin loci. J Mol Biol 127:141.

Russell LB, Russell WL, Popp RA, Vaughan C, Jacobson KB (1976). Radiation-induced mutations at mouse hemoglobin loci. Proc Natl Acad Sci USA 73:2843.

Wagner TE, Hoppe PC, Jollick JD, Scholl DR, Hodinka RL, Gault JB (1981). Microinjection of a rabbit β-globin gene into zygotes and its subsequent expression in adult mice and their offspring. Proc Natl Acad Sci USA 78:6376.

Whitney JB III, Martinell J, Popp RA, Russel LB, Anderson WF (1981). Deletions in the α-globin gene complex in α-thalassemic mice. Proc Natl Acad Sci USA 78:7644.

Whitney JB III, Russell ES (1980). Linkage of genes for adult α-globin and embryonic α-like globin chains. Proc Natl Acad Sci USA 77:1087.

DISCUSSION

DR. PATTERSON: It is my understanding that there are some thalassemias in humans that have been looked at by DNA technology methods which do not lack the genes involved. Apparently the genes are not turned on. Is there any information or any evidence regarding the mechanism of that problem?

DR. ANDERSON: Yes. There are a number of different mutations that have now been determined. There are point mutations which produce termination codons. There are point mutations that produce a frame shift mutation. Then there are mutations that have now been found in beta-plus thalassemias which are mutations in the intron-exon junction region. We can define the exact base sequence, the exact base in a patient, which has produced a defect in processing so that an abnormal message is produced. So, in an increasing number of thalassemias the exact molecular defects are known.

DR. PATTERSON: Actually what I was thinking about is whether there are thalassemias in which there are not demonstrable changes in the gene itself, or in the intervening sequences, but perhaps upstream which would affect gene regulation.

DR. ANDERSON: There is circumstantial evidence that such mutations exist, but as yet none have been identified.

Animal Models of Inherited Metabolic Diseases, pages 27-65
© 1982 Alan R. Liss, Inc., 150 Fifth Avenue, New York, NY 10011

ANIMAL ANALOGUES OF HUMAN INHERITED METABOLIC DISEASES:
MOLECULAR PATHOLOGY AND THERAPEUTIC STUDIES

Robert J. Desnick, Margaret M. McGovern,
Edward H. Schuchman, and Mark E. Haskins

Mount Sinai School of Medicine, New York, NY
10029 and University of Pennsylvania School of
Veterinary Medicine, and the University of Pennsylvania Genetics Center, Philadelphia, PA 19104

INTRODUCTION

During the past decade, efforts have focused on the
discovery and characterization of naturally occurring
animal models of human disease (Andrews et al., 1979;
Hommes, 1979; Capen et al., 1981). Animal analogues of a
variety of human "inborn errors of metabolism" have been
identified (Patterson et al., 1982). These models provide
the unique opportunity to investigate the molecular pathology of their human counterparts. Specifically, characterization of the underlying genetic defect and its resultant pathophysiologic consequences permits the rational
design and evaluation of various therapeutic strategies
which could not be assessed adequately in clinical trials
due to the limitations of human experimentation. Therefore, it is the purpose of this review to discuss selected
animal models of human lysosomal storage diseases, emphasizing the study of their molecular pathology and their
usefulness as prototype systems for the evaluation of novel
therapeutic strategies.

ANIMAL MODELS OF HUMAN LYSOSOMAL STORAGE DISEASES

Enzymatically Confirmed Models.

To date, over 30 human inborn errors of the lysosomal
apparatus have been identified (McKusick, 1978). Each is
inherited as an autosomal or X-linked recessive trait and
has been shown to result from the deficient activity of a

specific enzyme. At the metabolic level, the enzymatic deficiency causes a block resulting in either the accumulation of the substrate(s) [and precursor(s)] and/or the absence of a critical metabolic product; the metabolic abnormalities lead to the physiologic and phenotypic manifestations characteristic of the specific enzymatic defect.

Table 1 lists the animal models of human lysosomal storage diseases; the disorders are classified as glycogenoses, glycoproteinoses, glycosphingolipidoses or mucopolysaccharidoses on the basis of the primary accumulated substrate. Although other models of human lysosomal storage diseases have been described (Andrews et al., 1979; Hommes, 1979), the criteria for inclusion in Table 1 was the actual demonstration of the same enzyme deficiency as in the analogous human disorder. Each of these models is inherited as an autosomal recessive trait.

Recognition of the affected proband and/or identification of the proband's parents or heterozygous relatives has permitted the establishment of active breeding colonies for cows with Pompe disease (Richards et al., 1977) and α-mannosidosis (Hocking et al., 1972); goats with β-mannosidosis (Jones and Dawson, 1981); cats with G_{M1}-gangliosidosis type 2 (Baker et al., 1971), G_{M2}-gangliosidosis type 2 (Cork et al., 1977; Rattazzi et al., 1979), mucopolysaccharidosis Type I-H (Haskins et al., 1979a) and mucopolysaccharidosis Type VI (Haskins et al., 1979b; McGovern et al., 1981); dogs with Niemann-Pick disease (Bundza et al., 1979); as well as dogs (Suzuki et al., 1970) and mice (Duchen et al., 1980) with Krabbe disease. These models are the best characterized with respect to the clinical manifestations, natural history of the disease, morphologic pathology, and the nature of the metabolic defect [i.e., accumulated substrate(s) and deficient enzyme].

Recently Recognized Models.

Two new glycoprotein/oligosaccharide storage diseases have been described in animals. Nubian goats with a severe neurovisceral oligosaccharide storage disease recently have been shown to have deficient β-mannosidase activity (Jones and Dawson, 1981) and the lysosomal accumulation of a β-mannosyl-containing trisaccharide (Jones and Laine,

1981). This animal model is of particular interest since the analogous human disorder has not been identified to date. In addition to the well-characterized bovine model of α-mannosidosis (Hocking et al., 1972; Phillips et al., 1974), a second model has been identified in a domestic kitten which presented with neurologic manifestations, dysmorphic features and growth retardation (Burditt et al., 1980). Characterization of the residual acid α-mannosidase activity and urinary mannose-rich oligosaccharides suggested that the feline disease was similar to the severe form of human mannosidosis (Sung et al., 1977), whereas the bovine model was more analogous to the milder human variant (Desnick et al., 1976). Hopefully, a breeding colony for the feline disease can be established, since this model would be more convenient for therapeutic and other studies than the bovine analogue.

Three new models of human glycosphingolipidoses have been identified. Canine Gaucher type 2 disease has been described in several affected dogs in Australia. The deficiency of acid β-glucosidase and the accumulation of glucosyl ceramide and glucosyl psychosine have been demonstrated (Van de Water et al., 1979; Farrow et al., 1982). Efforts are currently underway to develop an enzymatic test to identify canine carriers of the Gaucher gene so that appropriate matings can be made and a colony established. A second model of human Krabbe disease (galactosyl ceramide: β-galactosidase deficiency) has been identified in mice with the "twitcher" mutation (Duchen et al., 1980). The availability of this model should permit intensive study of the globoid cell reaction which is the characteristic neuropathologic finding in the human disease. Analogues of the human neurodegenerative disorder, Niemann-Pick Type A disease, have been reported in Siamese cats (Wenger et al., 1980) and poodles (Bundza et al., 1979). These animals should provide insight into the interrelationships among the sphingomyelinase isozymes in health and disease.

Finally, a feline model of human mucopolysaccharidosis I-H (Hurler disease) due to deficient α-L-iduronidase activity has been identified and a breeding colony has been established (Haskins et al., 1979a). This is the second recognized analogue of a human mucopolysaccharidosis, the other being Type VI (Maroteaux-Lamy disease). The availability of these two models, one characterized by neurologic involvement (MPS I-H) and the other only by visceral

TABLE 1. Animal Models of Human Lysosomal Storage Diseases*

Disease	Enzymatic Defect	Species	Reference
Glycogenosis:			
Glycogenosis Type II (Pompe)	Acid α-Glucosidase	Shorthorn Cow	Richards et al., 1977
Glycoproteinoses:			
α-Mannosidosis	Acid α-Mannosidase	Angus Cow Domestic Cat	Hocking et al., 1972 Burditt et al., 1980
β-Mannosidosis	Acid β-Mannosidase	Nubian Goat	Jones & Dawson, 1981
Glycosphingolipidoses:			
G$_{M1}$-Gangliosidosis			
Type 2	Acid β-Galactosidase	Siamese Cat Friesian Calf Mixed Breed Dog	Baker et al., 1971 Donnelly et al., 1973 Read et al., 1976
G$_{M2}$-Gangliosidosis			
Type 2	β-Hexosaminidase A&B	Domestic Cat	Cork et al., 1977
Type 3	β-Hexosaminidase A, Partial Activity	Yorkshire Swine	Pierce et al., 1976

Table 1 - Continued

Gaucher Type 2	Acid β-Glucosidase	Silky Hair Terrier Dog	Van de Water et al., 1979
Krabbe	Galactosyl ceramide: β-Galactosidase	West Highland/ Cairn Terriers Twitcher Mouse	Suzuki et al., 1970 Duchen et al., 1980
Niemann-Pick Type A	Sphingomyelinase	Poodles Siamese Cat	Bundza et al., 1979 Wenger et al., 1980
Mucopolysaccharidoses:			
MPS I-H (Hurler)	α-L-Iduronidase	Domestic Cat	Haskins et al., 1979a
MPS VI (Maroteaux-Lamy)	Arylsulfatase B	Siamese Cat	Jezyk et al., 1977

*Includes only enzymatically confirmed models.

manifestations (MPS VI), should permit assessment of mucopolysaccharide metabolism in visceral and neural tissues as well as provide systems for the evaluation of various therapeutic endeavors.

It should be noted that many human lysosomal storage diseases await the discovery of their animal analogues. Veterinarians should be aware of the phenotypic and pathologic findings in various glycosphingolipidoses such as Fabry disease (angiokeratoma and vascular endothelial glycolipid deposition) and metachromatic leukodystrophy (neurologic symptoms of demyelination), in the glycoproteinoses such as Mucolipidoses I, II and III (dysostosis multiplex and facial dysmorphia), and in the remaining mucopolysaccharidoses, Types II, III, IV and VII (dysostosis multiplex, corneal clouding, facial dysmorphia and dwarfism). Once an affected animal is identified, efforts should be directed to identify other affected individuals, heterozygous parents and relatives in order to establish a breeding colony. These models provide the opportunity to characterize the molecular pathology of specific genetic defects and to evaluate the potential effectiveness of various therapeutic strategies for their human counterparts as illustrated below.

MOLECULAR PATHOLOGY OF LYSOSOMAL STORAGE DISEASES

Requisite to the use of animal models for the study of human disease is the necessity to establish the degree of homology between the human and animal counterparts. Obviously, an animal disease which has an identical molecular etiology to that of the corresponding human disorder will provide the ideal model for investigation of disease pathogenesis and treatment. For inborn errors of metabolism, an animal homologue would be one with the identical molecular defect at the genic level (e.g., the same or equivalent base substitution in the mutant gene). However, it is unlikely that any given animal model will share the precise gene mutation which occurs in the human disease. In fact, it is known that multiple mutations in the structural gene for any given protein can cause defective catalysis or function, as has been so well-demonstrated for the over 140 and 250 different mutations in the human molecules, glucose 6-phosphate dehydrogenase (Yoshida et al., 1971; Beutler and Yoshida, 1973; Yoshida and Beutler, 1978) and hemo-

globin (Bunn et al., 1977), respectively. Therefore, the
following section will review the nature of inherited
enzymatic defects with particular emphasis on the molecular
anatomy of structural genes and the types of mutations
which can alter the physical and functional properties of
the catalytic proteins encoded by these genes.

Nature of Inherited Enzymatic Defects.

Recent advances in molecular biology have revolution-
ized our concept of eukaryotic gene structure. Previously,
it was thought that a structural gene consisted of only the
deoxynucleotide sequence which was transcribed into mRNA
and then directly translated into the amino acid sequence
of the gene product. This concept has been revised by the
finding of deoxynucleotide sequences within and flanking
the structural gene which do not encode for the amino acid
sequence of the polypeptide product. As shown in Figure 1,
the intervening sequences (introns) separate the nucleotide
sequences (exons) which are ultimately translated into the
gene product. The flanking regions at the 5' and 3' ends
presumably contain the signals for the initiation of transcription and for RNA processing. The entire gene (both
introns and exons) is transcribed into a precursor RNA or
hnRNA (heterogeneous nuclear RNA) which then undergoes a
series of processing events to produce the mature mRNA,
which contains only the exon sequences. These processing
events include capping and polyadenylation at the 5' and 3'
ends, respectively, and excision (splicing) of the intron
sequences.

Various types of heritable mutations could result in a
defective enzymatic activity. These include mutations in
1) either the exon, intron or flanking regions of the
structural gene, 2) other genes controlling posttranslational modifications of the gene product, and 3) regulatory
genes controlling the synthesis of the active enzyme.

1) <u>Structural gene defects</u>. Missense (base substitutions), nonsense (chain terminating base substitutions) and frameshift (insertions or deletions) mutations
can occur in any intron, exon or flanking region of the
structural gene. A particular mutation can alter the
fidelity of transcription, RNA processing or translation,
depending on the specific site and type of mutation.

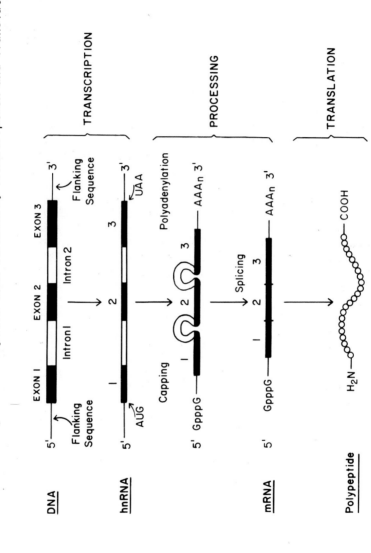

Figure 1. Current Concept of Eukaryotic Gene Structure, Transcription and Translation

Certain mutations (e.g., in the intron, intervening sequence junction or flanking region) may result in the quantitative deficiency, or absence, of normal gene product.

Qualitative mutations that alter the structure and function of the normal gene product result from single base substitutions in the exon portion of the gene. From the genetic code, it can be calculated that approximately 70% of single base substitutions in a DNA triplet located in an exon will change that codon to incorporate a different amino acid (missense mutations), about 25% of the substitutions will insert the same amino acid (degenerate mutations), and about 5% of substitutions will code for chain termination of the nascent polypeptide sequence (nonsense mutations). Although the rate of gene product synthesis remains relatively normal, missense and nonsense mutations in an exon can alter the kinetic, stability, or other properties of the enzyme, rendering it catalytically inactive or partially active. In the latter case, a mutation which results in a partially active enzyme permits purification of the residual activity and comparison of its properties with the normal enzyme. In this way, insight into the nature of the enzymatic defect can be obtained.

As illustrated in Figure 2, a normal structural gene will be transcribed and translated into a normal gene product with a specific sequence of amino acids that specifies a unique three-dimensional configuration. This configuration establishes at least three functional sites on the active enzyme molecule: the substrate binding site, the catalytic or active site, and at least one major antigenic site. There may also be sites for allosteric, coenzyme, and subunit interactions, etc. A single base substitution in an exon portion of the gene may alter an enzyme's structure in such a manner as to deleteriously affect one or more of these functional properties.

Nonsense or chain-terminating mutations in an exon result in an incompletely synthesized enzyme. If the nonsense mutation occurs early in the enzyme's amino acid sequence, the resultant polypeptide will not have sufficient structure for catalytic activity or immunologic recognition of its antigenic site(s) [i.e., cross-reacting material (CRM)-negative, Figure 2]. Missense mutations can modify the catalytic, substrate binding, cofactor binding or allosteric sites, resulting in kinetic mutations which

Figure 2. Effect of Various Single Base Substitutions on the Structure, Function and Stability of an Enzyme Protein

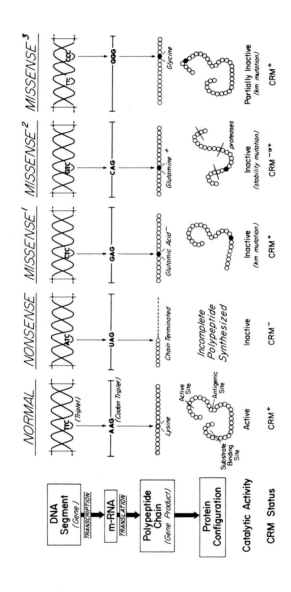

may partially or totally impair catalytic function. These mutations can be CRM-positive or negative depending on whether they alter the antigenic sites. Missense mutations also can affect the physical stability of the enzyme by altering its conformation or subunit interactions. Unstable proteins may be rapidly degraded by cellular proteases resulting in non-catalytic, CRM-negative mutations.

In the future, it is likely that these mutations will be characterized at the genic level using sophisticated nucleic acid and recombinant DNA techniques. The precise molecular defects (e.g., specific base substitutions, deletions, etc.) in each of the lysosomal storage diseases (and their subtypes and variants) will be identified, analogous to the recent accomplishments in the dissection of the molecular pathology of the human hemoglobinopathies and thalassemias (Kan et al., 1975; Wetherall and Clegg, 1979; Kantor et al., 1980; Proudfoot et al., 1980). At present, such studies are not possible for the lysosomal storage diseases since none of the genes have been isolated and cloned.

Recently, a variety of strategies have evolved for the isolation of eukaryotic genes which are expressed at extremely low levels. One approach involves the use of synthetic oligonucleotides for priming the synthesis of a cDNA specific for the gene in question or, alternatively, to directly screen cloned cDNA libraries for a segment corresponding to the gene's mRNA (Wallace et al., 1980). The first step toward this goal is the determination of the amino acid sequence of each enzyme and the construction of a DNA oligonucleotide probe. The availability of an oligonucleotide probe also would permit the analysis of CRM-negative mutations by establishing the absence, presence or quantity of mRNA and DNA present in cells of the mutant genotype (Szostak et al., 1979). Such studies would identify gene deletions or mRNA processing defects.

Since the exact molecular defects in the human lysososmal storage diseases cannot be determined at the genic level as yet, efforts have focused on the characterization of the enzymatic defects, particularly in those disorders with detectable residual activity. Information concerning the nature of a mutation which results in a partially active enzyme can be obtained by comparison of the kinetic and physical properties of the normal and residual activities. An increased K_m (decreased substrate binding) or a decreased V_{max} (reduced product formation due to defective product release or enzyme instability) would lead to abnormal substrate accumulation. In addition, the incorporation of an inappropriate amino acid, particularly if charged differently, may significantly alter the enzyme's configuration and render it unstable and susceptible to degradation by endogenous proteases; it is anticipated that most stability mutations would be catalytically inactive and CRM-negative. Of the enzymatic defects characterized to date, most residual activities have had markedly increased K_m values or both increased K_m and decreased V_{max} values. The latter presumably reflects mutations which alter substrate binding as well as render the enzyme less stable.

Missense or nonsense mutations in the structural gene exons may also alter the enzyme's ability to interact normally with critical small molecules, such as allosteric effectors and cofactors. A number of human inborn errors have been identified that involve enzymes requiring the binding of a specific vitamin cofactor for the normal expression of enzymatic activity (Fleisher and Gaull, 1980). These mutations often fall into two groups - those that respond to cofactor supplementation therapy and those that do not. Presumably, the former mutations represent defects in the coenzyme binding site of the enzyme that increase the K_a for the coenzyme, whereas the latter group represents defects that severely deform the coenzyme binding or other crucial sites. Similarly, multimeric enzyme proteins may be inactive if subunit assembly cannot occur due to a mutation in the structural gene coding for one polypeptide of a heteromultimeric enzyme or for the common subunits of a homomultimer.

2) <u>Posttranslational defects</u>. Missense or nonsense mutations in genes controlling the posttranslational modifications of the enzyme protein also may cause catalytic deficiencies. For example, one type of posttranslational modification involves processes which control the subcellular compartmentalization of an enzyme, including the cleavage of a peptide leader sequence (Blobel <u>et al</u>., 1979; Maccecchini <u>et al</u>., 1979), the synthesis of a specific membrane binding or transport protein, or the addition of specific oligonucleotide moieties. Such abnormalities have been elegantly demonstrated for the β-glucuronidase iso-

zymes in mice (Paigen, 1979), and more recently, for the defective lysosomal localization of many hydrolases in Mucolipidoses II and III (Hasilik et al., 1981; Reitman et ali., 1981). In the former, a defect in the protein responsible for the microsomal localization of β-glucuronidase has been described (Ganshow and Paigen, 1967). In Mucolipidoses II and III, the deficient activity of an enzyme, UDP-N-acetyl-glucosaminylphosphotransferase (Hasilik et al., 1981; Reitman et al., 1981), results in the failure to form the mannose-6-phosphate residues on the oligosaccharide moieties of most lysosomal hydrolases; the mannose-6-phosphate recognition signal appears to mediate the intracellular trafficking of lysosomal enzymes to the lysosomal apparatus (Kaplan et al., 1977; Sando and Neufeld, 1977; Ullrich et al., 1978; Bach et al., 1979; Natowicz et al., 1979; Hasilik and Neufeld, 1980; Sly, 1980). The absence of this signal results in the multiple deficiency of lysosomal hydrolases intracellularly and the extracellular accumulation of these enzymes.

3) <u>Regulatory gene defects</u>. Finally, mutations in regulatory genes controlling initiation, temporal modulation, or rates of enzyme synthesis could occur. These mutations may be in genes distant from the structural gene locus. Alternatively, such mutations could be in the 5' flanking region of the structural gene which presumably contains "promoter sequences" required for initiation of transcription (RNA polymerase recognition and/or binding). Although there are no well-documented examples of human enzymatic defects resulting from regulatory gene mutations, it is likely that these occur in nature, but presumably represent lethal mutations. However, a partial defect of a regulatory gene might be viable and result in an enzymatic deficiency.

Characterization of the Enzymatic Defects in the Human and Animal Diseases.

To date, studies of the molecular pathology in animal models of human lysosomal storage diseases have focused at the level of the metabolic defect. In each animal model disease listed in Table 1, the homology of the metabolic defect has been documented by the demonstration of the same enzymatic deficiency as in the corresponding human disorder. Several of these animal models have enzymatic

TABLE 2. Comparison of the Properties of Residual Activities in the Liver from Human and Animal Models of Lysosomal Storage Diseases

Disease	Residual Activity	pH	Kinetics	Thermo-stability	Mol. Wt.	Cations, Cofactors Effectors	IEF*/ Electrophoretic Migration	Cross Reacting Material	References**
Mannosidosis:									
Human	2-8%	N*	+ Km	↓	N	N	N	+	1
Bovine	15%	N	+ Km	↓	N	N	N	+	2
Feline	2%	N	N	N		N			3
G_{M1}-Gangliosidosis Type2:									
Human	2-18%	N	+ Km		N		Electro-positive	+	4
Feline	10%	N	+ Km	↓			Electro-positive	-	5
Canine	1%	N	N	N	N		N		6
Mucopolysaccharidosis VI:									
Human	4-15%	N	N	N	N		N	+	7
Feline	6-10%	N	+ Km	↓			Electro-negative		8

* N = normal; IEF = isoelectric focusing
** 1. Desnick et al., 1976; 2,3. Burditt et al., 1978, 1980; 4. Norden and O'Brien, 1975; 5. Holmes and O'Brien, 1978; 6. Rittmann et al., 1980; 7. Shapira et al., 1975; 8. Vine et al., 1981.

defects with residual activities which permit further comparison of their mutations with those in the human diseases. Interestingly, residual activities occur in both the human and animal counterparts of the following disorders: mannosidosis, G_{M1}-gangliosidosis and mucopolysaccharidosis Type VI. Comparison of the kinetic, physical and immunologic properties of these defective enzymes revealed that none of these animal models were homologues, but rather, were analogues of their human disease counterparts. These studies are summarized in Table 2 and are discussed below.

α-Mannosidosis. The residual α-mannosidase activities in both the bovine and human disorders had increased K_m values, decreased thermostabilities and cross-reacted with antibodies to the respective normal enzymes, consistent with a structural gene mutation (Burditt et al., 1978). The only difference between the human and bovine residual enzymes was the amount of activity detected (∿ 2-8% vs. ∿ 15% of normal, respectively). In contrast, the residual activity in feline mannosidosis was only 2% of normal levels and had similar physical and kinetic properties to the normal feline enzyme (Burditt et al., 1980). Although the immunologic properties of the residual feline enzyme were not investigated, it was suggested that the residual activity was the result of a structural gene mutation that led to enhanced susceptibility of the enzyme to proteolysis or an alteration in some property which decreased catalytic activity; a regulatory gene mutation, although less likely, was also considered (Burditt et al., 1980). Further purification and characterization, including CRM studies, are required to discriminate among these possibilities.

G_{M1}-Gangliosidosis. The feline model of G_{M1}-gangliosidosis has 10% residual hepatic activity which has an altered K_m toward both the natural and artificial substrates, is thermolabile, migrates less anodally and is not recognized (CRM-negative) by the antibody raised against normal feline β-galactosidase (Holmes and O'Brien, 1978). In contrast, the canine enzyme has 1% of normal hepatic activity, normal kinetic and physical properties and an amount of CRM directly corresponding to the amount of activity (Rittmann et al., 1980). Thus, the feline mutation is consistent with a structural gene mutation, but the nature of the canine mutation is unclear; possible mutations include mRNA processing, regulatory gene as well as structural gene defects. Discrimination of the different possibilities may require isolation of the gene and characterization of its transcriptional and translational integrity.

Mucopolysaccharidosis Type VI. Characterization of the residual activity in feline mucopolysaccharidosis Type VI illustrates the importance of investigating the molecular pathology of the defective enzyme in order to design rational therapeutic strategies. Affected cats accumulate dermatan sulfate in their tissues and urine due to the deficient activity of the lysosomal hydrolase, arylsulfatase B (ASB; EC 3.1.6.1). Analogous to the human disorder, 6-10% of normal ASB activity was present in the leukocytes, fibroblasts and liver of MPS VI cats (Jezyk et al., 1979; Haskins et al., 1979b).

Partially purified residual MPS VI enzyme differed from its normal counterpart in electrophoretic mobility, kinetic properties, stability and molecular weight (Vine et al., 1981). Compared to the partially purified normal hepatic enzyme, the MPS VI ASB activity had at least a 100-fold greater K_m value and was markedly more thermo-, cryo-, and pH-labile. In addition, the molecular weight of the native MPS VI residual activity was approximately half that of the native normal feline enzyme as determined by gel filtration, polyacrylamide gel electrophoresis, and sucrose density-gradient centrifugation (McGovern et al., 1982). These results, and the demonstration that the normal feline enzyme was a homodimer, suggested that the mutation in the structural gene for feline ASB altered the gene product such that it was unable to maintain its normal dimeric subunit conformation. Although the defective enzyme retained partial activity, the inability for subunit association (e.g., dimerization) presumably rendered the MPS VI enzyme protein more defective catalytically and markedly unstable.

It is notable that patients with MPS VI also have about 4-15% of normal ASB activity in liver, cultured fibroblasts and leukocytes (Stumpf et al., 1973; Fluharty et al., 1974; Beratis et al., 1975; Shapira et al., 1975). In contrast to the defective ASB activity in the feline disease, the human hepatic residual activity was similar to the normal human enzyme in pH optimum, apparent K_m, electrophoretic mobility, and thermostability at 60°C. Immunologic studies of the human MPS VI enzyme demonstrated that the ratio of immunoreactive protein to residual activity was 6.7 (Shapira et al., 1975). Thus, it can be concluded that the structural gene mutations which cause the defective ASB activities in human and feline MPS VI differ in their molecular nature. The implications of these findings relate to the development of therapeutic strategies. Obviously, if the molecular defects in the feline and human ASB deficiencies differ, a specific therapeutic approach, based on the molecular pathology of the animal disease, may not be useful for human disorder.

Molecular Pathology and Establishment of Breeding Colonies.

It is notable that the mutations causing bovine and feline mannosidosis as well as canine and feline G_{M1}-gangliosidosis are different, emphasizing the heterogeneity which can occur in the gene defects for the same disease in different species. Molecular genetic heterogeneity resulting from different allelic mutations in the same structural gene within the same species also is well recognized. The fact that recessively inherited enzymatic defects usually result from different allelic mutations (e.g., A = wild type allele; a^1, a^2, a^3,..a^n = different recessive mutations in the "A" structural gene which render the gene product non-functional) has important implications for the selection of mates when establishing an animal model breeding colony. For example, consider the situation where four affected animals of a newly recognized inborn error have been discovered. Although all four were found in distant geographic areas, two were the product of separate consanguineous matings, while the parents of the other two were not related. It is likely that in each of the consanguineous animals, the same mutant allele was inherited from each parent and, therefore, they are each homozygous for the same recessive allele, or homoallelic. Furthermore, since the two consanguineous animals were not related to each other, it is most likely that they are homoallelic for different mutant alleles (i.e., a^1a^1 and a^2a^2).

In the remaining two non-consanguineous animals, it is most likely that each inherited two different mutant allelic forms of the gene and, therefore, are heterozygous for the recessive alleles, or heteroallelic. Since both of the non-consanguineous animals were discovered in distant locales, it is likely that they were each heteroallelic for different alleles (i.e., a^3a^4, a^5a^6). Thus, breeding colonies should be optimally planned to keep each mutant allele homozygous. For affected animals that are the product of consanguineous matings, this objective should be achieved easily. For diseased animals that are presumably heteroallelic, this goal is difficult since it is not usually possible to differentiate among the a^1a^1, a^1a^2 or a^2a^2 genotypes. This is particularly true if the mutant enzyme is catalytically inactive or immunologically undetectable (CRM-negative). Should the defective enzyme have residual activity or a certain amount of CRM, enzymatic and immunologic studies of the progeny of heteroallelic parents may indicate that the two alleles have segregated, permitting appropriate mate selection.

In the future, it is anticipated that the application of recombinant DNA techniques will permit the specific identification of different mutant alleles at the genic level. In this way, it will be possible to determine if the enzymatic defects which do not have residual activity or immunologically detectable protein are homoallelic or heteroallelic. However, at present, such studies can only be accomplished in models with residual activity and/or CRM. Thus, veterinarians establishing breeding colonies should be aware of these considerations and make every attempt to characterize the mutations so that homoallelic lines can be established and maintained.

DEVELOPMENT AND EVALUATION OF THERAPEUTIC STRATEGIES IN MAMMALIAN MODEL SYSTEMS

Considerable attention has been focused on the development of strategies to treat patients with inherited metabolic diseases. Theoretically, the ideal cure for these diseases would be the insertion of the segment of DNA coding for the normal gene product. Therapeutic intervention at the level of the primary genetic defect, or gene therapy, is presently precluded by our inability to insert a gene and effect its normal expression. However, recent developments in recombinant DNA methodology and their rapid application to _in vitro_ gene product production have signaled that we are on the threshhold of future technical accomplishments which may lead to "gene transfer" as a means to replace defective human genes.

To date, therapeutic endeavors to ameliorate the molecular pathology of selected inherited metabolic diseases have primarily involved gene product therapy and manipulations at the level of the metabolic or cellular defect. These efforts have included cofactor supplementation, allotransplantation, enzyme replacement, plasmapheresis and surgical bypass procedures (for a comprehensive review, see Desnick and Grabowski, 1981). Several of these strategies have been evaluated in the animal models of the lysosomal storage diseases. These studies illustrate the value of animal model systems to obtain critical information regarding the ability of selected therapeutic strategies to alter the biochemical abnormalities and clinical course of these diseases.

Enzyme Replacement Therapy.

During the past decade, investigators have been intrigued by the possibility of enzyme therapy for various inborn errors of metabolism, particularly the lysosomal storage diseases. The rationale for enzyme therapy in these diseases evolved from two fundamental observations: a) the identification of lysosomes as the subcellular site of pathology, and b) the elucidation of the basic role of the lysosome in cellular catabolism. Thus, it was reasoned that, after endocytosis, exogenously supplied enzyme would be brought into contact with accumulated substrate by fusion of the various components of the lysosomal apparatus.

Human trials of enzyme replacement therapy have met with several difficulties, including the inability to serially evaluate the physiologic, immunologic and biochemical factors affecting the fate of the administered enzyme. Suitable animal models, such as β-glucuronidase deficient mice and G_{M2}-gangliosidosis cats, have provided the means to evaluate and manipulate the factors that maximize enzyme stability and tissue distribution prior to human trials. These studies also provided data regarding potential toxic and immunologic complications.

For example, the tissue and subcellular fate as well as immunologic safety of intravenously administered bovine β-glucuronidase have been studied extensively in C3H/HeJ Gus^h β-glucuronidase deficient mice (Thorpe et al., 1974;

Thorpe et al., 1975; Steger and Desnick, 1977). A selective inactivation assay provided the means to conveniently
differentiate the bovine enzyme from residual murine activity (Thorpe et al., 1974). Following intravenous injection, bovine β-glucuronidase was rapidly cleared from the
murine circulation ($T_{1/2} \sim 3$ min) with almost exclusive
enzyme uptake by the hepatic lysosomes. These observations, and similar findings in early human trials, identified the need to develop entrapment strategies to deliver
the enzyme to non-hepatic sites of pathology.

Intravenous administrations of bovine β-glucuronidase
entrapped in positively- and negatively-charged liposomes
and in autologous murine erythrocytes were evaluated to
determine the ability of these carrier vehicles to target-
deliver and protect the entrapped enzyme (Thorpe et al.,
1975; Steger and Desnick, 1977). These studies have shown
that enzyme entrapped in negatively-charged liposomes
prolonged the hepatic retention of enzymatic activity
compared to that of unentrapped enzyme (8 days vs. 1 day)
and allowed delivery of enzyme to the kidney. Although
positively-charged liposomes were capable of delivering
enzyme to liver with a longer retention time (~ 11 days),
they were noted to cause temporary labilization of the
lysosomal membrane resulting in the intracellular release
of endogenous lysosomal hydrolases (Desnick et al., 1977).
Furthermore, immunologic studies demonstrated that administration of the enzyme-loaded liposomes elicited an immune
response to both the liposome carrier and the entrapped
enzyme (Hudson et al., 1979). Although liposomes have been
proported to be ideal vehicles for the delivery of enzyme
to specific tissues (Gregoriadis, 1978), these animal model
studies illustrated the potential physiologic complications
of these enzyme carriers prior to clinical use.

Compared to unentrapped enzyme, intravenously administered erythrocyte-entrapped β-glucuronidase was retained
in the murine circulation four times longer with more
efficient delivery of enzyme to renal and splenic tissues.
Ultrastructural examination revealed that the major site of
erythrocyte-entrapped enzyme uptake was in Kupffer cells,
not hepatocytes, indicating that this method of entrapment
may be useful for diseases with substrate accumulation in
the reticuloendothelial system (e.g., Type 1 Gaucher disease). In marked contrast to enzyme administered unentrapped or in liposomes, erythrocytes loaded with the hetero-

logous bovine β-glucuronidase did not elicit an immune response following repeated intravenous administrations (Fiddler et al., 1977).

These studies also demonstrated that intravenously administered enzyme, whether entrapped in liposomes or erythrocytes, or unentrapped, was unable to cross the blood-brain barrier and gain access to the central nervous system. Thus, it was recognized that efforts to treat diseases with neurologic involvement required the development of strategies to reversibly open the blood-brain barrier for neuronal enzyme uptake. Using the feline model of G_{M2}-gangliosidosis, Rattazzi et al. (1979, 1980) evaluated the effectiveness of hyperbaric oxygen and intracarotid air micro-embolism as methods to reversibly open the blood-brain barrier. Following exposure to hyperbaric oxygen, β-hexosaminidase A was injected into the femoral or carotid vein and neural uptake was determined. In order to prolong the half-life of exogenous enzyme in the circulation and maximize its central nervous system exposure, hepatic clearance of the enzyme was partially inhibited by the infusion of receptor-blocking mannosaccharides (i.e., mannans). This inhibition resulted in a 3 to 5-fold increase in neural enzyme uptake over that observed without blockage of the hepatic uptake receptors. However, hyperbaric treatment followed by the intracarotid administration of large doses of enzyme resulted in the neural uptake of only about 1% of injected enzyme.

More encouraging results were obtained in preliminary experiments of intracarotid air micro-embolization. Following the injection of small volumes of air, mannans and β-hexosaminidase A were administered intravenously into normal or G_{M2}-gangliosidosis cats (Rattazzi et al., 1979; Rattazzi, 1980). One hour after enzyme injection, the exogenous β-hexosaminidase A activity reached 20-30% of the endogenous level in normal feline brain, suggesting that air micro-embolization or similar mechanical methods to open the blood-brain barrier will permit access to neuronal sites of substrate deposition by nonselective extravasation of plasma containing the administered enzyme. More recently, these investigators have improved their techniques, permitting increased amounts of injected enzyme to reach the central nervous system (see Rattazzi et al. and Baker et al., this volume). Clearly, animal models are essential for the development and evaluation of novel therapeutic strategies for human neurologic disorders.

Allotransplantation.

An intriguing means for transferring normal genetic information into individuals with certain structural and metabolic gene defects is allotransplantation (Matas et al., 1978a; Matas et al., 1978b; Hirschhorn, 1980; Desnick and Grabowski, 1981). This approach exploits the grafting of cells, tissues or organs containing the normal DNA for the production of functional gene products in the recipient.

Experimental transplantation designed to correct inborn errors of metabolism has been undertaken in only a few animal disorders. Mukherjee et al. (1973) reported that orthotopic liver grafts resulted in increased UDP-glucuronyl transferase activity and markedly decreased the hyperbilirubinemia in Gunn rats. Subsequently, Sutherland and co-workers (1977) administered isolated liver cells into the portal vein of Gunn rats and demonstrated decreased levels of plasma bilirubin.

Animal model studies have provided the rationale for allogenic bone marrow transplantation for disorders in which the primary disease pathology results from defects in lymphocytes, phagocytes, erythrocytes or platelets. For example, cyclic neutropenia, which occurs in both man and dogs, is thought to be due to a regulatory defect which affects the pluripotential stem cells. Marrow transplantation in dogs with this disease resulted in normal granulocytopoiesis and corrected the neutrophil defect (Dale and Graw, 1974). It should also be noted that bone marrow stem cells are the progenitors of other mesodermal cell types, including Kupffer cells and osteoclasts. Thus, successful transplantation of normal stem cells will provide a continuous source of differentiated cells for the correction of disorders in which the differentiated cell is the target site of disease pathology. For example, congenital severe osteopetrosis is a recessively inherited disorder of humans characterized by the progressive deposition of bone matrix leading to blindness, deafness, anemia, frequent fractures, increased susceptibility to infection and progressive hepatosplenomegaly. Studies of the molecular pathology of the murine analogue for this disease revealed that the

abnormal resorption was the result of an intrinsic osteo-
clast defect (Loutit and Sansom, 1976). Moreover, allogenic bone marrow transplantation in affected mice lead to
the amelioration of the disease (Walker, 1975; Loutit and
Sansom, 1976). Based on the murine model studies, bone
marrow transplantation was undertaken in several patients
with the human disease with therapeutic benefit (Sorell et
al., 1979; Coccia et al., 1980).

Successful bone marrow transplantation and correction
of the enzymatic defect have been accomplished in murine
acatalasemia and murine β-glucuronidase deficiency. In
acatalasemia, catalase deficiency in peripheral leukocytes
leads to an inability to kill certain types of bacteria
resulting in recurrent infections. Acatalasemic mice,
which are abnormally sensitive to injections of exogenous
hydrogen peroxide, were marrow transplanted and the defect
corrected as demonstrated by increased blood catalase
levels and increased survival after hydrogen peroxide
challenges (Sutherland et al., 1980). Marrow transplantation in murine β-glucuronidase deficient mice, using total
body irradiation to make space for the graft, resulted in
successful grafting and increased levels of β-glucuronidase
activity in liver and plasma (Slavin and Yatziv, 1980).

More recently, bone marrow transplantation has been
proposed as a therapeutic strategy for the treatment of a
variety of human inherited enzymatic deficiency diseases
(Hobbs, 1981). The proponents of this strategy have transplanted patients with several lysosomal storage diseases;
the early results in one recipient with MPS I-H (Hurler
disease) have been reported (Hobbs et al., 1981). The
rationale for bone marrow transplantation in this and other
lysosomal disorders is based on the concept that a continuous supply of normal circulating phagocytes will be capable of correcting the defective lysosomal catabolism in
these storage diseases. It is presumed that monocytes will
penetrate a variety of tissues and short-lived neutrophils
will exocytose their lysosomal hydrolases, thus providing a
continuous supply of normal enzyme. Furthermore, in disorders with primary liver involvement, the disease course
may be altered by the replacement of Kupffer cells containing the active enzyme. This hypothesis seems reasonable
for disorders in which reticuloendothelial cells and other
bone marrow cells are the primary sites of pathology, such
as Gaucher Type 1 disease and MPS Types IV and VI. How-

ever, it is doubtful that inborn errors with primary neuronal substrate accumulation (e.g., Tay-Sachs disease, metachromatic leukodystrophy or MPS Types I-H, II, IIIA, IIIB, IIIC, IIID or VII) would benefit from marrow transplantation, since it is unlikely that adequate numbers of marrow-derived cells can gain access to the neural cellular sites of pathology. Therefore, studies in appropriate animal models should be conducted to evaluate the capability of marrow engraftment to alter the course of lysosomal storage diseases with primary neurologic involvement. In this regard, one important animal model experience should be noted.

Jolly et al. (1976) have described the biochemical and clinical findings in a freemartin with mannosidosis. In this "experiment of nature" a calf with mannosidosis received an in utero marrow graft from a normal littermate. The level of α-mannosidase activity in leukocytes of the chimeric calf was in the heterozygote range. In addition, the calf had a marked decrease in the number of vacuolated lymphocytes, and a reduced level of accumulated mannose-rich oligosaccharides in visceral tissues. However, the level of substrate accumulation was not significantly reduced in the brain and the calf exhibited the typical neurologic manifestations and course of the disease. These results are instructive since they indicate that the marrow chimera did not alter the neurologic course of this lysosomal storage disease. Clearly, animal models provide the opportunity to fully assess the effectiveness and limitations of marrow transplantation. Such studies should provide essential data for subsequent human trials.

Enzyme Manipulation.

As noted above, several of the human and animal lysosomal storage diseases have defective enzymes with residual activity. Thus, efforts to purify and characterize the residual activities in these diseases may lead to the development of novel therapeutic strategies designed to manipulate and enhance the function and/or stability of the defective enzyme. For example, characterization of the residual enzymatic activities in bovine mannosidosis and feline MPS VI have led to clinical trials of enzyme manipulation therapy as discussed below.

The finding that zinc cations stimulated normal plant, mammalian and human acid α-mannosidase activity (Snaith, 1975; Phillips et al., 1974), as well as residual α-mannosidase in tissues and fluids from bovine and human mannosidosis (Desnick et al., 1976; Jolly et al., 1980), stimulated the trial of cofactor supplementaton in bovine mannosidosis. Following oral zinc supplementation, a modest increase in the activity of the residual acid α-mannosidase was observed in bovine liver, kidney and pancreas (organs in which zinc accumulates). A concomitant decrease in the levels of mannosyl-oligosaccharides also was observed in these tissues. However, in the brain of the treated calf, the residual enzymatic activity and oligosaccharide content were not changed. These findings indicated that the effect of zinc supplementation may be confined to tissues that accumulate zinc and that inadequate zinc uptake by tissues of the nervous system may have precluded a therapeutic effect.

As described above, characterization of the physical and kinetic properties of the residual ASB activity in feline MPS VI indicated that the mutation in the structural gene for the feline enzyme altered the gene product such that it was unable to maintain its normal dimeric conformation (Vine et al., 1981, 1982; McGovern et al., 1982). Although the defective enzyme retained partial activity, the inability for subunit association presumably rendered the enzyme protein more defective catalytically and markedly unstable. These findings stimulated the evaluation of thiol-active reagents as stabilizers. In the presence of dithiothreitol (DTT) or cysteamine, the residual feline MPS VI activity was dimerized (Vine et al., 1982) resulting in increased activity. Since DTT and cysteamine have been safely administered as experimental therapeutic agents in patients with cystinosis (Thoene et al., 1976; Aaron et al., 1971; Goldman et al., 1971; Depape-Brigger et al., 1977; Girardin et al., 1979; Yudkoff et al., 1981), the therapeutic use of these compounds was evaluated in the feline model.

Initially, in vitro studies were undertaken to determine if thiol-induced dimerization could enhance the MPS VI residual ASB activity in leukocytes and catabolize the accumulated substrate. Following incubation of fresh heparinized whole blood with DTT or cysteamine, the leukocyte residual ASB activity was increased up to 11- and

20-fold, respectively, and, most importantly, the accumulated dermatan sulfate was degraded. Based on these encouraging in vitro results, in vivo trials were conducted. Intravenously administered DTT resulted in an immediate, but transient, increase in leukocyte residual ASB activity and had little, if any, effect on the leukocyte dermatan sulfate levels. In contrast, cysteamine infusion not only enhanced the residual leukocyte activity for at least 1 hour, but also resulted in the clearance of leukocyte dermatan sulfate; the accumulated substrate was reduced to 35% of the pre-infusion level shortly after administration and remained at about 45% of the pre-infusion level for the 120 minute period studied. The differential effectiveness of these thiol-reducing reagents may have been due to the rapid inactivation (i.e., oxidation, plasma clearance, etc.) of DTT whereas cysteamine, an aminothiol, may have been protected by its preferential uptake by lysosomes (Thoene et al., 1976). The effectiveness of cysteamine and the fact that cystamine (the disulfide of cysteamine) enhanced the residual leukocyte activity in vitro suggests that the disulfide may be of therapeutic value since it is reduced to cysteamine, presumably by glutathione or other reducing agents (Thoene et al., 1976). In contrast to cysteamine, cystamine is odorless and colorless, which should facilitate its palatable inclusion in the feline diet for the evaluation of long-term therapy in feline MPS VI.

PROSPECTUS

It is anticipated that the study of animal models of inborn errors of metabolism will have a dramatic impact on the future development and evaluation of effective therapies for a variety of human enzyme deficiency diseases. Therefore, resources should be provided for continued efforts directed toward the discovery of new models and the establishment of breeding colonies. Requisite to the use of these model systems is the characterization of the molecular nature of the enzymatic defect in each newly discovered animal disorder. In the future, application of recombinant DNA techniques will permit the identification of the precise genetic alteration in each mutant allele. These molecular genetic studies will establish whether the animal model is an analogue or homlogue of the human disease. This information will not only provide insight into the molecular pathology of the disease, but will also permit selection of appropriate breeding mates with the same or different genic lesions and the rational design of therapeutic strategies at the cellular and enzymatic level. Selected models of inherited metabolic disorders should also provide the unique opportunity to intorduce and evaluate the effectiveness of various gene therapy strategies. Clearly, the future application of human gene therapy will be predicated on the results of critical experiments performed in these animal model systems.

ACKNOWLEDGEMENTS

The authors wish to thank Mrs. Linda Lugo for her expert clerical assistance.

This work was supported in part from grants (AM 25759, GM 20138 and AM 25279), from the National Institutes of Health and a grant (1-578) from the March of Dimes Birth Defects Foundation. MMMcG and EHS are the recipients of NIH predoctoral fellowships (1T32HD07105).

REFERENCES

Aaron K, Goldman H, Scriver CR (1971). Cystinosis; new observations: 1. Adolescent (type III) form. 2. Correction of phenotypes in vitro with dithiothreitol. In Caroon NAJ, Raine DN (eds): "Inherited Disorders of Sulphur Metabolism," Baltimore: Williams and Wilkins, p 150.

Andrews EJ, Ward BL, Altman NJ (1979). "Spontaneous Animal Models of Human Disease, Volume II." New York: Academic Press.

Bach G, Bargel R, Cantz M (1979). I-cell disease: Deficiency of extracellular hydrolase phosphorylation. Biochem Biophys Res Commun 91:976.

Baker HJ, Lindsey JR, McKhann GM, Farrell, DF (1978). Neuronal G_{M1} gangliosidosis in a Siamese cat with β-galactosidase deficiency. Science 174:838.

Beratis NG, Turner BM, Weiss R, Hirschhorn K (1975). Aryl-sulfatase B deficiency in Maroteaux-Lamy syndrome: Cellular studies and carrier identification. Pediatr Res 9:475.

Beutler E, Yoshida A (1973). Human glucose-6-phosphate de-hydrogenase variants: A supplementary tabulation. Ann Hum Genet Lond 37:151.

Blobel G, Walter P, Chang CN, Goldman BM, Erickson AH, Lingappa VR (1979). Translocation of proteins across membranes: The signal hypothesis and beyond. Symp Soc Exp Res 33:9.

Bundza A, Lowden JA, Charlton KM (1979). Niemann-Pick disease in a poodle dog. Vet Pathol 16:530.

Bunn HF, Forget BG, Ranney HM (1977). "Human Hemoglobins." Philadelphia: W.B. Saunders.

Burditt LJ, Phillips NC, Robinson D, Winchester BG, Van de Water NJ, Jolly RD (1978). Characterization of the mutant alpha-mannosidase in bovine mannosidosis. Biochem J 175:1013.

Burditt LJ, Chotai K, Hirani S, Nugent PG, Winchester BG (1980). Biochemical studies on a case of feline manno-sidosis. Biochem J 189:467.

Capen CC, Hackel DB, Jones TC, Migaki G (1981). In "Hand-book: Animal Models of Human Disease." Registry of Comparative Pathology, Armed Forces Institute of Pathology, Washington, DC.

Coccia PF, Krivit W, Cervenka J, Clawson CC, Kersey JH, Kim TH, Nesbit ME, Ramsay NKC, Warkentin PI, Teitel-baum SL, Kahn AJ, Brown DM (1980). Successful bone marrow transplantation for infantile malignant osteo-petrosis. N Engl J Med 302:701.

Cork LC, Munnell JF, Lorenz MD, Murphy JV, Baker HJ, Rat-tazzi MC (1977). G_{M2} ganglioside lysosomal storage disease in cats with β-hexosaminidase deficiency. Science 196:1014.

Dale DC, Graw RG (1974). Transplantation of allogenic bone marrow in canine cyclic neutropenia. Science 183:83.

Darling PR, McHowell J, Gawthorne JM (1981). Skeletal muscle α-glucosidases in bovine generalized glycogenosis Type II. Biochem J 198:409.

DePape-Brigger D, Goldman H, Scriver CP, Delvin E, Mainne O (1977). The in vivo use of dithiothreitol in cystinosis. Pediatr Res 11:124.

Desnick RJ, Sharp HL, Grabowski GA, Brunning RD, Sung JH, Quie PG, Ikonne JU (1976). Mannosidosis: Clinical, ultrastructural, immunologic and biochemical studies. Pediatr Res 10:985.

Desnick RJ, Fiddler MB, Thorpe SR, Steger, LD (1977). In Chang TMS (ed): "Biomedical Applications of Immobilized Enzymes and Proteins," New York: Academic Press, p 227.

Desnick RJ, Grabowski GA (1981). Advances in the treatment of inherited metabolic diseases. In Harris H, Hirschhorn K (eds): "Advances in Human Genetics," New York: Plenum Press, p 281.

Donnelly WF, Sheahan BJ, Kelly M (1973). Beta-galactosidase deficiency in G_{M1} gangliosidosis of Friesian calves. Res Vet Sci 15:139.

Duchen LW, Eicher EM, Jacobs JM, Scaravilli F, Teixeira F (1980). Hereditary leucodystrophy in the mouse: The new mutant twitcher. Brain 103:695.

Farrow BRH, Hartley WJ, Pollard AC, Grabowski GA, Fabbro D, Desnick RJ (1982). Gaucher disease in the dog. In Desnick RJ, Grabowski GA, Gatt S (eds): "Gaucher Disease: A Century of Delineation and Research," New York: Alan R. Liss, Inc.

Fiddler MB, Hudson LDS, Desnick RJ (1977). Enzyme therapy VIII: Immunologic evaluation of repeated administration of erythrocyte-entrapped β-glucuronidase to β-glucuronidase deficient mice. Biochem J 168:141.

Fleisher LD, Gaull GE (1980). Enzyme manipulation by specific megavitamin therapy. In Desnick RJ (ed): "Enzyme Therapy in Genetic Diseases:2," New York: Alan R. Liss, Inc.

Fluharty AL, Stevens RL, Sanders DL, Kihara H (1974). Arylsulfatase B deficiency in Maroteaux-Lamy syndrome cultured fibroblasts. Biochem Biophys Res Commun 59:455.

Ganschow R, Paigen K (1967). Separate genes determining the structure and intracellular location of hepatic glucuronidase. Proc Natl Acad Sci USA 58:938.

Girardin EP, DeWolfe MS, Crocker JFS (1979). Treatment of cystinosis with cysteamine. J Pediatr 94:838.

Goldman H, Scriver CR, Aaron K, Delvin E, Canlas R (1971). Adolescent cystinosis: Comparisons with infantile and adult forms. Pediatrics 47:979.

Grabowski GA, Walling L, Desnick RJ (1980). Human mannosidosis: In vitro and in vivo studies of cofactor supplementation. In Desnick RJ (ed): "Enzyme Therapy in Genetic Diseases:2," New York: Alan R. Liss, p 319.

Gregoriadis G (1978). Liposomes in therapy of lysosomal storage diseases. Nature 275:695.

Hasilik A, Waheed A, von Figure K (1981). Enzymatic phosphorylation of lysosomal enzymes in the presence of UDP-N-acetylglucosamine. Absence of the activity in I-cell fibroblasts. Biochem Biophys Res Commun 98: 761.

Hasilik A, Neufeld EF (1980). Biosynthesis of lysosomal enzymes in fibroblasts. Phosphorylation of mannose residues. J Biol Chem 255:4946.

Haskins ME, Jezyk PF, Desnick RJ, McDonough SK, Patterson DF (1979a). Alpha-L-iduronidase deficiency in a cat: A model of mucopolysaccharidosis I. Pediatr Res 13:1294.

Haskins ME, Jezyk PF, Patterson DF (1979b). Mucopoly-saccharide storage disease in three families of cats with arylsulfatase B deficiency: Leukocyte studies and carrier identification. Pediatr Res 12:1203.

Hirschhorn R (1980). Treatment of genetic diseases by allo-transplantation. In Desnick RJ (ed): "Enzyme Therapy in Genetic Diseases:2," New York: Alan R. Liss, p 429.

Hobbs JR (1981). Bone marrow transplantation for inborn errors. Lancet 2:735.

Hobbs JR, Barrett AJ, Chambers D, James DCO, Hugh-Jones K, Byron N, Henry K, Lucas CF, Rogers TR, Benson PF, Tansley LR, Patrick AD, Mossman J, Young EP (1981). Reversal of clinical features of Hurler's disease and biochemical improvement after treatment by bone marrow transplantation. Lancet 2:709.

Hocking JD, Jolly RD, Batt RD (1972). Deficiency of α-mannosidase in Angus cattle. Biochem J 128:69.

Holmes EW, O'Brien JS (1978). Feline G_{M1}-gangliosidosis: Characterization of the residual liver acid β-galactosidase. Am J Hum Genet 30:505.

Hommes FA (1979). "Models for the Study of Inborn Errors of Metabolism," Amsterdam: Elsevier/North Holland Biomedical Press.

Hudson LDS, Fiddler MB, Desnick RJ (1979). Enzyme therapy X: Immunological evaluation of repeated administration of liposome-entrapped protein in C3H/HeJ mice. J Pharm Exp Ther 209:507.

Jezyk PF, Haskins ME, Patterson DF, Mellman WJ, Greenstein M (1977). Mucopolysaccharidosis in a cat with aryl-sulfatase B deficiency: A model of Maroteaux-Lamy syndrome. Science 198:834.

Jolly RD, Thompson KG, Murphy CE, Manklelow BW, Bruere AN, Winchester BG (1976). Enzyme replacement therapy - an experiment of nature in a chimeric mannosidosis calf. Pediatr Res 10:219.

Jolly RD, Van de Water NS, Janmaat A, Slack PM, McKenzie PG (1980). Zinc therapy in the bovine mannosidosis model. In Desnick RJ (ed): "Enzyme Therapy in Genetic Diseases:2," New York: Alan R. Liss, p 305.

Jones M, Laine RA (1981). Caprine oligosaccharide storage disease. J Biol Chem 256:5181.

Jones MZ, Dawson G (1981). Caprine β-mannosidosis: Inherited deficiency of β-D-mannosidase. J Biol Chem 256: 5185.

Kan YW, Holland J, Dory A, Varmus H (1975). Demonstration of non-functional β-globin mRNA in homozygous β-thalassemia. Proc Natl Acad Sci 72:5140.

Kantor JA, Turner PH, Nienhuis AW (1980). Beta-thalassemia: Mutations which affect processing of the β-globin mRNA precursor. Cell 21:149.

Kaplan A, Fischer D, Aclord D, Sly W (1977). Phosphohexosyl recognition is a general characteristic of pinocytosis of lysosomal glycosidases by human fibroblasts. J Clin Invest 60:1088.

Loutit JF, Sansom JM (1976). Osteopetrosis of microphthalmice - a defect of the haemopoietic stem cell? Calc Tiss Res 20:251.

Maccecchini ML, Rudin Y, Blobel G, Schatz G (1979). Import of proteins into mitochonrdria: Precursor forms of the extramitochondrially-made Fi-ATPase subunits in yeast. Proc Natl Acad Sci USA 76:343.

Matas AJ, Simmons RL, Desnick RJ (1978a). Transplantation in metabolic disease. In Buchwald H, Varco RL (eds): "Metabolic Surgery," New York: Grune and Stratton, p 177.

Matas AJ, Desnick RJ, Najarian JS, Simmons RL (1978b). Clinical and experimental transplantation in enzymatic deficiency disease. Surg Gyn Ob 146:975.

McGovern MM, Vine DT, Haskins ME, Desnick RJ (1981). An improved method for heterozygote detection in feline and human mucopolysaccharidosis VI, arylsulfatase B deficiency. Enzyme 26:206.

McGovern MM, Vine DT, Haskins ME, Desnick RJ (1982). Arylsulfatase B: Comparative physical and kinetic properties of the feline and human isozymes. J Biol Chem, in review.

McKusick V (1978). "Mendelian Inheritance in Man," Baltimore: The Johns Hopkins University Press.

Mukherjee AB, Krasner J (1973). Induction of an enzyme in genetically deficient rats after grafting of normal liver. Science 182:68.

Natowicz MR, Chi MMY, Lowry OH, Sly WS (1979). Enzymatic identification of mannose 6-phosphate on the recognition marker for receptor-mediated pinocytosis of β-glucuronidase by human fibroblasts. Proc Natl Acad Sci USA 76:4322.

Noren AG, O'Brien JS (1975). An electrophoretic variant of β-galactosidase with altered catalytic properties in a patient with G_{M1}-gangliosidosis. Proc Natl Acad Sci USA 72:240.

Paigen K (1979). Acid hydrolases as models of genetic control. Ann Rev Genet 13:417.

Patterson DF, Haskins ME, Jezyk PF (1982). Models of human genetic disease in domestic animals. In Harris H, Hirschhorn K (eds): "Advances in Human Genetics," New York: Plenum Press.

Phillips NC, Robinson D, Winchester BG (1974). Human liver α-mannosidase activity. Clin Chim Acta 55:11.

Pierce KR, Kosanke SD, Bay WW, Bridges CH (1976). G_{M2}-gangliosidosis: Porcine cerebrospinal lipodystrophy. Am J Pathol 83:419.

Proudfoot NJ, Shander MH, Manley JL, Gefler ML, Maniatis T. (1980). Structure and in vitro transcription of human globin genes. Science 209:1329.

Rattazzi MC, Appel AM, Nestu JA (1979). Towards enzyme therapy in G_{M2}-gangliosidosis: Visceral organ and CNS uptake of human β-hexosaminidase in normal cats. Am J Hum Genet 30:59A.

Rattazzi MC, Lanse SB, McCoullough RA, Nestu JA, Jacobs EA (1980). Towards enzyme replacement in G_{M2}-gangliosidosis: Organ disposition and induced central nervous system uptake of human β-hexosaminidase in the cat. In Desnick RJ (ed): "Enzyme Therapy in Genetic Diseases: 2," New York: Alan R. Liss, Inc., p 179.

Rattazzi MC (1980). In Lowden S, Callehan M (eds): "Lysosomes and lysosomal storage diseases," Toronto: Academic Press.

Read DH, Harrington D, Keenan TW, Hinsman E (1976). Neuronal-visceral G_{M1}-gangliosidosis in a dog with β-galactosidase deficiency. Science 194:442.

Reitman ML, Varki A, Kornfeld S (1981). Fibroblasts from patients with I-cell disease and pseudo-Hurler polydystrophy are deficient in uridine 5'-diphosphate-N-acetylglucosamine, glycoprotein N-acetylglucosaminyl-phosphotransferase activity. J Clin Invest 67:1574.

Richards RB, Edwards JR, Cook RD, White RR (1977). Bovine generalized glycogenosis. Neuropathol Appl Neurobiol 3:45.

Rittmann LS, Tennant LL, O'Brien JS (1980). Dog G_{M1}-gangliosidosis: Characterization of the residual liver acid beta-galactosidase. Am J Hum Genet 32:880.

Sando GN, Neufeld EF (1977). Recognition and receptor-mediated uptake of a lysosomal enzyme, α-L-iduronidase, by cultured human fibroblasts. Cell 12:619.

Shapira E, DeGregorio RR, Matalon R, Nadler HL (1975). Reduced arylsulfatase B activity of the mutant enzyme protein in Maroteaux-Lamy syndrome. Biochem Biophys Res Commun 62:448.

Slavin S, Yatziv S (1980). Correction of enzyme deficiency in mice by allogenic bone marrow transplantation with total lymphoid irradiation. Science 210:1150.

Sly WS (1980). Saccharide traffic signals in receptor-mediated endocytosis and transport of acid hydrolases. In Svennerholm L, Mandel P, Dreyfus H, Urban PF (eds): "Structure and Function of the Gangliosides," New York: Plenum Publishing Corp, p 433.

Snaith SM (1975). Characterization of jack-bean α-D-mannosidase as a zinc metaloenzyme. Biochem J 143:83.

Sorell M, Rosen JF, Kapoor N, Kirkpatrick D, Chaganti RSK, Pollack MS, Dupont B, Goossen C, Good RA, O'Reilly RJ (1979). Bone marrow transplant for osteopetrosis in a 10 year old boy. Pediatr Res 13:481A.

Steger LD, Desnick RJ (1977). Enzyme therapy VI: Comparative in vivo fates and effects on lysosomal integrity of enzyme entrapped in negatively- and positively-charged liposomes. Biochim Biophys Acta 464:530.

Stumpf DA, Austin JH, Craker AC, LaFrance M (1973). Mucopolysaccharidosis type VI (Maroteaux-Lamy syndrome). Am J Dis Child 126:747.

Sung JH, Hayano M, Desnick RJ (1977). Pathology of the nervous system in mannosidosis. J Neuropath Exp Neurol 36:807.

Sutherland DER, Matas AJ, Steffes MW, Simmons RL, Najarian JS (1977). Transplantation of liver cells in an animal model of congenital enzyme deficiency disease: The Gunn rat. Transplantation Proceedings, Vol IX, no 1, p 317.

Suzuki Y, Austin J, Armstrong D, Suzuki K, Schlenkr J, Fletcher T (1970). Studies in globoid leukodystrophy: Enzymatic and lipid findings in the canine form. Exp Neurol 29:65.

Szostak JW, Stiles JI, Tye BK, Chiu P, Sherman F, Wu R (1979). Hybridization with synthetic oligonucleotides. In Wu R (ed): "Methods in Enzymology, Vol 68," New York: Academic Press, p 419.

Thoene JG, Oshima RG, Crawhall JC, Olson DL, Schneider JA (1976). Cystinosis: Intracellular cystine depletion by aminothiols in vitro and in vivo. J Clin Invest 58:180.

Thorpe SR, Fiddler MB, Desnick RJ (1974). Enzyme therapy IV: A method for determining the in vivo fate of bovine β-glucuronidase in β-glucuronidase deficient mice. Biochem Biophys Res Commun 61:1464.

Thorpe SR, Fiddler MB, Desnick RJ (1975). Enzyme therapy V: In vivo fate of erythrocyte-entrapped β-glucuronidase in β-glucuronidase deficient mice. Pediatr Res 9:918.

Ullrich K, Mersmann G, Weber E, von Figura K (1978). Evidence for lysosomal enzyme recognition by human fibroblasts via a phosphorylated carbohydrate moiety. Biochem J 170:643.

Van de Water NS, Jolly RD, Farrow BRH (1979). Canine Gaucher disease - the enzymic defect. Aust J Exp Biol 57:551.

Vine DT, McGovern MM, Haskins ME, Desnick RJ (1981). Feline mucopolysaccharidosis VI: Purification and characterization of the residual arylsulfatase B activity. Am J Hum Genet, in press.

Vine DT, McGovern MM, Schuchman EH, Haskins ME, Desnick RJ (1982). Enhancement of residual arylsulfatase B activity in feline mucopolysaccharidosis VI by thiol-induced subunit association. J Clin Invest, in press.

Walker DG (1975). Bone resorption restored in osteopetrotic mice by transplants of normal bone marrow and spleen cells. Science 190:784.

Wallace RB, Johnson MJ, Hirose T, Miyake T, Kawashima EH, Itakura K (1980). The use of synthetic oligonucleotides as hybridization probes. II. Hybridization of oligonucleotides of mixed sequence to rabbit β-globin DNA. Nucleic Acids Res 9:879.

Wenger DA, Sattler M, Kendoh T, Snyder SP, Kingston RS (1980). Niemann-Pick disease: A genetic model in Siamese cats. Science 208:1471.

Wetherall DJ, Clegg JB (1979). Recent developments in the molecular genetics of human hemoglobin. Cell 16:467.

Yoshida A, Beutler E, Motulsky AG (1971). Table of human glucose-6-phosphate dehydrogenase variants. Bull Wld Hlth Org 45:243.

Yoshida A, Beutler E (1978). Human glucose-6-phosphat dehydrogenase variants: A supplementary tabulation. Ann Hum Genet Lond 41:3 47.

Yudkoff M, Foreman JN, Segal S (1981). Effect of cysteamine therapy in nephrotic cystinosis. N Engl J Med 304: 141.

DR. JEZYK: How much enzyme do you think you have to get into the patient so that enzyme replacement is worthwhile?

DR. DESNICK: I think we are going to have to look at each disorder individually in order to determine how much normal enzyme is necessary to correct the metabolic defect. It is difficult to extrapolate from the tissue culture studies into the human being, as you are well aware, but I think our animal model studies will give us some insights.

DR. RATTAZZI: May I comment on Dr. Jezyk's question? I think the answer depends on the organ, the enzyme and the substrate. We can replace 100 percent of β-hexosaminidase in the liver of GM2 gangliosidosis cats, and in 48 hours we have a complete depletion of the stored ganglioside and globoside. We can also replace 100 percent of the enzyme in brain, but we don't get that kind of effect. There is a time factor. There is an uptake specificity factor. There is, also, a ratio of enzyme replaced to substrate stored. So, I don't think you can give a general answer to this problem. You have to look organ by organ.

DR. BAKER: I wish to reinforce Dr. Rattazzi's comment. The substrate specificity is very important to consider when you talk about residual activity. Dr. Desnick, I presume you are talking about residual activity against synthetic as opposed to natural substrate? It is very common to find a 10 percent residual activity against a simple substrate like 4-methylumbelliferyl with absolutely no detectable activity against the natural substrate.

DR. DESNICK: Yes, but if there is activity with the artificial substrate, it would be unusual to find absent natural substrate activity.

DR. T. C. JONES: Three or four years ago the Advisory Committee of the Registry of Comparative Pathology discussed the idea that technology in molecular biology was advancing so rapidly that very soon we would be in a position of being able to do genetic engineering and attack some of the metabolic disorders. We were encouraged to push this idea to stimulate people to develop animal models of metabolic disorders. We decided to do what we could to publicize this idea, and this was basically one of the, or maybe the basic thought, in organizing this symposium. Dr. Desnick, you put the use of animal models in such beautiful terms and in such specific ways that all I can say is just thank you so much. It was beautifully done, and it is exactly what I had in mind, when you talked about therapeutic strategies and applying modern technologies to the treatment of disease and the necessity of using animal models. I repeat, you said it very well. Few could express it like you have. You have done it superbly, and I thank you.

DR. DESNICK: Thank you.

DR. O'BRIEN: I liked it too. But I am curious just for my own information the extent to which the recombinant DNA in the field of lysosomal storage disease has progressed. Have molecular clones been prepared against any of these enzymes?

DR. DESNICK: Not to my knowledge.

DR. O'BRIEN: How about antisera against all of them? Has that been reported?

DR. DESNICK: Yes, there are antisera to a number of these enzymes.

DR. O'BRIEN: So, hopefully, we should start seeing the clones being announced in the next year or so.

DR. DESNICK: That would be nice, but a year or so may be optimistic.

Animal Models of Inherited Metabolic Diseases, pages 67-90
© **1982 Alan R. Liss, Inc., 150 Fifth Avenue, New York, NY 10011**

GENETIC ANALYSIS IN THE DOMESTIC CAT AS AN ANIMAL
MODEL FOR INBORN ERRORS, CANCER AND EVOLUTION

Stephen J. O'Brien, William G. Nash,
Cheryl A. Winkler, and Roger H. Reeves
Section of Genetics
Laboratory of Viral Carcinogenesis
National Cancer Institute
Frederick, MD 21701

The domestic cat has an established viral etiology of
leukemia and sarcoma and a well defined epidemiology of feline
leukemia virus (FeLV) associated antigens and antibody
distribution in cat households studied throughout the world
(Hardy et al., 1980). The cellular genetic organization of
those genes known to be operative in the onset of feline
leukemia and related phenomena would, we believe, be an
important subject for the understanding of neoplastic
development in cats as well as in related mammalian species.
An important class of genes to be considered in such an
analysis would be the endogenous retroviral gene sequences
(RD114 and FeLV) present in some Felis species including the
domestic cat. Earlier studies by Benveniste & Todaro (1974)
and by Benveniste et al. (1975) suggested that certain Felis
species have acquired virogenes from primates and rodents
(RD114 and FeLV, respectively) by cross species infection and
fixation subsequent to evolutionary divergence of mammalian
orders.

The domestic cat has also served as a model for several
inborn errors known to have homologous counterparts in man. A
list of a number of heritable biochemical disorders identified
in cats is presented in Table 1. We also present the specific
enzyme defect identified. Several of these cat diseases have
served as useful objects for enzyme therapy and treatment of
homologous human diseases. More extensive discussion of the
diseases and various technologies are presented in this volume
and elsewhere (Desnick, 1981).

Table 1
HUMAN HEREDITARY DISEASES WITH FELINE MODELS

Disease	Protein affected	Reference
Hemophilia	factor VIII	Cotter et al. (1978)
Hemophilia B (Christmas disease)	factor IX	Dodds (1978)
Factor XII (Hageman deficiency)	factor XII	Green and White (1977)
Chediak-Higashi Syndrome	unknown	Kramer et al. (1977)
Arterial Thrombosis (experimental)	unknown	Schaub et al. (1977)
Nieman-Pick Disease	lysosomal sphingomyelinase	Wenger et al. (1980)
Maroteaux-Lamy Syndrome (mucopolysaccharidosis-VI)	arylsulfatose B	Jezyk et al. (1977)
Hurler's Syndrome (Mucopolysaccharidosis-I	α-L-iduronidase	Haskins et al. (1979)
GM$_1$ Gangliosidosis	β-galactosidase	Baker et al. (1971)
GM$_2$ Gangliosidosis	β-hexosaminidase A	Cork et al. (1977)
Ehler's Danlos Syndrome	collagen fibrillogenesis	Patterson and Minor (1977)
Dermatosporaxis (bovine)	NH$_2$ procollagen peptidases	Counts et al. (1980)

An unfortunate gap in the use of mammalian animal models is the paucity of species with genetic maps extensive enough for consideration of genetic analysis. The genetic maps of man and mouse each contain over 300 defined and genetically localized loci representing the collective efforts of scores of laboratories for each species (Lalley, 1980; Womack, 1980). We have elected to develop the domestic cat to the point of feasible genetic analysis in several steps. These include: (1) Identification of polymorphic morphological and biochemical loci; (2) Genetic mapping of these genes by sexual and parasexual techniques; (3) Placement of neoplasia related genes on the map, and (4) Placement of the genes involved in inborn errors on the map; and (5) Comparative genetic analysis of homologous loci in mouse, cat and man. We present here a summary of our progress to date in genetic analysis of the cat.

POLYMORPHIC MORPHOLOGICAL LOCI.

Approximately 25 mutant loci have been described in the domestic cat, fifteen of which are polymorphic in feral cat populations and which contribute in various combinations to the over 100 breeds of cats presently being maintained (Robinson, 1977). Table 2 is a list of the morphological loci

Table 2
MORPHOLOGICAL LOCI OF THE CAT WHICH VARY BETWEEN BREEDS

Name of Gene	Alleles	Name of Gene	Alleles
agouti	A,a	Cornish rex	R,r
brown	B,b,b^e	Devon rex	Re,re
albino	C,c^b,c^s,c^a,c	Oregon rex	Ro,ro
dilute	D,d	Whitespotting	S,s
melanin inhibitor	I,i	sphinx	Sp,sp
long hair	L,l	tabby	T,T^a,t^b
manx	M,m	white	W,w
orange	O,o	wire hair	Wh,wh

Adapted from Robinson (1977)

Table 3
POLYMORPHIC BIOCHEMICAL LOCI:
ALLELE DISTRIBUTION AND TEST FOR
CONFORMITY OF GENOTYPE FREQUENCY TO
HARDY-WEINBERG EQUILIBRIUM (HWE)

Locus	No. cats	Allele frequency	Frequency of heterozygotes		HWE χ^2
			observed	expected (HWE)	
1. ADA	33	a = 0.55 b = 0.39 c = 0.06	0.67	0.53	4.2
2. ES1	33	a = 0.08 b = 0.78 c = 0.14	0.30	0.35	3.4
3. ES5	45	a = 0.78 b = 0.22	0.35	0.34	0.77
4. FUCA	29	a = 0.89 b = 0.11	0.21	0.20	0.41
5. GDH2	23	a = 0.52 b = 0.48	0.50	0.49	0.001
6. GPI	56	a = 0.95 b = 0.05	0.07	0.10	3.2
7. HB( )	35	s = 0.63 d = 0.37	N.D.	0.47	N.D.
8. ME1	33	a = 0.94 b = 0.06	0.0	0.11	N.D.
9. PEPA	31	a = 0.61 b = 0.39	0.65	0.48	3.7
10. PFK	23	a = 0.85 b = 0.15	0.13	0.25	5.9
11. PGD	54	a = 0.38 b = 0.62	0.46	0.47	0.01
12. PGM3	27	a = 0.74 b = 0.26	0.44	0.38	0.6

which vary at appreciable frequencies in cats (Robinson, 1977). One of these, 0, is presumably X-linked, since its heterozygous expression in females produces the calico or tortoise shell phenotype due to mosaic X-inactivation (Centerwall & Benirschke, 1973). For an excellent treatment of the interaction of these morphological loci to produce various cat breeds, the reader should consult Robinson (1977).

POLYMORPHIC BIOCHEMICAL LOCI.

A sample of 56 adult cats from rural farm cat population trapped in 1978 in Pennsylvania, Maryland, and Virginia was examined for allelic variation at 55 biochemical loci (O'Brien, 1980). The soluble proteins and enzymes were visualized by histochemical enzyme development following gel electrophoresis of crude extracts of kidney, liver, red blood cells, and serum (O'Brien et al., 1980; Harris & Hopkinson, 1976). Of the 55 loci which were scored, 43 were invariant and 12 were polymorphic (22 percent) for at least two alleles. The allele designations and their frequencies of polymorphism in the population sample are presented in Table 3. Monomorphic loci are listed by O'Brien (1980). The gene designations conform to the recommendations for the homologous human enzymes of the International System for Human Nomenclature ISGN (Shows et al., 1979).

The genotypic frequencies at the polymorphic loci were each distributed in conformity with the expectation of the Hardy-Weinburg equilibrium. The average heterozygosity over all loci in the population was 0.07, which is similar to estimates in other mammalian species including mice and man (Powell, 1976; Nevo, 1978; Rice & O'Brien, 1980; Harris & Hopkinson, 1972). The polymorphic loci in Tables 1-3 represent the total genetic variation available today for sexual genetic analysis of the domestic cat .

DERIVATION OF A SYNTENIC MAP OF THE CAT BY SOMATIC CELL GENETICS.

Interspecific somatic cell hybrids provide an important technology for gene mapping because it is possible to generate hybrids which preferentially segregate the chromosomes of one parental species (for example, the cat) in different combinations among the hybrid clones. Concordant expression and loss of two genetic markers (antigens, isozymes, etc.) form the basis for identification of a syntenic group in the segregant parent. The syntenic groups, which are analogous to linkage groups derived from sexual genetic crosses (Ruddle et al., 1971), presumably represent groups of loci which reside on individual chromosomes. The empirical definition of a syntenic group of multiple loci depends upon two important observations: (1) the concordant appearance of the markers in a hybrid panel, and (2) substantial discordancy with all the other markers followed in the same cross. In addition, concordant segregation of gene markers and specific chromosomes identified by banding techniques permits the assignment of the syntenic groups to individual chromosomes. These parasexual techniques have provided detailed genetic maps of man, mouse, and several primates in cumulative studies over the past decade (Womack, 1980; McKusick & Ruddle, 1977; Ruddle & Creagan, 1975; Pearson et al., 1981; Lalley, 1980).

We have derived a feline syntenic map based upon concordant segregation of isozyme markers in 645 primary hybrid colonies and 158 subclones derived from 20 fusions of 9 different types between rodent cells and cat cell lines or fresh tissue. Each of these hybrids were found to retain the entire rodent genome and to segregate feline chromosomes in different combinations (O'Brien, 1976; O'Brien & Nash, 1982). The hybrid clones were each expanded to between 10^7 and 10^8 cells, harvested, and electrophoretically typed for presence or absence of feline isozymes (31 loci). Multiple cell fusions were employed to circumvent phenotyping difficulties inherent in certain individual crosses, such as similar electrophoretic mobilities of isozymes in cat x mouse hybrids which could be resolved in cat x hamster hybrids. Table 4 presents a list of the biochemical loci typed in these hybrids, their genetic symbol, tissue distribution, and derived chromosomal location.

Seventeen syntenic groups have been defined in this analysis (O'Brien & Nash, 1982) and these are presented in Table 5. Twelve of the seventeen groups have been assigned to specific feline chromosomes by karyologic analysis of representative hybrid clones. Thirty-three primary hybrids and 41 secondary subclones were karyotyped, and the frequency of each feline chromosome on a background of rodent (mouse or

Table 4
BIOCHEMICAL LOCI OF THE CAT

IUPAC-Enzyme	Gene IUB No.	Symbol	Chromosome	Tissues Present	Absent
Erythrocyte Acid phosphatase-1	3.1.3.2	ACP1	A3	R,K,C,L	
Tissue acid phosphatase-2	3.1.3.2	ACP2	A2	C	
Adenosine deaminase	3.5.4.4	ADA	-	K,C	R
Adenylate kinase-1	2.7.4.3	AK1	-	R,K,C,L	
Esterase-D	3.1.1.1	ES5	A1	K,C,R	
Glyceraldehyde-3-phosphate dehydrogenase	1.2.1.12	GAPD	B4	C	
Glyoxylase-1	4.4.1.5	GLO1	B2	K,R,C	
Glucose-6-phosphate dehydrogenase	1.1.1.49	G6PD	X	K,R,C	
Glucose phosphate isomerase	5.3.1.9	GPI	-	R,K,L,C	
Glutathione reductase	1.6.4.2	GSR	-	K,C,R	
Hexosaminidase-A	3.2.1.30	HEXA	B3	K,L,C	R
Hexokinase-1	2.7.1.1	HK1	D2	K,C	R

(Cont'd)

Table 4 (Cont'd)

Enzyme	IUPAC-IUB No.	Gene Symbol	Chromosome	Tissues Present	Absent
Hypoxanthine-guanine phosphoribosyl transferase	2.4.2.8	HPRT	X	C,K	
Isocitrate dehydrogenase-1 (soluble)	1.1.1.42	IDH1	C1	K,C	R
Lactate dehydrogenase-A	1.1.1.27	LDHA	A2	K,R,C,L	
Lactate dehydrogenase-B	1.1.1.37	LDHB	B4	K,R,C	
Malate dehydrogenase-1 (soluble)	1.1.1.37	MDH1	A3	K,R,C	
Malic enzyme-1 (soluble)	1.1.1.40	ME1	B2	K,C	
Mannose phosphate isomerase	5.3.1.8	MPI	B3	K,R,C	
Purine nucleoside phosphorylase	2.4.2.1	NP	B3	K,C	R
Peptidase A	3.4.11*	PEPA	-	K,C	R
Peptidase B1	3.4.11*	PEPB1	B4	K,R,C	
Peptidase S	3.4.11*	PEPS	B1	C	
6-Phosphogluconate dehydrogenase	1.1.1.44	PGD	C1	R,K,L,C	
Phosphoglucomutase-1	2.7.5.1	PGM1	C1	K,C,R	

(Cont'd)

Table 4 (Cont'd)

Enzyme	IUPAC-IUB No.	Gene Symbol	Chromosome	Tissues Present	Absent
Phosphoglu-comutase-3	2.7.5.1	PGM3	B2	K,C	R
Pyrophospha-tase, inorg.	3.6.1.1	PP	D4	K,C	R
Pyruvic kinase	2.7/1/40	PKM1	B3	C	
Superoxide dismutase-1	1.15.1.1	SOD1	C2	C	
Superoxide dismutase-2	1.15.1.1	SOD2	B2	L,K,R,C	
Triosephos-phate iso-merase	5.3.1.1	TPI	B4	R,K,C	
Other Loci:					
Orange	-	O	X	coat color	
Balb virus restriction-1	-	BVR1	X	C	

*Tissues where enzyme is expressed: R-red blood cells; K-kidney; L-liver; C-culture cells.

Chinese hamster) chromosomes was determined. Figure 1 presents karyotypes of RAG mouse and Chinese hamster E36 cells, as well as hybrid cells with certain feline chromosomes so indicated. Our results, which have been presented in detail (O'Brien & Nash, 1982; O'Brien et al., 1980), provide the basis for chromosome assignment of 26 feline enzyme

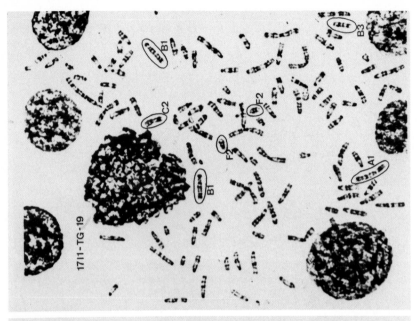

Fig. 1A

Fig. 1B

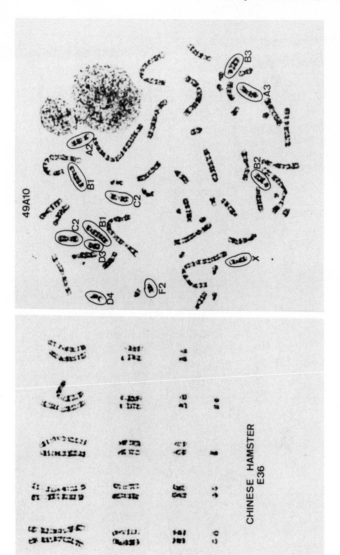

Fig. 1C

Fig. 1D

CHINESE HAMSTER
E36

Table 5

FELINE GENETIC MAP.
(*Felis catus*), N = 19

Feline Linkage Group	Feline Chromosome	Gene
1.	A1	ESD
2.	A2	LDHA, ACP2
3.	A3	MDH1, ACP1
4.	B1	PEPS
5.	B2	ME1, PGM3, GLO, SOD2
6.	B3	NP, MPI, PKM2, HEXA
7.	B4	TPI, PEPB1, LDHB, GAPD
8.	C1	PGM1, PGD, IDH1
9.	C2	SOD1
11	D.4	PP
10.	D2	HK
19.	X	G6PD, HPRT, BVR1, 0
	-	ADA
	-	GPI
	-	GSR
	-	PEPA
	-	AK1

structural genes (Table 4 and 5). The remaining five syntenic groups each contain a single isozyme marker, ADA, GPI, GSR, PEPA and AK1. We have been unable to provide precise chromosome assignments for these markers for technical reasons.

COMPARATIVE GENETIC MAPPING IN MAMMALS.

The construction of the feline genetic map permits the direct comparison to the genetic maps of homologous loci previously derived in man, in primates, and in the mouse (Pearson et al., 1981). Figure 2 presents a chromosome by chromosome comparison of 31 mapped feline genes and their homologous human counterparts. The genes are arranged in order of their location on human chromosomes, since the subchromosomal locations of the cat genes are largely unknown.

Figure 2

COMPARATIVE LINKAGES OF CAT AND MAN

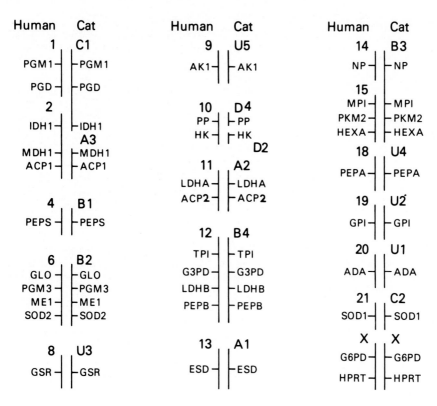

A striking observation of this comparison between human and feline linkages is the similarity between the two species. Of the 17 groups compared in Figure 2 (several with 2-4 loci), only 3 differences between the species are evident. First, in man, IDH1 is linked to MDH1 and ACP1 on chromosome 2, while in cats, IDH1 is linked to PGM1 and PGD (chr. Cl). A discordance of IDH1 and MDH1-ACP1 is also observed in maps of chimpanzee, gorilla, orangutan and rhesus monkey which possess no metacentric homologue to human chromosome 2 (Pearson et al., 1981). In the chimpanzee, this genetic material is contained on 2 acrocentric chromosomes (chimp chr. 12 and 13) homologous to human chromosome arms 2p and 2q. Apparently, human chromosome two was derived from a rather recent end-to-end fusion between the telomeres of the more ancestral primate telocentric chromosomes. The second exception is that NP is linked to PKM2-MPI-HEXA (chr. B3) in cats, while in man NP is on a separate chromosome (chr. 14) from PKM2-MPI-HEXA (chr. 15) (Lalley, 1980). The linkage association of NP with PKM2-MPI and HEXA is conserved in pigs and rhesus monkeys, but is broken (with respect to NP only) in chimpanzee and man (Pearson et al., 1981), indicating that dual chromosomes for these markers are a recent primate acquisition. The third exception is the placement of HK1 and PP on two chromosomes (D2 and D4, respectively) in the cat while these groups are linked in both mouse and man. The separation of these markers may be a recent Felidae development.

Comparative gene mapping data is of importance in two ways: first as an indicator of chromosomal subregions which have remained tightly linked, possibly by selective pressure throughout evolution. In addition, the various syntenic groups can be used as markers of evolutionary progression and thereby order the divergence of various species in evolutionary time. This sort of data and logic has been applied to analyses of chromosome banding in closely related Drosophila species (Wallace, 1966) and to primate evolution of syntenic groups (de Grouchy et al., 1978). The second importance of comparative gene mapping lies in its ability to predict gene locations in one species (like man) after genes have been located in another. For example, several of the genes which participate in various inborn errors have been mapped to certain chromosomes in man (Table 1). In those cases where the feline homologue has been identified (Figure 2), we are inclined to look for the feline enzyme locus on that chromosome as well. Conversely, the location of certain feline genes not yet identified in man would have some predictive value in analysis of human loci. An example of this would be the loci which participate in development of FeLV mediated leukemia in cats (Hardy et al., 1980).

DEFINING THE FELINE MAJOR HISTOCOMPATIBILITY COMPLEX.

A major histocompatibilitiy complex (MHC) responsible for surgical allograft rejection and subsequent induction of alloantibodies has been defined in a number of laboratory mammals with the glaring exception of the domestic cat (Gotze, 1977). The participation of the MHC in development of the immune response, resistance to leukemias, susceptibility to various disease and transplant rejection, makes this locus a high priority in the study of feline genetics. We have initiated a breeding colony of 40 cats at the NIH Animal Center in Poolesville, Maryland for purposes of sexual genetic experiments (Winkler, 1981). Reciprocal skin grafts (approximately 40 cm^2) have been performed between 12 pairs of cats which differ by 0, 1, or 2 haplotypes (Winkler, 1981). Incompatible grafts are generally rejected in approximately 11 days or less. Serial, weekly bleeds of cats were monitored for alloantibody using a (feline) complement dependent microcytotoxicity assay. Of seven cats which had rejected at least two grafts from donor animals, three have produced cytoxic antibodies (Table 6). We anticipate the use of these and additional alloantisera to characterize the MHC of the cat. It may be important, in a genetic sense, to note that human chromosome 6, where HL-A resides, has 4 isozyme markers whose homologues are also linked in the cat on feline B4 (Figure 2). One might expect then by analogy to locate the feline MHC to this chromosome as well.

ORGANIZATION OF ENDOGENOUS RD114 VIROGENES IN THE FELINE GENOME.

An endogenous type C RNA tumor virus (RD114 retrovirus) is a permanent resident in the cellular DNA of all domestic cats (Benveniste & Todaro, 1974). The virus is generally quiescent; however, it can be induced to expression by treatment of cultured cat cells with halogenated pyrimidines. The virus is present in multiple copies (10-20 per haploid genome) and represents a fascinating model for the evolution and function of such endogenous virogenes.

Table 6

CYTOTOXICITY OF RECIPIENT ANTISERA ON DONOR CATS

Donor	Recipient	No. Allografts Rejected	% Cytotoxicity of Donor Lymphocytes* [Antisera Dilution (-1)]					
		Bleed Date	1	2	4	8	16	32
415	519	1-9-81	1	<10	<10	<10	<10	<10	<10
519	415	1-9-81	2	<10	<10	<10	<10	<10	<10
445	542	3-13-81	2	>90	>90	70	40	<10	<10
542	445	3-3-81	3	80	80	70	50	30	<10
SL	1A	2-17-81	2	<10	<10	N.T.	N.T.	N.T.	N.T.
1A	SL	2-17-81	2	<10	<10	N.T.	N.T.	N.T.	N.T.
1B	SHN	2-17-81	0	<10	N.T.	N.T.	N.T.	N.T.	N.T.
SN	1B	2-17-81	2	90	70	50	20	20	<10
248	480	12-15-81	0	<10	<10	<10	<10	<10	<10
480	248	12-15-81	1	<10	<10	<10	<10	<10	<10
1F	1D	1-9-81	1	<10	<10	<10	<10	<10	<10
1D	1F	1-9-81	2	<10	<10	<10	<10	<10	<10
R.S.[o]	Rabbit, pooled			100	100	100	100	80	50

*Cytotoxicity with homologous sera and complement controls was lesss than 10%. Cytotoxicity with the rabbit anti-cat lymphocyte serum was <10% in the absence of cat complement and 100% in the presence of cat complement.

[o]R.S. Lymphocytes were pooled from three Random Source cats.

The development of molecular cloning technologies including Southern blot hybridization of cell DNA (Southern, 1975) has provided us with an opportunity to examine directly the multiple RD-114 virogenes in cell DNA virtually by direct observation. Extrachromosomal DNA was prepared by the Hirt method (Hirt, 1967) from human cells acutely infected with RD114. This material, when hybridized in situ with a reverse transcribed ^{32}P-labeled cDNA probe, shows a high concentration of linear proviral DNA 8.8 kilobases long and a less abundant amount of proviral circles (Fig. 3a). Digestion of proviral linear forms with a variety of restriction endonucleases has permitted the derivation of a restriction map of the proviral genome (Fig. 3).

We have also used Southern blot hybridization to examine RD-114 sequences in cat cell DNA and in cat x mouse somatic cell hybrids. Hybridization of RD-114 specific probes to feline DNA reveals a highly complex pattern of bands, while no sequences are detected in the murine RAG cell line (Fig. 3b). The complex feline pattern is simplified in somatic cell hybrids which have segregated cat chromosomes and depends upon the feline chromosome constitution of the hybrid cell. This suggests that endogenous RD-114 sequences are distributed on multiple feline chromosomes and, further, that they may be assigned to specific chromosomes by segregation analysis. For example, the restriction patterns in two of the hybrids in Figure 3b, 17I1TG14 and 17I1TG25, are identical except for a 3.1 kb band which is present in hybrid 14 but absent from hybrid 25. Hybrid 25 contains the same feline chromosomes as hybrid 14 except for cat chromosome B4, which is present in 14 but absent from 25. This suggests that the 3.1 kb fragment may originate from RD-114 sequences located on chromosome B4, and that the other fragments, which are common to hybrids 14 and 25, are not located on this chromosome. A comprehensive analysis of a panel of somatic cell hybrids containing different arrays of feline chromosomes is being developed for assigning each of the viral DNA fragments to specific feline chromosomes.

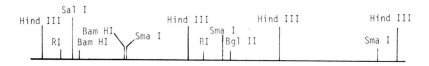

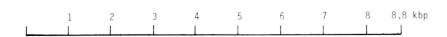

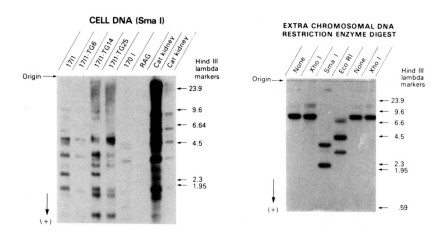

Figure 3. Top - Restriction enzyme map of linear cDNA from an extrachromosomal preparation of RD114 infected human cells. Autoradiogram of unrestricted and restricted RD114 cDNA is presented in lower right. Lower left is a restriction analysis of cellular feline DNA, murine RAG cells, and hybrids of RAG x cat with different feline chromosome complements.

CONCLUSIONS.

The data presented here provide a biochemical genetic baseline for genetic analysis of the cat. Thirty-one enzyme structural genes plus two previously mapped X-linked loci, orange O coat color (Centerwall & Benirske, 1973) and BVR1, a retrovirus restriction locus (O'Brien, 1976), have been placed in 17 syntenic groups which represent chromosomal linkage groups of the cat. This genetic map combines with several additional types of genetic data previously reported to make the cat a workable model for mammalian genetic analysis. These advances include: (1) the description in feral and domesticated cats of over twenty loci polymorphic for morphological traits, many of which are homozygous recessive in different combinations in over 100 cat breeds registered throughout the world (Robinson, 1977); (2) the detection of common allozyme variation at twelve biochemical loci studied in a feral cat permitting sexual genetic analysis of these variants (O'Brien, 1980); (3) the feasibility of fertile sexual genetic crosses between Felis catus and both Felis bengalensis, the leopard cat (Benveniste & Todaro, 1975), and Felis chaus, the jungle cat (Robinson, 1977), thereby providing additional interspecies genetic variation. Twenty-five biochemical loci tested to date vary in interspecies backcrosses between Felis catus and Felis bengalensis including both polymorphic (in either species) or monomorphic (but electrophoretically different) enzyme structural loci (S.J. O'Brien, unpublished observations). Finally, the prolific breeding of cats and the existence of small "households," where sizable cat families are maintained, provide a rich source for consanguinous matings and isolated population demes, which have been of use to date in epidemiological studies (Hardy et al., 1980; Essex, 1975).

The genetic map of the cat is remarkably similar, with respect to linkage arrangements to the map of homologous loci of man and Pongidae primates despite evolutionary divergence of these species for 80 million years. This conservation of linkage association is retained to a limited extent in rodent evolution on the sub-chromosomal level, but not on the gross chromosomal level, where numerous chromosomal exchanges have been evident. The comparative similarity of primates and felids provide an unexpected opportunity for alignment of genetic linkage groups in the two diverse mammalian orders.

REFERENCES

Baker HJ, Lindsey JR, McKhann GM, Farrell DF (1971). Neuronal GM1 in a Siamese cat with beta-galactosidase deficiency. Science 174:838-839.

Benveniste RE, Todaro GJ (1975). Segregation of RD114 and FeLV related sequences in crosses between domestic cat and leopard cat. Nature 257:506-508.

Benveniste, RE, Todaro GJ (1974). Evolution of C-type viral genes: inheritance of exogenously acquired viral genes. Nature 252:456-459.

Benveniste RE, Sherr CJ, Todaro GJ (1975). Evolution of type C viral genes: origin of feline leukemia virus. Science 190:886-888.

Centerwall WR, Benirschke K (1973). Male tortoiseshell and calico cats. J Hered 62:272-278.

Cork LC, Munnel JF, Lorenz MD, Murphy JV, Baker HJ, Rattazzi MC (1977). GM2 ganglioside lysosomal storage disease in cats with beta-hexosaminidase deficiency. Science 196:1014-1017.

Cotter SM, Brenner RM, Dodds WJ (1978). Hemophilia A in three unrelated cats. J Am Med Assoc 172:166-168.

Counts DF, Byers PH, Holbrook KA, Hegreberg GA (1980). Dermatosporaxis in a Himalayan cat: I Biochemical studies of dermal collagen. J Invest Dermatol 74:96-99.

de Grouchy J, Turleau C, Finaz C (1978). Chromosomal phylogeny of the primates. Ann Rev Genet 12:289-328.

Desnick RJ, Grabowski GA (1981). Advances in the treatment of inherited metabolic diseases. Adv Hum Genet 5:281-367.

Dodds WJ (1978). Inherited bleeding disorders. Canine Pract 5:49-58.

Essex M (1975). Horizontally and vertically transmitted oncornaviruses of cats. Adv Cancer Res 21:175-248.

Gotze D. (1977). "The major histocompatibility system in man and animals." New York: Springer-Verlag.

Green RA, White F (1977). Feline factor XII (Hageman) deficiency. Am J Vet Res 38:893-895.

Hardy WD, Essex M, McClelland AJ (1980). "Feline Leukemia Virus." New York: Elsevier/North Holland.

Harris H, Hopkinson DA (1972). Average heterozygosity per locus in man: an estimate based upon incidence of enzyme polymorphisms. Ann Hum Genet 36:9-20.

Harris H, Hopkinson DA (1976). Handbook of Enzyme Electrophoresis in Human Genetics. Amsterdam: North-Holland Publishing Co.

Haskins ME, Jezyk PF, Desnick RJ, McDonough SK, Patterson DF (1979). Mucopolysacchariodosis in a domestic short-haired cat--a disease distinct from that seen in the Siamese cat. J Am Vet Med Assoc 175:384-387.

Hirt B (1967). Selective extraction of polyoma DNA from infected mouse cell cultures. J Mol Biol 26:365-369.

Jezyk PF, Haskins ME, Patterson DF, Mellman WJ, Greenstein M (1977). Mucopolysaccharidosis in a cat with arysulfatase B deficiency: a model of Maroteaux-Lamy syndrome. Science 198:834-836.

Kramer JW, Davis WC, Prieur DJ (1977). The Chediak-Higashi syndrome of cats. Lab Invest 36:554-562.

Lalley PA (1980). Human gene map of biochemical markers. Genetic Maps 1:255-264.

McKusick VA, Ruddle FH (1977). The status of the gene map of human chromosome. Science 196:390-405.

Nevo E (1978). Genetic variation in natural populations: patterns and theory. Theoret Pop Biol 13:121-177.

O'Brien SJ (1976). Bvr-1, a restriction locus of a type C RNA virus in the feline cellular genome: identification, location, and phenotypic characterization in cat x mouse somatic cell hybrids. Proc Natl Acad Sci USA 12:4618-4622.

O'Brien SJ (1980). The extent and character of biochemical genetic variation in the domestic cat. J Hered 71:2-8.

O'Brien SJ, Nash WG (1982). Comparative mapping in mammals: chromosome map of the domestic cat. Science, in press.

O'Brien SJ, Nash WG, Simonson JM, Berman EJ (1980). Establishment of a biochemical genetic map of the domestic cat (Felis catus). In Hardy WD, Essex M, MacClelland AJ (eds): "Feline Leukemia Virus," New York: Elsevier-North Holland.

O'Brien SJ, Shannon JE, Gail MF (1980). A molecular approach to the identification and individualization of human and animal cell cultures: isozyme and allozyme genetic signatures. In Vitro 16:119-135.

Patterson DF, Minor RR (1977). Hereditary fragility and hyperextensibility of the skin of cats. A defect in collagen fibrillogenesis. Lab Invest 37:170-179.

Pearson PL, Roderick TH, Davisson MT, Lalley PA, O'Brien SJ (1981). Comparative mapping: report of the International Committee. Cytogen Cell Genet, in press.

Powell J (1976). Protein variation in natural populations of animals. In Dobzhansky T, Hecht MK, Steere WC (eds): "Evolutionary Biology," Vol. 8, p 69-119.

Rice MC, O'Brien SJ (1980). Genetic variation of laboratory outbred Swiss mice. Nature 283:157-161.

Robinson R (1977). "Genetics for Cat Breeders." New York: Pergammon Press, 2nd Ed.

Ruddle FH, Chapman VM, Ricciuti F, Murnane M, Klebe R, Meera-Khan P (1971). Linkage relationships of seventeen human gene loci as determined by man-mouse somatic cell hybrirds. Nature New Biol 232:69-73.

Ruddle FH, Creagan RP (1975). Parasexual approaches to the genetics of man. Ann Rev Genet 9:407-486.

Schaub RG, Meyers KM, Saude RD (1977). Serotonin as a factor in collateral blood flow inhibition following experimental arterial thrombosis. J Lab Clin Med 90:645-653.

Shows T, et al (1979). International system for human gene nomenclature. Cytogenet Cell Genet 25:96-116.

Southern EM (1975). Detection of specific sequences among DNA fragments separated by gel electrophoresis.

Wallace B (1966). "Chromosomes, Giant Molecules and Evolution". New York: WW Norton and Co.

Wenger DA, Sattler M, Kudoh T, Snyder SP, Kingston RS (1980). Niemann-Pick disease: a genetic model in Siamese cats. Science 208:1471-1473.

Winkler CA (1981) Preliminary characterization of the major histocompatibility complex in Felis catus. M.S. thesis, University of Maryland, College Park, Maryland.

Womack JE (1980). Biochemical loci of the mouse, Mus musculus. Genetic Maps 1:218-224.

DR. GUÉNET: Are the genes responsible for tail deformities or malformations located in the genetic map of the cat?

DR. O'BRIEN: The only gene that I know of is the Manx gene which is a dominant tailless mutation and a recessive lethal. We have not studied that, and it has not been mapped.

DR. DESNICK: You have clone panels of cat-mouse and cat-hamster hybrids. What other hybrid panels do you have, and would you make these available to those of us involved in mapping human genes? We might be able to use our systems for comparative mapping.

DR. O'BRIEN: Our panels change all the time. Right now we have an extremely powerful cat panel which consists of actually two and three tiers. We have four or five hybrids that we look at first, and then we make a decision on which tier to go to from the basis, because these are extremely well characterized. By well characterized, I mean that we have hybrids in which the karyotypes have been documented rigorously. The isozymes have been run as best we can. The DNA has been extracted, and the extracts have been aliquoted at milligram levels so that a lot of things can be done. I am basically developing these materials for collaborative work and for providing them to other investigators. Most of the work that I have done with humans has involved a gene called BEVI, which is a retrovirus integration site on chromosome 6. We have several hundred human hybrids which have been characterized, but they are not characterized to the extent I would like, but they should be in about two months. To answer your question about availability, I certainly would be happy to provide any materials to any of you who are interested in mapping a gene or in using them in whatever studies you might think are useful. We developed them for this reason. I have been well supported in terms of developing all these materials, and I think that I owe the scientific community the opportunity to use them.

DR. DESNICK: How stable are the cat chromosomes in your hybrids?

DR. O'BRIEN: That sort of depends. In primary clones, they are not very stable, but we have found that when you develop subclones, especially when you are at the secondary and tertiary level, many chromosomes will become fixed at a very high frequency, some of them as many as 2 and 3 per cell, but not all. It is just sort of an empirical thing. We simply have to watch it and see what happens.

DR. YUNIS: I would like to make only a suggestion about the chromosome B-2. It is very homologous to chromosome 6 in man which contains the genes of the major histocompatibility complex (MHC). I think perhaps an easier approach to identify the MHC in the cat would be to look for polymorphism of complement 4, using an electrophoretic technique with plasma. This may provide faster identification of the major histocompatibility complex in the cat, perhaps in chromosome B-2.

DR. O'BRIEN: First of all, we don't know that it is on chromosome B-2, yet; and second, I think that your point is well taken. However, the MHC is a very complex one. There are a lot of different components, and if you want essentially to develop a model system which involves that for the leukemia connection, for example, it is important that all different classes of phenotypes be studied. Now, the reason that we set up the grafting procedures and so forth is because I think it would be very presumptuous of me to get up and talk about the major histocompatibility complex in the mouse on the basis of some complement mapping. I think that it is important to do that, and I have not done it, simply because there are so many other things going on, but I certainly am considering putting such tests into the profiles. I think you would agree that sooner or later somebody has to do the cytotoxicity and the grafting if you really want to make the analogy with the MHC in homologous systems.

DR. YUNIS: But in man, for instance, the polymorphism of complement 4 is very pronounced, and it is possible to do a pretty extensive genotype of the complex without having to do HLA typing.

DR. O'BRIEN: I understand, and I agree with you. All I am saying is that in addition to that, sooner or later, somebody is going to have to do the cytotoxicity studies just because of the historical definition of the system.

SECTION II.
DETECTION OF ANIMAL MODELS OF HUMAN DISEASE

Animal Models of Inherited Metabolic Diseases, pages 93–116
© **1982 Alan R. Liss, Inc., 150 Fifth Avenue, New York, NY 10011**

SCREENING FOR INBORN ERRORS OF METABOLISM IN DOGS AND CATS.

Jezyk, P.F., Haskins, M.E., Patterson, D.F.
Sections of Medical Genetics and Pathology
School of Veterinary Medicine
University of Pennsylvania
Philadelphia, Pennsylvania 19104

The advantages of the dog and cat as models of human inborn errors of metabolism have been enumerated elsewhere (Jezyk, 1978; Patterson, Haskins and Jezyk, in press). The purpose of this report is to share our experiences in purposefully searching for such models using biochemical screening methods. Our program was originally designed to utilize the population of a large veterinary hospital which is staffed by veterinary specialists and operates primarily as a regional referral center. We also planned to screen litters of animals owned by cooperating breeders in the area, especially those with high rates of neonatal mortality. The success of this program has attracted additional referrals and samples from many area veterinarians, from other areas of the United States, and from other countries.

It thus appears that when appropriate diagnostic facilities are available, veterinarians will respond with an increased index of suspicion of metabolic dysfunction in sick animals. This in turn increases the probability of finding such abnormalities. As the screening program has developed, the relative frequency of positive findings has steadily increased with time. Increased ability to discern and separate the abnormal from the normal has also improved detection of more subtle abnormalities.

The basic methodologies utilized in our laboratory have been described elsewhere (Jezyk, 1978). This paper will, therefore, concentrate on the interpretation of these tests, the types of abnormalities that we have detected in this program, and our general approach to the recognition and utilization of canine and feline animal models.

Materials and Methods

Briefly, we utilize essentially the same methods used by many human metabolic screening laboratories. For initial screening, we prefer fresh urine samples, as the highest concentration of metabolites from most inborn errors is found in the urine. Samples from young animals are often collected on Whatman 3MM paper and dried before analysis. We have prepared kits with instructions for collecting and mailing such samples which we distribute to veterinarians or breeders. A series of spot tests are performed on all liquid samples (Thomas and Howell, 1973). All samples are screened for amino acids, carbohydrates and organic acids by one-dimensional paper chromatographic procedures (Shih, 1973; Jezyk, 1978).

Abnormalities detected by these procedures are further investigated by a variety of techniques. Amino acids are fractionated and quantitated by automated ion-exchange chromatography using a single-column, lithium buffer system (Blazer-Yost and Jezyk, 1979). Organic acids are isolated by solvent extraction, converted to trimethylsilyl derivatives, and separated by gas-liquid chromatography (Cohn et al, 1978; Tanaka, 1980). They are identified by comparisons to known standards separated under the same conditions and/or calculation of their methylene unit values after separation on two different columns (Tanaka, 1980, Goodman, 1980) or by gas chromatography-mass spectrometry (Cohn et al, 1978). Paper chromatography has thus far proved sufficient to identify any monosaccharides detected.

Glycosaminoglycans are precipitated with cetylpyridinium chloride, recovered and separated by electrophoresis on cellulose acetate (Wessler, 1968, Jezyk et al, 1977).

Results:

General

In their book on metabolic screening tests, Thomas and
Howell (1973) point out that such tests are basically
designed to be indicators of alterations in certain
metabolic pathways, and not in themselves diagnostic of
any given disorder. They also stress the fact that while
many of the tests employed are extremely simple, correct
interpretation of results requires considerable skill and
experience. This is certainly true in screening samples
from dogs and cats. There are sufficient differences in
certain physiologic parameters and metabolic pathways in
these animals that complicate application of some tests
developed for screening human samples. For example, when
present in high concentrations, creatinine reacts with
nitroprusside reagent to form a salmon-colored derivative.
This color may be confused with the magenta given by
sulfhydryl-containing amino acids. Dogs and cats generally
have more concentrated urines than humans, with the specific
gravity of cat urines often being greater than 1.070, and
their urine creatinine concentrations usually 3 to 4 times
greater. Nursing puppies also have a high incidence of
glycosuria and lactosuria (Jezyk, 1978) and positive tests
for reducing substances are common.

A "false" positive nitrosonaphthol test is often
obtained in animals with gastrointestinal problems. There
have been several reports of increased excretion of
tyrosine metabolites in human disorders associated with
pancreatic insufficiency, e.g., cystic fibrosis, and/or
bacterial overgrowth (van der Heiden, et al, 1971).
Chalmers et al, 1979, have in fact published a report
that increased excretion of p-hydroxyphenylacetate
can be used to diagnose bacterial overgrowth in patients
with intestinal disorders. We have determined the organic
acid content of several such urines and have indeed found
them to contain increased concentrations of several
tyrosine metabolites (Jezyk and Burrows, unpublished data).
We have also had urines from animals with neurologic disorders that give weakly positive reactions in this test in
which we are unable to demonstrate increased amounts of
tyrosine metabolites using our routine extraction and

derivatization procedures. We are continuing to investigate the nature of the substance(s) in such urines responsible for this reaction.

In the following sections, abnormalities in various constituents that have been detected in the program are tabulated and several of these will be discussed. When considering the number of positive results, it should be kept in mind that only about 6000 animals have been tested. This includes about 2000 beagle puppies from a colony of dogs raised for sale as research animals. Samples were collected during the first and third weeks of life from surviving members of all litters born during a one-year period. The initial samples collected during this screening were all urines on filter papers, with liquid urines and/or plasmas obtained only if abnormalities were detected on the first samples. While this gave us valuable experience in interpretation of chromatograms, the yield of positive results was very low. The only abnormalities detected which could be reasonably linked to an inborn error was marked prolinuria and citrullinuria in several members of one litter (Jezyk, 1978).

Abnormalities in urinary and/or plasma amino acids

Interpretation of amino acid chromatograms has proved to be one of the most difficult areas in the screening program. Examples of what we consider to be within the realm of normal for amino acid excretion by cats and dogs of various ages are shown in Fig. 1 to illustrate this problem. The variation is considerably greater than that seen in man, particularly due to variations in diet. Differences in metabolic pathways and/or control of these pathways also is important. For example, cats often have large amounts of a sulfur-containing amino acid, felinine, in their urine, but lack of excretion of this compound does not appear to be abnormal. Its excretion is reportedly related to diet (Greaves and Scott, 1960). As cats are obligate carnivores, their diet usually includes large amounts of carnosine and anserine and they therefore have very large amounts of histidine and 1-methylhistidine in their urines, as do many dogs. They, like dogs (Blazer-Yost and Jezyk, 1979), also excrete large amounts of methylated basic amino acids, primarily dimethylarginines.

TABLE 1

Abnormalities in urinary and/or plasma amino acids
detected by University of Pennsylvania Veterinary
Metabolic Screening Laboratory

Abnormality	Associated Defect
cystinuria +/- dibasic aminoaciduria	renal tubular defect-cystinuria
generalized aminoaciduria	renal tubular defect-Fanconi syndrome
ornithinuria + -emia	ornithine:2-oxoacid aminotransferase deficiency-gyrate atrophy of choroid and retina
tyrosinuria + -emia	soluble + mitochondrial tyrosine aminotransferase deficiency - (Tyrosinemia Type II ?)
citrullinuria	(arginosuccinate synthetase deficiency ?)
branched-chain amino-aciduria + -emia	(Maple Syrup Urine Disease?)
alaninuria + -emia	deranged pyruvate metabolism - various causes
glutaminuria + -emia	hyperammonemia - secondary to portal caval anomalies, liver disease, (urea cycle defects ?)

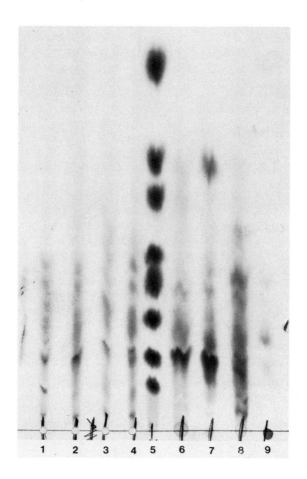

Fig. 1   Paper chromatogram of urinary and plasma amino
         acids from clinically normal dogs and cats.
Conditions as described in materials and methods 1-4:
canine urines; 5: amino acid standard containing, from
top to bottom, leucine, methionine, tyrosine, alanine,
glutamate, serine, lysine and cystine; 6 and 7: feline
urines, the spot near valine in 7 is felinine;
8: canine urine; 9: canine plasma.

We have detected a number of abnormalities in urinary and/or plasma amino acids. These are summarized in Table 1 and several examples are shown in Fig. 2.

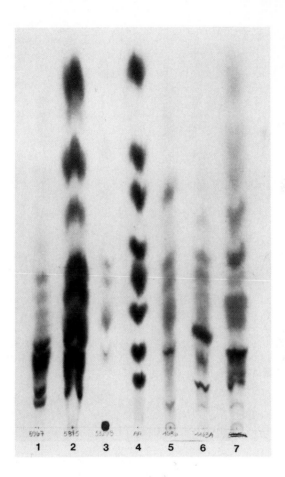

Fig. 2   Paper chromatogram of urinary and plasma amino
          acids from animals with various abnormalities.
1: urine from a canine with cystinuria; 2: urine from canine
with Fanconi syndrome; 3: plasma from a canine with hyperammonemia; 4: amino acid standard as in Fig. 1. 5: urine
from a canine with tyrosinemia; 6: urine from a canine with
hyperammonemia showing marked glutaminuria; 7: urine from a
feline with ornithinemia.

One of these animals, a dog with tyrosinemia, will be discussed here as an example of the recognition of such a disorder and the progression to elucidation of the under- lying defect. This dog was seen by one of our dermatolo- gists during a consulting trip to a clinic in the midwest. The patient was a six month-old female German Shepherd puppy with chronic ophthalmologic and dermatologic problems. Her ocular problems had been diagnosed as a chronic kera- titis with corneal ulceration and congenital cataracts. The skin lesions consisted primarily of ulcerations of the keratinized tissue on her external nares and the pads of her feet. Routine hematologic and serum biochemical parameters were within normal ranges. Due to the life-long nature of the problem and its unresponsiveness to previous therapy, the dermatologist biopsied the lesions and obtained urine on filter paper and serum for metabolic screening. Chromatography showed markedly increased tyrosine (Fig. 2) and a large spot on the organic acid chromatogram (Fig. 3). Quantitative analysis of the serum amino acids confirmed that it was in fact tyrosine and that the concentration was approximately 35 times the upper limit of the reference range. The owner of the dog was then contacted, the nature of the problem explained to him, and arrangements were made to acquire the dog for our colony. When she arrived, more urine was collected and the organic acids were analyzed by GLC. Large amounts of tyrosine metabolites were found, primarily p-hydroxyphenyllactate. The clinical and bio- chemical features of the disorder in this dog therefore closely resembled those of the Richner-Hanhart syndrome, or Tyrosinemia Type II of man (Fellman et al, 1969; Goldsmith, 1978; Hunziker, 1980) and of hereditary tyrosinemia of mink (Christensen et al, 1979; Marsh and Goldsmith, 1981). A biopsy was then performed and a sample of liver obtained for determination of tyrosine aminotransferase activities. Unlike Tyrosinemia Type II, in which there is a specific defect in the soluble form of this enzyme, decreased activity of both soluble and mitochondrial forms of this enzyme were found (Jezyk, Emeigh and Balsai, unpublished results). This raises some interesting questions as to the source of the large quantities of tyrosine metabolites detected in the urine. The postulated pathway to these compounds in afflicted people involves increased formation of p-hydroxyphenyl- pyruvate (PHPPA) in mitochondria, which can only be degraded in the cytoplasm (Fellman et al, 1969). The increased PHPPA may cause substrate inhibition of cytosolic PHPPA dioxygenase and result in its increased conversion to other metabolites. Additionally it has been suggested that PHPPA is formed in excess by other tissues, accumulates and is excreted by the kidney (Fellman et al, 1972). In this dog the postulated pathway does not appear to be tenable, as both soluble and mito-chondrial tyrosine amino transferase activities are decreased. It appears, however, that the soluble form also has a decreased affinity for tyrosine, which may result in a shift in intracellular substrate concentrations similar to that produced by the absence of the cytosolic form in the human condition.

The type of problems that may be encountered in interpretation of screening results by inexperienced personnel can be illustrated by an example from early in our program. A young toy poodle was seen by a local practitioner with a seizure disorder that began at 10 weeks of age. A urine sample was obtained for screening. Due to the small size of this dog and its poor condition, only a very small urine sample was available and spot tests were not performed. No major abnormalities were found at the time, however, large spots corresponding to ampicillin and its metabolites were noted on the amino acid chromatogram. The dog died shortly thereafter and its brain was obtained for histopathology. Within the next ten days, the other two members of this dog's litter also had seizures and were taken to other veterinarians. We managed to learn of this through contact with their breeder and obtained immediate pre-mortem plasma samples from both. Paper chromatography of these samples indicated a moderate increase in branched-chain amino acids, which was confirmed by ion-exchange chromatography of one sample. However, at about that time, the histo-pathology of the brain from the first animal became avail-able and was interpreted as having lesions classic for canine distemper, a paramyxoviral infection. The matter was therefore not pursued further. Some months later, ion-exchange chromatograms of dog samples were reviewed with a technician from a human amino acid laboratory. She remarked that the pattern of the plasma amino acids from the poodle appeared similar to that in maple syrup urine disease (MSUD). The amino acids in the remaining samples were then separated by ion-exchange chromatography and found to be similar to the original. Alloisoleucine, a hallmark of maple syrup urine disease (Norton et al, 1962), was then identified in the urine from the original dog. Unfortunately, not enough of any sample remained to determine the organic acid content. No maple syrup odor was noted in the initial urine sample, but this would have been masked by the large amount of ampicillin present, which has a pungent thiol odor. The distemper in the first dog may well have been a secondary phenomenon, as it has been established that immunologic function is impaired in patients with other organic acidurias (Rosenberg, 1978).

While screening of any given given population usually results in a low yield of positive results, it becomes much more attractive when an abnormality has been shown to exist in some members of the population. The greatest number of abnormalities in amino acid excretion have been found while screening wild and captive maned wolves for cystinuria after it was established that the disease existed in some captive animals (Bush and Bovee, 1978; Bovee et al, 1980), and screening of basenji dogs for the Fanconi syndrome subsequent to its recognition, (Easley and Breitschwendt, 1976; Bovee et al, 1978a, 1978b; Bovee et al, 1979). Studies on these latter animals will be reported by Dr. Bovee and his collaborators at this meeting (Bovee et al, this Symposium). Both of these screening programs grew from the initial clinical recognition of the syndromes.

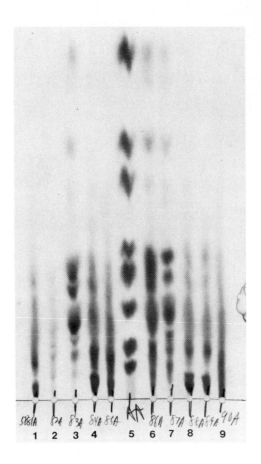

Fig. 3   Paper chromatogram of urinary amino acids
          from a series of Basenji dogs.
          1, 2, 9, 10, 11: normal; 3, 4: cystinuria;
          5, 7, 8: generalized aminoaciduria;
          6: amino acid standard as in Fig. 1.

Abnormalities in urinary and/or plasma organic acids.

TABLE 2

Abnormalities in urinary and/or plasma organic acids
detected by University of Pennsylvania Veterinary
Metabolic Screening Laboratory

Abnormality	Associated Defect
Methylmalonic aciduria	(methylmalonyl Co A mutase deficiency ?)
Lactic aciduria + -emia	(deranged pyruvate metabolism)
p-hydroxymandelic aciduria	(deranged catecholamine metabolism ?)
p-hydroxyphenyllactic, p-hydroxyphenylpropionic, p-hydroxyphenylpyruvic aciduria + -emia	soluble and mitochondrial tyrosine aminotransferase deficiency - (Tyrosinemia Type II ?)

Few models of diseases involving excessive accumulation and/or excretion of organic acids have been described.
A dog with methylmalonic aciduria has been previously
reported by our laboratory (Jezyk, 1978). We recently
recognized a new disorder characterized by an organic
aciduria in a group of Irish Setter dogs. The first of
these dogs was screened because of apparent visual
abnormalities. The initial sample from this dog gave
a strongly positive acetest reaction for ketone bodies
and a large spot on the organic acid chromatogram,
corresponding to lactic acid (Fig. 3). A positive reaction
for ketone bodies in canine urine is rare, as dogs have
been shown to be extraordinarily resistant to fasting
ketosis (deBruijne et al, 1981). These latter studies
demonstrated the ability of dogs to withstand many days
of fasting before sufficient ketones accumulate to produce
ketonuria, unlike the situation in man, where relatively
short periods of fasting may result in ketonuria.
Positive acetest reactions are a fairly common finding in
human urines submitted for metabolic screening.

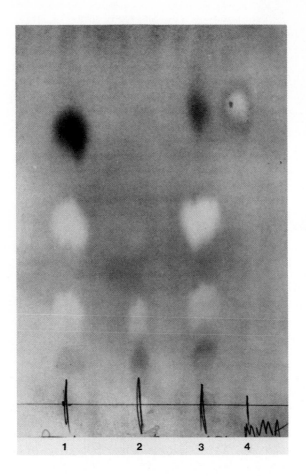

Fig. 4   Paper chromatogram of urinary organic acids
          from three dogs. Conditions as described in
materials and methods. 1: urine from a dog with
lactic aciduria; 2: urine from a clinically normal dog;
3: urine from a dog with tyrosinemia; 4: methylmalonic
acid standard.

The sample was then analyzed for organic acids by gas-liquid chromatography, confirming the presence of lactate, ketone bodies and smaller amounts of several other acids, including p-hydroxyphenylacetate. Urines were then obtained from several closely related dogs and others with similar findings were identified. In addition to the usual screening tests, we quantitatively determined the urinary lactate excretion of these dogs using an enzymatic method (Gutmann and Wahlefeld, 1974; Fernandes and Blom, 1976). We have previously established reference ranges for lactate excretion and shown this method to be useful for detecting disorders of lactate excretion, demonstrating consistent increases in basenji dogs with the Fanconi syndrome (Jezyk, Newman and Siddall, unpublished results). By testing only 48 animals, we have identified 5 definitely affected animals and several that may be affected.

The affected dogs in this highly inbred kindred that we have had the opportunity to study thus far have few obvious clinical signs associated with the disorder. The initially suspected visual problems turned out to be spurious, and no visual deficits have been detected in other dogs. Affected dogs have a mild metabolic acidosis, but no signs of hepectic or renal dysfunction. The owner of several affected dogs reports otherwise unexplained periods of depression, decreased appetite and weight loss in these dogs. Such an episode has been associated with increased lactate excretion in one animal. All affected animals detected thus far have been young adults and the long-term consequences of the disorder are yet to be understood. At no time have the affected animals' measured plasma lactates been elevated sufficiently to account for the degree of lactate excretion. This disorder may therefore involve a defect in renal handling of the lactate. Such a disorder has recently been reported in a retarded child (Jaeken et al, 1980). The etiology of this syndrome is currently being investigated. Our initial studies of these animals involve measurement of pertinent metabolites in response to a series of loading tests and examination of the in vivo metabolism of glucose, using heavy isotope-labeled glucose and gas chromatography-mass spectrometry of the metabolites.

Abnormalities in urinary glycosaminoglycans

TABLE 3

Abnormalities in urinary glycosaminoglycan excretion
detected by University of Pennsylvania Metabolic
Screening Laboratory

Abnormality	Associated Defect
Dermatan sulfaturia	Arylsulfatase B deficiency - Feline MPS VI
Dermatan and heparin sulfaturia	Iduronidase deficiency - Feline MPS I
Keratan sulfaturia	? (Canine MPS IV ?)
Chondroitin sulfaturia	Rapid growth, hypothyroidism, various dwarfisms, metabolic bone diseases, (enzyme defects?)

The program has been most successful in uncovering
models of the mucopolysaccharidoses, which will be discussed
in detail at this meeting by Dr. Haskins (Haskins et al,
this Symposium). Our major screening test for these
compounds, the toluidine blue spot test (Berry and Spinanger,
1960) is extraordinarily simple to perform and quite dis-
criminating. We have had no known instances of false
negatives, i.e., we have been able to detect all animals
in our colonies that have been proven to be affected by
enzymatic assay. We do get a fairly high percentage of
"false" positives. Some of these urines contain large
amounts of compounds not subsequently detected by glycosaminoglycan electrophoresis, e.g., nucleic acids or glycoprotein.
Many animals have chondroitin sulfaturia. This has been
seen in conditions in which there is increased turnover of
bone, such as rapid growth, hypothyroidism, metabolic bone
diseases, and in some animals which had clinical features
consistent with a storage disorder. We have investigated
several of these latter animals and have been unable to
demonstrate lysosomal storage and/or accumulation of
labelled GAGs by cultured fibroblasts incubated with

radiolabelled sulfur. These animals may have metabolic
disorders involving other constituents of the ground
substance and/or bony matrix, and the glycosaminoglycanuria
is probably a secondary event. Hopefully, we will be able
to better define the defect in such animals at some future
time.

Abnormalities in urinary monosaccharides

TABLE 4

Abnormalities in urinary monosaccharide excretion
detected by University of Pennsylvania
Metabolic Screening Laboratory

Abnormality	Associated Defect
Glucosuria	diabetes mellitus, Fanconi syndrome, stress
Lactosuria	nursing puppies, (Type II glyco-genosis ?)
Galactosuria	Liver disease
Fructosuria	Unknown

We have found relatively few disorders of carbohydrate
excretion. We, of course, see glucosuria in animals with
diabetes mellitus and animals with the Fanconi syndrome.
It is also common to see glucose in the urine of sick cats.
Cats generally appear to have significant hyperglycemia in
response to stress, great enough to exceed the renal
threshhold and produce glucosuria. Lactosuria is common
in nursing animals and was also consistently seen in a
young cat that we believe, though failed to prove, suffered
from Type II glycogenosis (lysosomal α-glucosidase
deficiency). Lactosuria has been reported to be a feature
of this disease in man (Tsai and Marshall, 1979).

Early in the program we screened a number of animals with cataracts and/or lens luxations and found one to have tremendous galactosuria. We were able to study this dog and found him to have an abnormal galactose tolerance test, but normal activities of all galactose-metaboizing enzymes in red cell extracts. Routine serum chemistries revealed indications of active hepatocellular disease. On careful questioning of the owners, it was determined that the dog liked milk and was given a large dish each evening. The urine sample that we had screened had been collected during the period after the dog was given the milk. It is well established that there is galactose intolerance in liver disease, and galactose tolerance tests have been used as a measure of liver function (Bauer, 1906; Rommel et al, 1968). This illustrates the need for a good clinical history and complete workup when assessing metabolic screening results. All animals that we see because they are suspected of having a metabolic disorder on the basis of screening tests are given a thorough physical examination, have a good history taken (including pedigree information) and have routine serum chemistries and a complete blood count performed as a minimum data base. Other tests, such as radiographs, ophthalmologic examination, etc., are performed as indicated.

DISCUSSION

As in human medicine, more abnormalities have been detected when there has been a clinical suspicion of a metabolic origin or component to a disease process than in general screening. After several years experience, we can only confirm the initial hypothesis that prompted the screening program: that naturally occurring models of metabolic disease in domestic animals can best be identified in a setting where veterinary specialists see animals at risk for such diseases. While such models have certainly been identified without formal metabolic testing programs, the presence of such a program greatly increases the probability of such an event.

The distribution of types of disease diagnosed by the Veterinary Screening Laboratory has differed markedly from those diagnosed in another laboratory supervised by one of the authors (P.J.) at Children's Hospital of Philadelphia. We find less disorders of amino and organic acid metabolism and more lysosomal storage diseases. This is at least in part due to the skew in age of animals screened. Except for occasional samples from breeders, it is unusual to obtain samples from animals less than six weeks old. One would therefore expect that most animals afflicted with severe defects in amino or organic acid metabolism to have succumbed by that time. Disorders of this type that we have identified tend to have non-systemic manifestations, e.g., gyrate atrophy of the choroid and retina in a cat associated with hyperornithinemia attributable to a deficiency of ornithine: 2-oxoacid aminotransferase (Valle et al, 1981).

Within just a few years of undertaking this screening program, we have far exceeded our initial expectations in terms of the number of abnormalities detected. Unfortunately, some provocative findings have had to be ignored for lack of time and personnel, or their further investigation at least postponed. Collaboration with other investigators has been fruitful in pursuing some of these findings and we continue to solicit such collaboration. Major research programs have resulted from our findings and we stress the importance of pursuing investigation and utilization of models identified in our program. Simple identification of a model is hardly sufficient, utilization of the model being the goal, as is illustrated in Dr. Haskins' paper on our studies of the feline models of mucopolysaccharide storage diseases (Haskins et al, this Symposium).

ACKNOWLEDGEMENTS

This work was supported by NIH grant AM 25759 and Genetics Center Grant GM 20138.

REFERENCES

Bauer R (1906). Über die Assimilation von Galaktose uns Milchzucker beim Gesunden und Kranken. Wien med Wschr 56:20.

Berry HK, Spinanger J (1960). A paper spot test useful in the study of Hurler's syndrome. J Lab Clin Med 55:136.

Blazer-Yost B, Jezyk PF (1979). Free amino acids in the plasma and urine of dogs from birth to senescence. Am J Vet Res 40:832.

Bovee KC, Joyce T, Reynolds R, Segal S (1978a). Spontaneous Fanconi syndrome in the dog. Metabolism 27:45.

Bovee KC, Joyce T, Reynolds R, Segal S (1978b). The Fanconi syndrome in Basenji dogs: A new model for renal transport defects. Science 201:1129.

Bovee KC, Joyce T, Blazer-Yost B, Goldschmidt MS, Segal S (1979). Characterization of renal defects in dogs with a syndrome similar to the Fanconi syndrome in man. J Am Vet Med Assoc 174:1094.

Bovee KC, Bush M, Dietz J, Jezyk P, Segal S (1980). Cystinuria in the maned wolf of South America. Science 212:919.

Bush M, Bovee KC (1978). Cystinuria in a maned wolf. J Am Vet Med Assoc 173:1159.

Chalmers RA, Valman HB, Liberman MM (1979). Measurement of 4-hydroxyphenylacetic aciduria as a screening test for small bowel disease. Clin Chem 25:1791.

Christensen K, Fischer P, Knudsen KEB, Larsen S, Sorensen H, Venge O (1979). A syndrome of hereditary tyrosinemia in mink. Can J Comp Med 43:333.

Cohn RM, Updegrove S, Yandrasitz JR, Rothman R, Tomer K (1978). Evaluation of continuous solvent extraction of organic acids from biological fluids. Clin Biochem 11:126.

deBruijne JJ, Altzuler N, Hampshire J, Visser TJ, Hackeng WHL (1981). Fat mobilization and plasma hormone levels in fasted dogs. Metabolism 30:190.

Easley JR, Breitschwerdt EB (1976). Glucosuria associated with renal tubular dysfunction in three Basenji dogs. J Am Vet Med Assoc 168:938.

Fellman JH, Vanbellinghen PJ, Jones RT, Koler RD (1969). Soluble and mitochondrial forms of tyrosine amino-transferase. Relationship to human tyrosinemia. Biochemistry 8:615.

Fellman JH, Buist NRM, Kennaway NG, Swanson RE (1972). The source of aromatic ketoacids in tyrosinemia and phenylketonuria. Clin Chim Acta 39:243.

Fernandes J, Blom W (1976). Urinary lactate excretion in normal children and in children with enzyme defects of carbohydrate metabolism. Clin Chim Acta 66:345.

Goldsmith LA (1978). Molecular biology and molecular pathology of a newly described molecular disease-Tyrosinemia II (the Richner-Hanhart syndrome). Expl Cell Biol 46:96.

Goodman SI (1980). An introduction to gas chromatography - mass spectrometry and the inherited organic acidemias. Am J Hum Genet 32:781.

Greaves JP, Scott PP (1960). Urinary amino-acid pattern of cats on diets of varying protein content. Nature 187:242.

Gutmann I, Wahlefeld AW (1974). L-(+)-lactate determination with lactate dehydrogenase and NAD. In Bergmeyer HU (ed): "Methods of Enzymatic Analysis." New York: Academic Press, p 1464.

Hunziker N (1980). Richner-Hanhart syndrome and tyrosinemia Type II. Dermatologica 160:180.

Jaeken J, DeCock P, Proesmans W, Corbeel L, Eggermont E, Eeckels R, Monnens L, Bakkeren J (1980). Defective tubular resorption of pyruvic and L-lactic acid. N Engl J Med 303:706.

Jezyk PF, Haskins ME, Patterson DF, Mellman WJ, Greenstein M (1977). Mucopolysaccharidosis in a cat with arylsulfatase B deficiency: A model of Maroteaux-Lamy syndrome. Science 198:834.

Jezyk PF (1979). Screening for inborn errors of metabolism in dogs and cats. In Hommes FA (ed): "Models for the study of inborn errors of metabolism," Amsterdam: Elsevier/North Holland, p 11.

Marsh RF, Goldsmith LA (1981). Animal models - Tyrosinemia II. Comp Pathol Bull 13:2.

Norton PM, Roitman E, Snyderman SE, Holt LE, Jr. (1962). A new finding in maple syrup urine disease. Lancet 1:26.

Patterson DF, Haskins ME, Jexyk PF (1982). Models of human genetic disease in domestic animals. Adv Hum Genet: in press.

Rommel K, Bernt E, Schmitz F, Grimmel K (1968). Enzymatic Galaktosebestimmung im Blut und oraler Galaktose-Toleranztest. Klin Wschr 46:936.

Rosenberg L (1978). Disorders of propionate, methylmalonate, and cobalamin metabolism. In Stanbury JB, Wyngaarden JB, Fredrickson DS (eds): "The Metabolic Basis of Inherited Disease." New York: McGraw Hill, p 411.

Shih VE (1973). "Laboratory Techniques for the Detection of Hereditary Metabolic Disorders." Cleveland: CRC Press.

Tanaka K, Hine DG, West-Dull A, Lynn TB (1980). Gas-chromatographic method of analysis for urinary organic acids. 1. Retention indices of 155 metabolically important compounds. Clin Chem 26:1839.

Thomas GH, Howell RR (1973). "Selected Screening Tests for Genetic Metabolic Diseases." Chicago: Year Book Medical Publishers.

Tsai MY, Marshall JG (1979). Screening for urinary oligo-saccharides and simple sugars by thin-layer chromatography. Med Lab Sci 36:85.

Valle DL, Boison AP, Jezyk PF, Aguirre G (1981). Gyrate atrophy of the choroid and retina in a cat. Invest Ophthalmol Vis Sci 20:251.

van der Heiden C, Wauters EAK, Ketting D, Duran M, Wadman SK (1971). Gas chromatographic analysis of urinary tyrosine and phenylalanine metabolites in patients with gastrointestinal disorders. Clin Chim Acta 34:289.

Wessler E (1968). Analytical and preparative separation of acidic glycosaminoglycans by electrophoresis in barium acetate. Anal Biochem 26:439.

DR. PATTERSON: Just a question to the group. I have wondered for some time whether anyone else is running a screening laboratory of the type Dr. Jezyk described. I suspect Dr. Jezyk's laboratory was the first one of its kind in a veterinary school, even though these kinds of tests have been done for quite a few years, especially in children's hospitals. Does anyone know of other veterinary institutions that are doing similar things?

DR. J. SMITH: Several years ago, we screened blood samples for red cell defects. We looked at about three or four thousand samples (mostly dogs, some cats and a few other species) for glucose-6-phosphate dehydrogenase (G6PD) and glutathione using routine blood samples without any histories. We did find one dog that was partially G6PD deficient. That type of screening would not be as fruitful as testing animals that seemed to be at risk for disorders such as Dr. Jezyk has done.

DR. JEZYK: Yes, we have had far and away the greatest success in finding metabolic diseases when the animals have been worked up for other disorders. The clinicans get frustrated when they cannot find any of the usual causes such as infection, and then they come to us for help. I think part of the problem with looking for these diseases in veterinary medicine has been the fact that, for some reason, most of the people who come into school seem to be scared by biochemistry. I think a lot of them come from farm backgrounds; at least they have in the past, and when you start talking about biochemistry and metabolism, they just get turned off by the whole thing. Even now it is difficult to describe to many clinicians what you are looking for in terms of these diseases.

DR. J. SMITH: You primarily directed your work at urine. Are you using any blood components in your screening program?

DR. JEZYK: I also would like to tell you that, in addition to the very few samples that we have screened, we have done it with very little personnel. Our entire program consists of Dr. Haskins, Dr. Patterson and myself, one biochemistry technician, one cytogenetics technician, and that is it. So, all of these things that we do, or as far as we pursue a defect, we do it ourselves. We don't have a large amount of help to do it, and we have avoided looking for anything else. Urine is chosen primarily because we are looking for abnormal metabolites, and due to the lack of renal resorptive mechanisms for most of these metabolites, the easiest place to look for them is in urine.

DR. CORK: In what percentage of the cases that you have seen, have you been able to acquire the breeding stock and resolve the genetics?

DR. JEZYK: We have been reasonably successful. I am not sure I could tell you exactly what percentage it is, because we see a lot of defects that for lack of time, for lack of clinician follow-up or for other reasons, we don't really pursue. Of the ones that we have actively pursued, we have about an 80 percent success rate in obtaining either the animals, or related animals, for breeding purposes.

DR. WOOD: Have you ever pursued large animal defects by screening large animal samples?

DR. JEZYK: We have chosen not to for a number of reasons. One is that I don't have enough technical help to do it. And as we are looking exclusively for models, we feel that dogs and cats have certain advantages over large animals.

DR. O'BRIEN: In your travels through urines of the cat and dog, have you come across, or has anyone a decent assay for pregnancy in either of those animals?

DR. JEZYK: No, you cannot assay for pregnancy in the dog because the hormonal changes that go on in the normal bitch who has just gone through estrus are essentially the same as those who are pregnant, and you cannot really tell them by any of the hormone assays, at least those that we have available.

DR. O,BRIEN: Is that also true in the cat?

DR. JEZYK: I am not as sure. I think I would have to defer to Dr. Seager. It is probably true.

DR. DESNICK: You have provided a very comprehensive review of the approaches to the detection of inherited metabolic defects in animals. I would like to re-emphasize one of your points--that we should pay particular attention to dysmorphology, findings such as inclusions in bone marrow or peripheral cells, evidence of bony alterations like dysostosis, organomegaly, etc. In suspect animals, specimens can be shipped to laboratories such as Dr. Jezyk's for biochemical studies. In addition, many suspect animals die in the hospital. Autopsy studies may reveal pathologic findings. It is important that we freeze fresh tissues so that appropriate biochemical assays can be performed. Also efforts should be made to contact the owners and identify parents and siblings. We can ship the samples to those who do have the laboratory procedures once we have the index of suspicion.

DR. JEZYK: Early in the program we sat down and wrote

a protocol for those occasions when we have an animal that we strongly suspect has a metabolic disease, and it is going to die. We defined the minimum number of things that we have to do, such as taking samples for histology, taking samples for EM, taking samples to freeze for enzyme assays later, appropriate blood samples, etc. If you have a check-list all drawn up, you know you are going to get all these things on a potentially important animal. You may end up discarding a lot of them, but when the animal does come along that has something, then you will have the appropriate samples, and you can go back and complete the workup.

DR. HEGREBERG: Have you developed an approach for screening for cystic fibrosis in your laboratory?

DR. JEZYK: That is an interesting question. We thought about screening for cystic fibrosis, but one of the problems is if you look at all of the lesions that you see in man associated with cystic fibrosis, and you start look-ing at animals, you see a lot separately, but not really an awful lot that ties together. So while we thought very seriously about doing that, we have come across so many other things and are so busy that we have decided that if we do run across one, hopefully we will recognize it. However, we haven't gone about looking for them in any systematic way.

DR. HIGAKI: I was interested in your comments about gyrate atrophy of the choroid and retina. Are there any clinical markers? Are the affected animals blind?

DR. JEZYK: The animal that we had, and unfortunately, we have only had the one, was a stray cat that had been picked up off the street and was brought in to me just for a routine checkup. The owner complained that the animal seemed blind. On physical examination of the fundus, one could see that there was a generalized retinal atrophy that looked a little different from the types that we usually see, and there are certainly a large number of retinal atrophies in animals, so I decided to screen the animal. No other markers were present.

DR. HIGAKI: Are there published reports of this condi-tion? I am aware of a single case in a cat reported by Dr. Valle.

DR. JEZYK: That one is this cat. We sought outside collaboration in this case as Dr. Valle had the assays al-ready established in his laboratory. One thing we have learned is that you cannot do everything in your own labora-tory.

Animal Models of Inherited Metabolic Diseases, pages 117–132
© 1982 Alan R. Liss, Inc., 150 Fifth Avenue, New York, NY 10011

AN EFFECTIVE MASS-SCREENING PROGRAM FOR ANIMAL MODELS OF
THE INHERITED BLEEDING DISORDERS[*]

W. Jean Dodds, DVM

Division of Laboratories and Research
New York State Department of Health
Empire State Plaza
Albany, NY 12201

The inherited bleeding disorders represent one of the
most successfully developed and exploited categories of
animal models of human disease (Dodds, 1979, 1981). The
Second International Registry of Animal Models of Hemorrhagic and Thrombotic Diseases (Dodds, 1981) contains 94 en-
tries of which 46 are inherited diseases comprising a total
of 17 different mutants. These include coagulation factor,
platelet function and complement deficiencies, and antico-
agulant drug resistance or sensitivity. Most of these
models have been discovered in dogs and many investigators
have actively searched within the canine population for
additional or new models. The preferential selection of
this species probably reflects a combination of circumstances. Companion animals live in close daily contact with
their owners and thus diseases are more likely to be noticed and treated. Also economic factors are less important considerations when it comes to providing appropriate
veterinary care for a beloved pet. Research scientists who
study animal models need a subject large enough to obtain
serial blood samples for diagnostic and/or investigative
purposes and one that can be readily handled and treated.
The common practice to line breed and inbreed purebred
animals, especially dogs, facilitates transmission and
recognition of all types of genetic defects (Jolly et al,
1981; Dodds et al, 1981). The program we developed at

[*]Supported in part by Grant HLO9902 awarded by the National
Heart, Lung, and Blood Institute, National Institutes of
Health, PHS/DHHS.

Albany has been effective and relatively easy to establish because we are involved as purebred dog owners, breeders and exhibitors in addition to being veterinarians and research scientists. Individuals who breed and own purebred dogs have a particular emotional attachment and financial commitment to their animals. Consequently, they are often reluctant to part with their pets especially if they are to be subjected to biomedical experimentation. Thus, it is essential that the scientist's credibility and concern for the welfare of his/her research animals be established. In the past 20 years, this approach has led to the discovery and characterization in animals of all but two of the known bleeding disorders of man (Dodds, 1981).

The first cases of animals with hemophilia and von Willebrand's disease were discovered just over 40 years ago (Dodds, 1979). Since then a productive and well-recognized research literature has grown from studies of these animals. The following summary discusses some of the newer models that have been discovered but are as yet uncharacterized at the biochemical level, and focuses on canine models of the of the hemophilias and von Willebrand's disease as examples for the effective implementation of a mass-screening program for these defects within the purebred dog population (Dodds et al, 1981; Jolly et al, 1981).

The first new model is a form of familial thrombopathia common amongst purebred basset hounds throughout North America (Dodds, 1981). In addition to our laboratory, two other groups have been studying this disorder. It affects at least five major bloodlines of present-day basset hounds and current estimates suggest that the defect arose as a genetic mutation in a common ancestor(s) over 25 years ago. The most interesting fact about this model, however, is that there is no known human counterpart with exactly the same defect in platelet function. While the condition appears to be inherited as an autosomal incompletely dominant trait - as are many of the other bleeding disorders and most human thrombopathias - the specific defect is unique. It shares some characteristics common to other rare platelet defects such as Glanzmann's thrombasthenia, Bernard-Soulier syndrome and essential athrombia, but is biochemically and morphologically distinct based on the current available data. The most striking finding of affected basset hound platelets is their failure to aggregate in response to even very high concentrations (1×10^{-3}M) of adenosine diphosphate (ADP) but in the presence of perfectly normal clot retraction. In the parallel situation for

Glanzmann's disease, defective ADP aggregation is accompanied by abnormal clot retraction and a specific deficiency of the platelet membrane glycoprotein that acts as an ADP-receptor (Raymond and Dodds, 1979). This receptor protein is normal in basset hound thrombopathia. The second important aspect of the model is that it permits study of the initial "shape-change" events of platelet activation without progression to the sequential primary and secondary aggregation and release phenomina normally observed. The functional block in affected basset hound platelets occurs after the induction of shape-change but before primary aggregation. The question remains to identify the specific defect(s) involved and to determine whether it expresses a malfunctioning alternate pathway of normal platelet physiology that could be common to other mammals or else is unique to the canine species.

The second interesting new model involves a large inbred family of borzoi (Russian wolfhound) dogs with dysfibrinogenemia (Dodds, 1981). The fibrinogen molecule synthesized by affected animals is a mutant which affects its active site (ie. thrombin clottability) without altering its other physical or immunologic properties. There have been many such defects described in man and each has been characterized and named according to the specific amino acid substitution found in the active site region of the protein. Most patients with dysfibrinogenimia do not have a serious bleeding diathesis and the defect is frequently discovered fortuitously during routine coagulation screening because of the long thrombin clotting time (Morse, 1978).

The borzoi defect represents the first documented animal model of dysfibrinogenemia. The breeder maintains a kennel of over 90 related dogs ranging in age from young pups to aged pets. She was unaware of the problem until an affected puppy experienced excessive bleeding following trauma. More close inspection of this dog and three of his littermates revealed a minor bleeding history at teething and from recurrent small decubital (elbow and hip) hematomas. The owner was then questioned carefully about the background of these dogs. In checking her records and blood-testing the entire kennel, the defect was traced back to a 12-year-old Russian import who was the foundation dam of all the present stock. This bitch and more than a dozen of her descendents had exhibited bleeding episodes varying in severity from mild to fatal over the past decade. All of the affected survivors were shown to have the same la-

boratory defect in functional fibrinogen activity. Several
other asymptomatic relatives were also found to have defective fibrinogen. Discovery of this defect is yet another
example of the benefits from nationwide awareness of veterinarians and breeders about our referral program.

The effectiveness of our mass-screening program for
the bleeding disease of purebred dogs (Dodds et al, 1981)
is exemplified by results of tests for the hemophilia and
von Willebrand's disease genes.

Hemophilia A, a deficiency of factor VIII coagulant
activity, is the most common, severe inherited bleeding
disorder of man and domestic animals. It has been recognized in practically every pure breed of dog, in mongrel
dogs, in cats, and in standardbred and thoroughbred horses
(Dodds, 1979). Like that of man, the disease in the dog
and cat can be expressed by a very severe, a moderately
severe, or a mild form of bleeding diathesis. Generally
the larger the animal the more severe will be the clinical
expression of the disease, and also the lower will be the
level of plasma factor VIII clotting activity.

In terms of the diagnosis of hemophilia A and heterozygote (carrier) detection, it has been known for years
that carrier females have about half of the amount of factor VIII clotting activity present in normal plasma from
the same species. In fact heterozygotes usually have
levels between 20 and 60% of normal. Carrier detection by
this assay method was helpful, both in man and animals, but
there was considerable overlap between the normal and abnormal ranges which reduced the accuracy of identification
to about 60 or 70%. About a decade ago, however, immunologic assays were developed that could detect what we now
call the factor VIII-related antigen in normal plasma.
This immunologic property of the factor VIII complex was
found to be normal in hemophilia but reduced or defective
in von Willebrand's disease.

Today this plasma system has been characterized to the
point where we know that factor VIII circulates in plasma
as a complex of two molecules: the factor VIII-coagulant
protein, which is deficient in hemophilia A and is under
X-chromosomal synthetic control; and a second protein, the
von Willebrand's factor protein, which is under autosomal
control and has a variety of properties.

One of the properties of the von Willebrand's factor
protein is its ability to cross-react with heterologous
antisera directed against the purified factor VIII component of plasma. We call this immunologic property of the

von Willebrand's factor protein, factor VIII-related antigen.

In human patients and in dogs, cats, and horses with
hemophilia it was universally found that their plasma contained normal or elevated amounts of von Willebrand's factor protein as measured by the factor VIII-related antigen
level. Nearly all of the several hundred canine and feline
hemophilic plasmas we have examined have had elevated
levels of factor VIII-related antigen.

These findings with respect to the von Willebrand's
factor protein greatly facilitated hemophilia carrier detection. The carrier individual was found not only to have
reduced amounts of coagulant activity, but also normal
amounts of von Willebrand's factor protein. Thus, the
ratio of factor VIII activity to antigen/von Willebrand's
factor protein was about 1:2. This fact has allowed
carrier detection in man and animals to be improved to the
point where it is reliable in 86 to 95% of cases (Jolly et
al, 1981; Dodds et al, 1981).

With respect to the dog populations we have studied,
the families are relatively inbred and so we can more
easily identify the carrier from the normal females within
a litter. We counsel dog breeders on this basis by recom-
mending that they breed only those females that are normal
by blood test and neuter the ones that test as carriers.
Retrospective analysis of results from this 9 to 1 ratio
of accuracy in carrier identification, indicates that we
have been successful in nearly all cases as very few hemophilic puppies have been produced.

The other form of hemophilia, which is much more rare,
is known as hemophilia B although the preferred name is
Christmas disease. It is caused by a deficiency of clotting factor IX activity and has exactly the same inheritance pattern as hemophilia A (ie. an X-chromosomal-linked
recessive trait).

Hemophilia B was originally described in the Cairn
terrier (Rowsell et al, 1960) and has subsequently been
found in eight other breeds of dogs and in a family of inbred British shorthair cats (Dodds, 1981). This is a relatively rare disease in man, and six of the nine canine mutants of Christmas disease have been described within the
last two years. What this points out is the increased
awareness of the existence of bleeding diseases within
animal populations. More and more pet owners and veterinarians are recognizing these conditions before the animals
die and are able to make the diagnosis and provide samples

from other family members for study.

The last example to be discussed is von Willebrand's disease, which is by far the most common inherited bleeding disorder of the dog and probably also of man (Dodds, 1981).

It is very difficult to estimate the frequency of this particular mutation in human populations. Some recent studies in so-called "normal" populations in Scandinavia, Great Britain, and North America have estimated that the gene may be as common as 15 to 20% (Stuart et al, 1979). By comparison we have now recognized this disease in 25 pure breeds of dogs as well as in mongrels. New cases are being discovered regularly. Suffice it to say that if you are interested in studying von Willebrand's disease in the dog, there are plenty of models around. In fact, many of them can be found at the local dog pound, particularly if you select Dobermans or Doberman crossbreds.

Animal models for von Willebrand's disease were first recognized in Poland-China swine (Hogan, Muhrer and Bogart, 1941). This defect has been very well-studied and exploited (Bowie et al, 1973; Griggs et al, 1974; Fass et al, 1979).

Von Willebrand's disease in man and animals is expressed in two forms (Fass et al, 1979; Dodds, 1981). One is an autosomal recessive disease in which only the homozygote has a bleeding diathesis but heterozygotes are detectable by a variety of deficiencies of plasma von Willebrand's factor activity. The other and more common form is an autosomal incompletely dominant trait in which there is varying expression or penetrance.

Porcine von Willebrand's disease is an autosomal recessive disorder in which heterozygotes are asymptomatic despite their demonstrable laboratory defects of von Willebrand's factor protein (Bowie et al, 1973; Fass et al, 1979). Homozygous animals are clinically affected, and have a relatively severe form of the disease. There are two colonies of pigs currently being maintained and studied. One is kept by Dr. Walter Bowie and colleagues at the Mayo Clinic in Rochester, MN (Bowie et al, 1973), and the other is kept by Dr. Kenneth Brinkhous and colleagues at Chapel Hill, NC (Griggs et al, 1974).

One of the most exciting recent discoveries with this particular model has been the observation that homozygous, affected pigs appeared to develop less atherosclerosis than did normal pigs (Fuster and Bowie, 1978; Bowie and Fuster, 1980). This stimulated a more thorough examination of the theory of atherogenesis in terms of the role of von Wille-

brand's factor in precipitating smooth muscle cell proliferation and the initial intimal hyperplasia associated with
atherosclerosis. Although there is controversy about the
findings with the pig model, studies of these animals have
contributed significantly to our current knowledge of the
pathogenesis of atherosclerosis.

Of the 25 breeds of dogs confirmed to have von Willebrand's disease, only two of them have the autosomal recessive form. These are the Scottish terrier and the
Chesapeake Bay retriever (Rosborough et al, 1980; Dodds et
al, 1981).

The Doberman pinscher is the second most popular dog
in North America today, and our original findings indicated
that 65% of the animals screened for this disease had reduced levels of von Willebrand's factor protein. About
12% of the total population had signs of excessive bleeding
when exposed to stress situations like intercurrent disease, hormonal imbalance, trauma, or surgical intervention. Today we have reduced the prevalence with two and
one-half years of intensive genetic counseling to 63%
(Dodds et al, 1981). So, we have a long way to go with
this breed.

In developing an accurate heterozygote detection
assay for von Willebrand's disease, we found, like Dr.
Jolly did with bovine mannosidosis (Jolly et al, 1981), a
skewed distribution between the normal and the abnormal
populations with a small, but defined area of overlap.
Despite this problem, we have been able to mount an effective program to identify heterozygotes and gradually eliminate them from the breeding population (Dodds et al,
1981).

The screening program is based upon measurements of
plasma factor VIII-related antigen by the Laurell electro-
immunoassay using monospecific anticanine factor VIII
(Rosborough et al, 1980; Dodds et al, 1981). The sensitivity or lower limit of detection of this method is about
7%. Thus, animals with levels at or less than 7% read as
undetectable. By using the more sensitive radioimmuno-
electrophoretic technique which detects as little as 0.01%
antigen, affected dogs could be classified into two groups.
Those individuals expressing the homozygous form of the
autosomal recessive disease had no detectable antigen,
whereas their heterzygous parents and all those with the
autosomal incomplately dominant form of von Willebrand's
disease had reduced but detectable amounts of antigen.

In order to establish the normal range for canine

factor VIII-related antigen, we measured levels in over 125 healthy purebred dogs of breeds in which von Willebrand's disease has yet to be recognized. The antigen levels of these animals ranged from 60-172%. We next compared values obtained for several thousand dogs of the six breeds in which von Willebrand's disease had an apparently high prevalence. These were the Scottish terrier, Pembroke Welsh corgi, Doberman pinscher, golden retriever, miniature schnauzer, and standard Manchester terrier. It was immediately apparent, when a histogram of the antigen levels for these breeds was compared to that of the normal population, that a portion of each affected breed had values less than 50% (Jolly et al, 1981). In the Scottish terrier breed, for example, about 3% of the more than 2000 animals examined were homozygous, affected and had no measurable antigen. Another 30% or so dogs had values below 50% and were either the obligatory heterozygous parents of homozygous pups or were considered to be heterozygous for the trait based on parental or family status with respect to the VWD gene. Retrospective analysis of the results for progeny from all four mating types indicates a greater than 92% accuracy of carrier detection by this blood test (Dodds et al, 1981).

In Pembroke Welsh corgis that have the incompletely dominant form of von Willebrand's disease, there is also a group of dogs with antigen levels less than 50% (Jolly et al, 1981). Of these, the clinically affected individuals had levels as low as zero (undetectable) and as high as 46%. In this breed, homozygosity for the von Willebrand's disease gene appears to be lethal, and heterozygosity may or may not be clinically expressed depending on other modifiers of expression or intercurrent stress and disease.

Data from the Doberman pinscher breed is the most striking (Jolly et al, 1981). About 3000 animals of this breed have been tested to date and there is a tremendous skew in the distribution of antigen levels. Over 40% of the animals tested had plasma factor VIII-related antigen levels between zero and 20% of the normal amount, and of those about one-third of them are clinically affected with von Willebrand's disease. Although a bleeding tendency has been recognized in heterozygotes with antigen levels as high as 48%, most clinically affected animals have much lower values.

As you might expect, the "founder effect" plays a major role in most of these purebred dog families. The very best, top winning show dogs are frequently involved in

passing on both desirable and undesirable genes. The need
to develop practical mass screening programs for undesirable genetic traits is thus underscored (Jolly et al, 1981).

Currently, we have screened about 8000 purebred dogs
for inherited bleeding disorders and about 6000 of these
were screened specifically for von Willebrand's disease.
Prior to the summer of 1979 we had screened 943 Scottish
terrier dogs for the von Willebrand's disease gene and
nearly 40% of them were abnormal. Since then we have
screened another 1569 dogs, but the disease prevalence in
those animals was only 16%, which in part is a result of
our screening and genetic counseling program (Dodds et al,
1981). The affected Scottish terrier is homozygous for the
gene and therefore an effective means of control is to en-
sure that heterozygous individuals are bred only to normal
mates. The progeny can then be tested for the gene to plan
for the next generation. Provided there is no misclassifi-
cation or misidentification of parental status, these
matings should not produce affected get. Thus breeders can
effectively select the most desirable show stock for subsequent generations.

Another byproduct of our screening program is the acquisition of new animals with bleeding disorders to be used
for research on the biochemical, genetic and physiologic
aspects of the problem (Dodds, 1981). With respect to
genetics, the von Willebrand's disease model has provided
a reliable means of checking the transmission of the gene
and the accuracy of diagnostic testing. For example, in
the Scottish terrier we have measured the factor VIII-
related antigen level of 177 puppies with two normal
parents as determined by the blood test. The results for
the offspring were 97% normal and 3% with antigen values
below 50%. These pups would have been misclassified as
heterozygotes on the basis of their blood test results.
Conversely, however, the other 97% were accurately identified as being normal for the gene. Similarly, in Dobermans
we have tested 121 progeny with two normal parents. Of
these 98% were classified as normal and 2% had values below
50%. For testmatings in which one parent was a heterozygote, we had 442 Scottie pups and the breakdown in the offspring was 58% normal and 42% carriers (heterozygotes) as
determined by the blood test. In the Doberman breed, out
of 353 offspring, 55% were normal and 45% were abnormal.
If both parents carried the von Willebrand's gene, the expected ratio of 25% normal and 75% abnormal also was
achieved in the three breeds examined: the Scottish

terrier, the Pembroke Welsh corgi and the Doberman pinscher (Dodds et al, 1981). The overall accuracy rate for hetero-zygote detection was 92% which is remarkable when one de-pends not only upon proper collection of samples without clots, proper processing of samples without hemolysis, proper shipment of samples without thawing, but also upon correct identification of the animals by their owners or breeders.

References

Bowie EJW, Owen Jr CA, Zollman PE, Thompson Jr JH, Fass DN (1973). Tests of hemostasis in swine: normal values and values in pigs affected with von Willebrand's disease. Am J Vet Res 34:1405.

Bowie EJW, Fuster V (1980).Resistance to atherosclerosis in pigs with von Willebrand's disease. Acta Med Scand (Suppl) 642:121.

Dodds WJ (1979). Hemorrhagic disorders. In Andrews EJ, Ward BC, Altman NH (eds): "Spontaneous Animal Models of Human Disease," Volume 1, New York: Academic Press, p 266.

Dodds WJ (1981). Second international registry of animal models of thrombosis and hemorrhagic diseases. ILAR News 24:R3.

Dodds WJ, Moynihan AC, Fisher TM, Trauner DB (1981). The frequencies of inherited blood and eye diseases as deter-mined by genetic screening programs. J Am An Hosp Assoc 17:697.

Fass DN, Bowie EJW, Owen Jr CA, Zollman PE (1979). Inheri-tance of porcine von Willebrand's disease: study of a kindred of over 700 pigs. Blood 53:712.

Fuster V, Bowie EJW (1978). The von Willebrand pig as a model for atherosclerosis research. Thromb Haemost 39: 322.

Griggs TR, Webster WP, Cooper HA, Wagner RH, Brinkhous KM (1974). Von Willebrand factor: gene dosage relationships and transfusion response in bleeder swine - a new bio-assay. Proc Natl Acad Sci USA 71:2087.

Jolly RD, Dodds WJ, Ruth GR, Trauner DB (1981). Screening for genetic diseases: principles and practice. In Corne-lius CE, Simpson CF (eds): "Advances in Veterinary Science and Comparative Medicine," Volume 25, New York: Academic Press, p 245.

Morse EE (1978). The fibrinogenopathies. Ann Clin Lab Sci 8:234.

Raymond SL, Dodds WJ (1979). Platelet membrane glycoproteins in normal dogs and dogs with hemostatic defects. J Lab Clin Med 93:607.

Rosborough TK, Johnson GS, Benson RE, Swaim WR, Dodds WJ (1980). Measurement of canine von Willebrand factor using ristocetin and polybrene diagnosis of canine von Willebrand's disease. J Lab Clin Med 96:47.

Rowsell HC, Downie HF, Mustard JF, Leeson JE, Archibald JA (1960). A disorder resembling hemophilia B (Christmas disease) in dogs. J Am Vet Med Assoc 137:247.

Stuart MJ, Miller ML, Davey FR, Wolk JA (1979). The post aspirin bleeding time: a screening test for evaluating hemostatic disorders. Br J Haematol 43:649.

DR. PATTERSON: We generally think of animal models in terms of their usefulness in determining pathogenesis or possibly treatment, but it occurred to me while I was listening that this may be a suitable subject for a study of selection. The high frequency of the gene for von Willebrand's disease (VWD) in humans and dogs suggests that there is something, perhaps a heterozygote advantage, that maintains this gene in the population at high frequency, even though it is deleterious in the homozygous state.

Of course, in the purebred dog the high gene frequency could simply be due to chance. It could be a result of genetic drift or perhaps founder effect, but when you see it in two different species, both dog and man, it certainly makes one think the phenomenon is real. Do you have any thoughts about that?

DR. DODDS: With respect to the question of a selected advantage of the VWD gene in the dog, I think the expression of canine VWD is primarily the result of a founder effect. Animals carrying the von Willebrand's disease gene are clearly less fit because manifestation of the disease by mucosal surface bleeding is precipitated by stress. Thus, affected dogs do poorly when challenged by such conditions as enteric viruses (parvo and corona viruses), hormonal imbalances and trauma. About half of the Doberman pinscher breed, for example, is prone to familial hypothyroidism, and it is interesting that nearly two-thirds of them also carry the gene for von Willebrand's disease. In this regard, clinical studies in man have reported that von Willebrand's factor levels are depressed in hypothyroidism and are increased in hyperthyroidism. We have just finished the first of several trials with normal dogs and Dobermans affected with von Willebrand's disease, in which we monitored their TSH response test and supplemented them either with T3 or T4 in the presence and absence of propranolol. Results of preliminary studies showed that thyroid supplementation of normal dogs did not change to their levels of von Willebrand's factor. By contrast, seven Doberman pinschers with von Willebrand's disease supplemented with thyroid whose von Willebrand's factor levels varied from less than 7 to 42 percent of normal expressed a difference in their temperament, hair coat and skin condition, and within four days von Willebrand's factor levels in 5 of the 7 had increased from 150 to 400 percent of the initial values. We do not understand what this means, at present, but there seem to be several factors that modify the expression of this gene in normal and abnormal individuals.

DR. O'BRIEN: I would like to amplify Dr. Patterson's question by simply asking with the data as high as 9000 animals you have an excellent opportunity to find out whether or not there is any evidence for selection by simply testing for Hardy Weinberg equilibrium, especially since you have all three genotypes. Have you attempted to do this, and if so, what is the answer?

DR. DODDS: That is a very good question which we have not yet addressed. The problem is that we have just developed a computer program to handle all the data and have as yet not been able to ask such questions. The data clearly need to be examined.

We have the same problem that Dr. Jezyk alluded to earlier. We are screening about 4500 animals annually with few personnel. All but two of the support staff are supported by NIH-funded research grants. The remaining two persons are funded by private sources such as the American Kennel Club and Geraldine R. Dodge Foundation. Thus, much of the data gathered by the genetics screening program have not been analyzed because of insufficient time to share between research productivity and the screening of purebred dog populations.

DR. O'BRIEN: I might add also that there are excellent controls, within the human population, in the number of polymorphic genes that have been detected in thousands of people.

DR. DODDS: Correct.

DR. GUÉNET: Do dog populations mate at random?

DR. DODDS: No. Dr. Patterson, perhaps you can elaborate on this point.

DR. PATTERSON: They certainly don't mate at random with respect to things like temperament and color and things of that sort, but it is possible that they mate at random with respect to some marker that is not selected by man.

DR. DODDS: You see, in purebred dogs, mating selections are based on a desired phenotype and to a lesser extent on temperament.

DR. PATTERSON: The little work that has been done on this shows that most enzyme polymorphism and hemoglobin types that don't have any deleterious effect do fit a Hardy Weinberg distribution. The genotypes do seem to be in equilibrium.

DR. DODDS: There is an interesting point I have noticed during my years of studying dog populations. When you screen litters from a heterozygous X normal mating, frequently the phenotypically ideal puppies, based on the owner's assessment, are the ones that are abnormal for the biomedical marker you are monitoring. I have a persistent impression that it is more often the best puppies in a litter that are abnormal for the mutant gene in question.

DR. O'BRIEN: If there is a selective distortion it simply could be artificial.

DR. DODDS: Basically, I agree with you.

DR. ZOOK: There is a recent paper describing a family of humans with both von Willebrand's disease and endocardial fibroelastosis (EFE). Have you noticed heart failure or lesions of EFE in dogs with von Willebrand's disease?

DR. DODDS: If you look at Dobermans for example, they have various myocardial anomalies, renal agenesis, temperament changes and von Willebrand's disease.

DR. ZOOK: But you have not observed EFE specifically?

DR. DODDS: No. There are a variety of reports in the literature of patients with von Willebrand's disease and some other disease. Actually the number of such reports may reflect a general interest in von Willebrand's disease and its diagnosis. When you look for a problem, you are more likely to find it.

DR. BUSS: In the measurements which you make to identify the heterozygote and the normal, is the variability of the measurement greater for the heterozygote than for the normal?

DR. DODDS: No, it is not. The error of the canine von Willebrand's factor assay is about 10 or 11 percent at any level from about 10 to 150 percent.

DR. T. C. JONES: Could you say something about the status of linkage studies with the other characteristics, and where do we stand on the study of DNA of the genes that are involved in coagulation defects?

DR. DODDS: To my knowledge there have been no linkage studies. We are interested, for example, in familial hypothyroidism to try to determine what effect this could have genetically or physiologically on the expression of von Willebrand's disease. There is nothing known about the DNA of the vWD gene. One of the really difficult problems in working effectively with these animal models is that we have too many models to study in depth. For example, we don't have the time or specific expertise to study the new model of canine dysfibrinogenemia. Several experts in fibrinogen structure and metabolism are interested in such a model, but find it difficult to support the maintenance and therapy necessary to keep a 100-pound dog alive that is bleeding repeatedly.

We have had five hemophilic dogs donated within the last month. The problem is where to get the money to support these colonies. You have to have experienced, specially-trained persons to keep the animals alive in order to study their diseases. Further, if you are treating them all the time, they are not available in pristine form for biochemical or physiological research.

DR. SNYDER: Do you conclude that the owner-breeder of the terrier is receptive to genetic counseling whereas those of Dobermans are not?

DR. DODDS: In working with dog breeders one soon realizes that every breed has owners with special personality traits. The only comment I can make is that the Doberman is so much more popular than the other breeds we've worked with, and that a lot of money and prestige is associated with having top-producing sires. How does one test them for the carrier state of the VWD gene when the owner is uncooperative or chooses to cover up their true status? The way this is done is to breed a VWD-normal bitch to such a male and then test the resultant progeny for the VWD trait. If some of the puppies are abnormal for the VWD gene, everybody will soon know that the particular stud involved is a carrier of VWD. This is widely discussed by competitors of the owner and so a major problem exists.

DR. LEADER: I want to make one comment, as a response to what Dr. Benirschke said this morning about the current onslaught that is being launched against the use of animals in biomedical research. We have a very strong point going for us in a group of this type. We are studying naturally occurring animal diseases, and they benefit man as animal models, but they, also, benefit the animals being studied because there have been a number of examples, including yours and Dr. Jolly's that I remember very specifically this afternoon, where there has been an enormous decrease in the prevalence of certain specific genetic diseases because of the studies that have been carried out. I think we must keep this in mind. Many of us eventually will be called on to speak about this issue before legislative bodies and other forums. Potentially adverse developments are occurring rapidly and it is a major responsibility for us to speak out on these issues.

DR. DODDS: I could not agree with you more. One of the reasons why we have been successful in having these animals donated is that we guarantee that none of them will be subjected to invasive experimentation and that they will be kept under ideal conditions for the rest of their natural lives. All we do is collect their blood for research studies of the biochemical defects involved; breed the dogs to study the genetics and expression in their progeny; treat them when indicated; and use them for a variety of experimental in vivo physiologic and treatment-oriented research. We also invite interested people and former owners to visit the facilities and see the animals.

Animal Models of Inherited Metabolic Diseases, pages 133-142
© 1982 Alan R. Liss, Inc., 150 Fifth Avenue, New York, NY 10011

MOUSE HEMOGLOBINOPATHIES: DETECTION AND CHARACTERIZATION
OF THALASSEMIAS AND GLOBIN-STRUCTURE MUTATIONS

J. Barry Whitney III, Ph.D.

Department of Cell and Molecular Biology
Medical College of Georgia
Augusta, Georgia 30912

When appropriate models of human genetic diseases are
desired but not known among research mammals, one approach
is to attempt to induce new mutations that cause the same
diseases in manageable laboratory animals. Screening for
mouse hemoglobin mutations has been quite successful, which
suggests that such an approach may also be feasible for a
variety of other human genetic diseases.

The advantages of mice (Mus musculus) for such studies
are manifold and include their short generation time,
moderate cost, manageability, the ease with which embryos
or isolated cells can be manipulated, their thorough
genetic characterization, and (at least for the moment) the
ready availability of a tremendous variety of genetic and
cytogenetic markers in living mice. The particular advantages of the hemoglobins include their easy availability in
good purity and in reasonable amounts from living, breed-
able mice for complete polypeptide characterization, and
the relative ease with which variant or mutant globin genes
can be characterized at the mRNA and DNA levels.

HUMAN HEMOGLOBINOPATHIES

Hemoglobin defects are among the best characterized of
the inborn errors of human metabolism. Two general classes
of mutations that directly affect the hemoglobins are
recognized. The first class includes mutations that affect
hemoglobin synthesis without affecting the structure(s) of
whatever hemoglobins may be present. This class includes

the thalassemias, defects in the synthesis of one or a group of related globin chains. Alpha thalassemias affect α-globin expression; beta thalassemias affect β-globin expression. Thalassemias can be of either the "zero" type or of the "plus" type. Persons with β^{+}-thalassemia make normal beta-globin, but in abnormally low amounts. Homozygotes for β^{0}-thalassemia make no beta globin whatsoever and are therefore severely anemic. Homozygotes for α-thalassemia-1 (α^{0}-thalassemia) sometimes survive to birth but die shortly thereafter.

The second general class includes mutations that affect the primary structure of a globin chain. A variety of abnormal hemoglobins have been detected both through studies of anemic patients and through widespread screening of diverse human populations. Each mutation affects the structure of only one of the globin chains; over 300 mutations are known that affect the alpha, beta, delta, $^{G}\gamma$, or $^{A}\gamma$ globins (I.H.I.C.; Hemoglobin 4: 215, 1980). For instance, hemoglobin G-Georgia has the amino acid leucine at position 95 of the alpha globin chain, instead of the normal proline. Hemoglobin S has valine at position 6 of the beta globin, instead of the normal glutamic acid. Normal hemoglobin genetic variations that have no clinical manifestations in the homozygote are quite rare.

In contrast, normal genetic variations in mouse hemoglobins are quite common while hemoglobinopathies, other than those resulting from induced mutations, have not been described. The normal genetic variations can provide useful markers of the expression (or non-expression) of individual globin genes, adding to the value of inbred laboratory mice for genetically controlled studies of the regulation of the expression of the clusters of globin genes.

NATURAL GENETIC VARIATION

Normal genetic variation in mouse hemoglobins is recognized among inbred strains as well as in wild mice (feral mice or exotic laboratory stocks). Electrophoretic analysis, especially when cystamine is employed (Whitney, 1978; Wegmann and Gilman, 1970), readily discriminates among some of the haplotypes at the Hbb hemoglobin beta locus. The term "haplotypes" is used instead of "alleles" because several genes that encode globins lie within each of the α- and β-globin gene complexes, on mouse Chromosomes 11 and 7, respectively. Hemoglobin α-chain, Hba, genetic variation is not detected by simple electrophoresis even though more than a dozen different haplotypes are now known.

ALPHA GLOBIN (Hba) GENETIC VARIATION

Popp (1962) recognized among mice with the same single beta genotype a strong difference in hemoglobin solubility in concentrated phosphate buffer, now recognized to be determined by the α-globin locus, called Hba. Differences in the hemoglobin crystal structures were also apparent. Hemoglobin solubility in 2.25 M or 2.8 M phosphate buffer reveals Hba genotypes which encode hemoglobins with solubilities that fall into at least four classes: high, high-intermediate, low-intermediate, and low (Russell and McFarland, 1974). Sequencing studies revealed that some mice have only one type of alpha globin while mice belonging to other fully-inbred strains have two different alpha globins, indicating that they have a duplicate α-globin structural gene (also the normal case in man). Substitutions at four (of 141) different positions within the alpha globin, α^{25}, α^{62}, α^{68}, and α^{78}, define five unique chains: for example, at these positions Chain 4 has valine, isoleucine, serine, and glycine, respectively, while Chain 5 has glycine, valine, asparagine, and alanine (Popp, Bailiff, Skow and Whitney, 1982). Chain 1 differs from Chain 5 only in having glycine at α^{78}.

That no Hba-dependent electrophoretic variation is seen among normal hemoglobins of the same β-globin type is consistent with all of the substitutions recorded being of neutral for neutral amino acids (valine, isoleucine, serine, threonine, alanine, glycine). Many of the substitutions are nonetheless detectable by isoelectric focusing (Whitney, Copland, Skow, and Russell, 1979). The existence of Chain 5 was first revealed by the fact that its hemoglobin, which has a solubility like that of Chain 1-containing hemoglobin, nonetheless has a higher isoelectric point because of the glycine for alanine substitution. Isoelectric focusing, in combination with solubility testing, defines at least 15 naturally-occurring Hba haplotypes (see Table I).

Hba Haplotype	α-Globin Chain(s)	Solubility	Strain or Stock
a	1	High	C57BL, 129
b	2,3	Low	SEC, BALB
c	1<4	Hi-Int.	SWR, C3H
d	1<2	Lo-Int.	SM, CBA
e	4	Int.	
f	5	High	CE, AKR
g	5,1	High	STAR, DBA
h	(5<4)	Hi-Int.	BDP, P, SEA
i	5<1	High	M. m. molossinus
j	(6)	Low	M. spretus
k	(1,3)		Various feral
(1)	(2)		Skive (Danish)
(m)	(1,5')	High	Induced mutant
(n)	(3,4)		Czech I
Other(s)		Low	M.m. brevirostris
Other	(new)		Canadian feral

Table I. Alpha Globin Genetic Variation in Mice.

Designations within parentheses are tentative -- for these, globin sequences have not been established by sequencing. Hba^e was reported only in strain NB, now extinct. All protein sequences have been determined by Popp and his collaborators (see Popp, Bailiff, Skow, and Whitney, 1982; and Russell and McFarland, 1974; for references). Hemoglobins containing α-chains listed separated by commas are present in approximately equal amounts; those separated by "<" are present in roughly a 1:2 ratio. Int. = Intermediate. Haplotypes a through i are carried by Jackson Laboratory inbred mice. New haplotypes i, j, k, l, and n were discovered in exotic stocks maintained by M. Potter (see Potter, 1981). Hba^k was found in Potter's Centreville Light stock (Whitney and Forrest, 1981) and the same or a similar haplotype in British (Newton, 1981) and Canadian (M. Petras, personal communication) feral mice. Other incompletely characterized new haplotypes exist in mice from Ontario (Petras and Popp, personal communication) and in Mus musculus brevirostris.

The entire sequence of the gene that encodes the BALB/c mouse alpha globin Chain 2 has been determined (Nishioka and P. Leder, 1979) and recombinant DNA clones have been prepared that collectively contain a 40 kilobase region that includes one alpha-like embryonic and two adult alpha globin genes (A. Leder et al., 1981). Normal DNA-level genetic polymorphism in this region, of an Eco Rl site believed to be 3' to the adult α-globin genes, has been reported (Whitney et al., 1981). Some of the genetic polymorphisms responsible for the known amino acid substitutions should also be detectable by restriction enzyme analysis. For example, the restriction enzyme Sau 3A should cut within AAGATCGCC sequence that presumably encodes the amino acids at α^{61}-α^{63} of Chain 4 (and other, new α-globins that may contain isoleucine at α^{62}).

BETA GLOBIN (Hbb) GENETIC VARIATION

Ranney and Gluecksohn-Waelsch (1955) described a genetic difference in mouse hemoglobins, some giving a "single" and some, a "diffuse" pattern on paper electrophoresis. The exact nature of this difference remained in some doubt until Gilman (1972) and Popp and Bailiff (1973) established that "diffuse" hemolysates contain a mixture of two different hemoglobins, "major" and "minor," with beta globins of different primary structure. About half of the inbred strains of mice carry the Hbb^d haplotype for diffuse hemoglobin and half, the Hbb^s genotype for single hemoglobin. That separate genes encode the two beta chains was confirmed by Konkel et al., 1978, 1979), who sequenced the two genes. The genomic map of the region containing both adult "diffuse" β-globin genes was presented by Jahn et al. (1980). That the Hbb^s genomic region contains two genes that encode the same β-globin was established by Weaver et al. (1981). Other Hbb genotypes are present in strain AU/SsJ (HbbP) and in other mouse stocks (Whitney, 1978; Gilman, 1974).

MOUSE GLOBIN GENE MUTATIONS

Screening by a variety of methods has been successful in recovering mouse hemoglobin mutations that have effects in the heterozygous carriers. Three independent mutations that block the synthesis of alpha globins and two mutations that affect mouse hemoglobin structures are currently available. In addition, an X-ray induced duplication of about 25% of Chromosome 7 that includes the beta locus complex, Hbb, also affects embryonic and adult hemoglobin expression (Popp, Skow, and Whitney, 1980).

At the Oak Ridge National Laboratory, initially 8621 offspring (Russell et al., 1976) and more recently another 6000 offspring (R.A. Popp, personal communication) of X-irradiated parents have been screened for hemoglobin mutations, using hemoglobin solubility and crystal structure and starch gel electrophoresis. Three alpha thalassemias, two of which proved heritable, the duplication in Chromosome 7, and several other somatic or non-heritable conditions were detected.

A third heritable α-thalassemia was the only hemoglobin abnormality discovered among 500 offspring of male mice treated with triethylenemelamine at The Jackson Laboratory (Whitney and Russell, 1980) when cellulose acetate electrophoresis was employed for screening.

Among 8288 offspring of strain DBA/2J males treated with procarbazine at the National Institute of Environmental Health Sciences, one or two possible mutations affecting minor hemoglobin mobility were recovered using starch gel electrophoresis (Johnson et al., 1981). More recently, this group has screened another 1974 offspring of males treated with ethylnitrosourea and has recovered a proven mutation that affects the structure of one of the two adult alpha globin chains (Johnson and Lewis, 1981, and personal communication).

Alpha Thalassemia Mutations

All three heritable α-thalassemias have similar effects upon their carriers. The adults have a microcytic anemia with anisocytosis (Popp and Enlow, 1977; Whitney and Russell, unpublished results) and unusual proportions of "diffuse" hemoglobins or presence of beta-tetramers (Hemoglobin H). Heterozygous embryos have a large amount of a β-like embryonic globin tetramer (y_4, analogous to Hb H or Hb Barts) (Whitney and Russell, 1979; Popp, Skow, and

Whitney, 1980). Homozygous embryos are inferred to die around the time of implantation (Popp, Bradshaw, and Skow, 1980).

The heterozygous adults have no α-globin synthesis directed by the mutant chromosome (Popp, Stratton, Hawley and Effron, 1979; Whitney, Martinell, Popp, Russell, and Anderson, 1981). Total α-globin synthesis and α-mRNA levels are reduced (Martinell, Whitney, Popp, Russell, and Anderson, 1981), though only to about 75% of normal. It has now been established that each of these three mutations, which inactivate both adult α-globin genes and an embryonic α-like globin gene, have actually deleted at least the 3 kilobase DNA segments that contain each adult α-globin gene, and presumably all of the material between these segments (Whitney et al., 1981), which would be about 12 kilobases (A. Leder et al., 1981). A detailed dicussion of these mutations appears elsewhere in this volume (W.F. Anderson).

Successful therapy of mouse α-thalassemia has been achieved, and an inverse demonstration also carried out, by transplantation methods (Russell, 1979) which are routinely employed in the study of mouse hereditary anemias. In the first case, C57BL/6J-congenic mice heterozygous for the $\underline{\text{Hba}}^{th-J}$ thalassemia were lethally irradiated and then given life-sparing transplants of bone marrow cells from normal mice of the C57BL/6J strain. In time, the blood picture of the recipients became entirely normal, as the donor stem cells repopulated their hemopoietic systems. Non-irradiated thalassemic recipients showed a slight acceptance of normal marrow cell transplants. In the inverse demonstration, a $\underline{\text{W}}/\text{W}^{V}$ recipient, with a genetically-determined macrocytic anemia (Whitney, 1981), was given marrow cells from a C57BL/6J-$\underline{\text{Hba}}^{th-J}$/+ thalassemic male. In time, the macrocytic anemia of the host was replaced by the microcytic anemia characteristic of the $\underline{\text{Hba}}^{th-J}$ heterozygote, and Hb H appeared in the blood. These two demonstrations emphasize the potential special values of congenic mice for the development and testing of methodologies useful for eventual gene replacement therapy with cloned normal genes (see Anderson, 1980), in particular, the free acceptance of congenic cells, as though they were reimplantations of the recipient's own cells, somehow made genetically normal, by $\underline{\text{W}}/\text{W}^{V}$ genetically-anemic, or by normal, lethally irradiated hosts.

Globin Structure Mutation

Using starch gel electrophoresis without cystamine, Johnson and Lewis (1981) find normally the doublet (minor/ major) hemoglobin pattern in samples from mice of the Hbb^d/ Hbb^s genotype. One of 1974 offspring of an ethylnitro- sourea-treated DBA/2J male gave an abnormal pattern, with each of the minor and major bands appearing as a doublet consisting of a strong band of each of the usual types and a weaker, slower-migrating band. The appearance of second components to each beta-dependent band suggested that an alpha-dependent electrophoretic mutant was present, in spite of the fact that electrophoretic variations due to mouse alpha chains had never been reported in nature despite extensive searches. Independent segregation from Hbb strengthened the idea of an Hba-dependent electro- phoretic mutant.

Homozygotes for the new mutation, denoted Hba^m in Table I, are healthy and reproduce well, as do Hba^m/Hba^{th-J} double heterozygotes for the mutant and the Jackson Labora- tory thalassemia -- effectively hemizygous for the new mutation. The DBA/2J father of the original mutant was tested and confirmed normal, therefore, of the Hba^g or Chain 1 plus Chain 5 type. Isoelectric focusing analysis indicates that Hba^m homozygotes do have a hemoglobin with Chain 1, but have none with Chain 5: instead, a new hemo- globin band of higher isoelectric point is found. The mutation maps genetically near wa-2. Our conclusion is therefore that ethylnitrosourea induced in the adult α-globin structural gene for Chain 5 a mutation that changed the structure encoded to one that gives an unnatu- rally high hemoglobin isoelectric point, but left the Chain 1 gene intact. More detailed analyses are now underway.

REFERENCES

Anderson, WF (1980). Regulation of globin gene expression at the molecular level. Ann NY Acad Sci 344:262.
Gilman, JG (1972). Hemoglobin beta chain structural varia- tion in mice: evolutionary and functional impli- cations. Science 178:873.
Gilman, JG (1974). Rodent hemoglobin structure: a compari- son of several species of mice. Ann NY Acad Sci 241: 416.

Jahn, CL, Hutchison, III, CA, Phillips, SJ, Weaver, S, Haigwood, NL, Edgell, MH (1980). DNA sequence organization of the β-globin complex in the BALB/c mouse. Cell 21:159.

Johnson, FM, Roberts, GT, Sharma, RK, Chasalow, F, Zweidinger, R, Morgan, A, Hendren, RW, Lewis, SE (1981). The detection of mutants in mice by electrophoresis: Results of a model induction experiment with procarbazine. Genetics 97:113.

Johnson, FM, Lewis, SE (1981). Electrophoretically detected germinal mutations induced in the mouse by ethylnitrosourea. Proc Natl Acad Sci 78:3138.

Konkel, DA, Maizel, Jr, JV, Leder, P (1979). The evolution and sequence comparison of two recently diverged mouse chromosomal β-globin genes. Cell 18:865.

Konkel, DA, Tilghman, SM, Leder, P (1978). The sequence of the chromosomal mouse β-globin major gene: homologies in capping, slicing, and poly(A) sites. Cell 15: 1125.

Leder, P, Hansen, JN, Konkel, D, Leder, A, Nishioka, Y, Talkington, C (1980). Mouse globin system: A functional and evolutionary analysis. Science 209: 1336.

Leder, A, Swan, D, Ruddle, F, D'Eustachio, P, Leder, P. (1981). Dispersion of α-like globin genes of the mouse to three different chromosomes. Nature 293:196.

Martinell, J, Whitney III, JB, Popp, RA, Russell, LB, Anderson, WF (1981). Three mouse models of human thalassemia. Proc Natl Acad Sci 78:5056.

Newton, MF (1981). A new Hba haplotype. Mouse News Letter 64:67.

Nishioka, Y, Leder, P (1979). The complete sequence of a chromosomal mouse α-globin gene reveals elements conserved throughout vertebrate evolution. Cell 18:875.

Popp, RA (1962). Studies on the mouse hemoglobin loci III. Heterogeneity of electrophoretically indistinguishable single-type hemoglobins. Journal of Heredity 75.

Popp, RA, Bailiff, EG (1973). Sequence of amino acids in the major and minor β chains of the diffuse hemoglobin from BALB/c mice. Biochim Biophys Acta 303:61.

Popp, RA, Bailiff, EG, Skow, LC, Whitney III, JB (1982). The primary structure of genetic variants of mouse hemoglobin. Biochem Genet (in press).

Popp, RA, Bradshaw, BS, Skow, LC (1980). Effects of alpha thalassemia on mouse development. Differentiation 17:205.

Popp, RA, Enlow, MK (1977). Radiation-induced α-thalassemia in mice. Am J Vet Res 38:569.

Popp, RA, Skow, LC, Whitney III, JB (1980). Expression of embryonic hemoglobin genes in α-thalassemic and ir β-duplication mice. Ann NY Acad Sci 344:280.

Popp, RA, Stratton, LP, Hawley, DK, Effron, K (1979). Hemoglobin of mice with radiation-induced mutations at the hemoglobin loci. J Mol Biol 127:141.

Potter, M (1981). Source and breeding characteristics of species and subspecies in the genus Mus. Mouse News Letter 64:64.

Ranney, HM, Gluecksohn-Waelsch, S (1955). Filter-paper electrophoresis of mouse hemoglobin: preliminary note. Ann Hum Genet 19:269.

Russell, ES (1979). Hereditary anemias of the mouse: a review for geneticists. Advances in Genetics 20:357.

Russell, ES, McFarland, EC (1974). Genetics of mouse hemoglobins. Ann NY Acad Sci 241:25.

Weaver, S, Comer, MB, Jahn, CL, Hutchison III, CA, Edgell, MH (1981). The adult β-globin genes of the "single" type mouse C57BL. Cell 24:403.

Wegmann, TG, Gilman, JG (1970). Chimerism for three genetic systems in tetraparental mice. Develop Biol 21:281.

Whitney III, JB (1978). Simplified typing of mouse hemoglobin (Hbb) phenotypes using cystamine. Biochem Genet 16:667.

Whitney III, JB (1981). Sl/Sl^d and W/W^v adult mice have fetal and neonatal levels of mouse minor hemoglobin. in Hemoglobins in Development and Differentiation. Alan R. Liss, Inc., NY.

Whitney III, JB, Copland, GT, Skow, LC, Russell, ES (1979). Resolution of products of the duplicated hemoglobin α-chain loci by isoelectric focusing. Proc Natl Acad Sci 76:867.

Whitney, JB, Forrest, B (1981). Hba: new genotypes. Mouse News Letter 64:53.

Whitney, III, JB, Martinell, J, Popp, RA, Russell, LB, Anderson, WF (1981). Deletions in the α-globin gene complex in α-thalassemic mice. Proc Natl Acad Sci 78 (12, in press).

Whitney III, JB, Russell, ES (1980). Linkage of genes for adult α-globins and an embryonic α-like globin chain. Proc Natl Acad Sci 77:1087.

SECTION III.
ANIMAL MODELS OF LYSOSOMAL STORAGE DISEASES

Animal Models of Inherited Metabolic Diseases, pages 145-163
© 1982 Alan R. Liss, Inc., 150 Fifth Avenue, New York, NY 10011

TWO MODEL LYSOSOMAL STORAGE DISEASES

R.D. Jolly

Department of Veterinary Pathology

Massey University, Palmerston North, New Zealand

INTRODUCTION

Lysosomal storage diseases are characterised by the storage of non-digestable material within lysosomes of a variety of cells within the body (Jolly, 1978 a). Whereas most are of genetic origin, others may be induced by ingestion or administration of chemicals. It is the purpose of this paper to describe two different types of storage disease with which we have worked, i.e. bovine mannosidosis and ovine ceroid-lipofuscinosis. Whereas the former disease is well defined, the latter is not. They are discussed in relation to their pathogenesis, veterinary importance and their application as models of analogous human disease.

MANNOSIDOSIS

Bovine mannosidosis occurs in cattle of Angus and related breeds. The genotype can be expected to occur wherever these breeds are used and it has been estimated that in New Zealand at least 10% of Angus cattle carried this lethal gene prior to instigation of a control program. At this gene frequency it was also estimated that 2,500 cases would occur each year in that country alone, which would make this the most common known genetic storage disease of humans or animals. Calves may die at birth but those that survive develop progressive ataxia and inco-ordination and die, usually within the first 12 months of life (Jolly, 1975, 1978 b). In this regard the disease appears more rapidly progressive than in human patients who may live into their second and third decade.

Pathologically there is vacuolation of neurons and a wide variety of other cell types throughout the body (Jolly, 1971; Jolly and Thompson, 1978). Ultrastructurally vacuoles are seen to be membrane bound vesicles that are empty other than for a small amount of amorphous material and membrane fragments. They are interpreted as being secondary lysosomes with most of their contents being leached out during fixation and preparation of sections for microscopy.

The storage material is oligosaccharide in nature, with up to 10 structures containing mannose and N-acetylglucosamine. Although the structures of all these have not been determined as they have for those in human mannosidosis (Yamashita *et al.*, 1980; Matsuura *et al.*, 1981), they are expected to be similar, but may contain extra molecules of N-acetylglucosamine (Lundblad *et al.*, 1975). These mannose-containing oligo-saccharides are the core structures of the heterosaccharide fractions of glycoproteins. Their occurrence in tissues and urine in this disease entity gave rise to the name mannosidosis (Öckerman, 1967; Hocking *et al.*, 1972) and implied that the basic enzyme deficiency would be that of acidic lysosomal α-mannosidase. This was confirmed for both the human and bovine diseases.

In calves with mannosidosis, the degree of deficiency of lysosomal α-mannosidase activity varies between tissues and body fluids measured. There are negligible amounts in plasma and leucocytes but 8 - 15% residual activity is believed attributable to the mutant enzyme in pancreas, brain, liver and other organs (Phillips *et al.*, 1977; Burditt *et al.*, 1978). The mutant enzyme is CRM+ve, heat labile and with slightly reduced substrate binding capacity. As with the normal enzyme, activity is increased by the addition of zinc ions to the assay mixture.

Heterozygous individuals have approximately 35 - 38% normal acidic α-mannosidase activity in plasma (Fig.1), neutrophils and lymphocytes and this observation has formed the basis of test and control programs in the pedigree nuclei of the Angus and Murray Grey breeds in New Zealand (Jolly *et al.*, 1974 a; Jolly, 1978 b) and the Angus breed in Australia.

Plasma/serum levels of enzyme are influenced by age up until maturity, plus a variety of ill-defined environmental influences. When plasma/serum is used, then

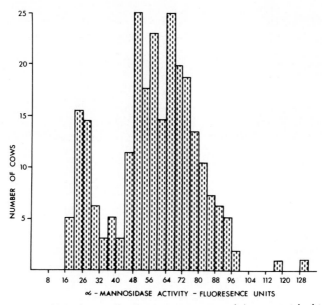

Fig. 1. Distribution of plasma α-mannosidase activity values in a herd of Angus cows. Animals are segregated into two populations representing those normal and heterozygous for the mannosidosis gene but there is an overlap between values from each population. The mean of the heterozygous values is 37% of the normal values and the normal value curve is positively skewed. Such skewness is characteristically noted in other populations irrespective of whether plasma, neutrophil or lymphocyte *a*-mannosidase activity values are plotted. (Redrawn from Jolly *et al.*, 1978 b with permission of the editor of the NZ Vet J).

tests are best interpreted within age and sex matched groups from the one herd (Jolly *et al.*, 1973; 1974 b; 1974 c). The environmental influences are less important when neutrophils are used (Jolly *et al.*, 1977) but the percentage of contaminating eosinophils may influence the assay (Healy, 1978). Plasma is preferred to serum as clotting may cause variations in enzyme activity with serum (Jolly *et al.*, 1973) due to variable losses from platelets (Gordon, 1975).

With plasma/serum, neutrophils or lymphocytes, the distribution of normal values is usually skewed and there is an overlap between low normal and high heterozygous values (Fig. 1; Jolly *et al.*, 1974 a; 1977; Thompson *et al.*, 1976; Jolly 1978 b). The large numbers of progeny of bulls, the short generation time of cattle and the ability to check results within large extended family groups helps overcome this disadvantage (Jolly, 1978 b). To date, approximately 100,000 animals have been screened for heterozygosity.

Bovine mannosidosis has also been exploited as a model of similar human diseases with particular emphasis on specific therapy. To interpret results of therapy in either experimental animals or human patients, it is necessary to understand the patterns of storage and excretion of storage oligosaccharides. This latter was determined in a longitudinal study involving quantitative measurements of these in organs of calves of different ages. It was found that storage of mannose-containing oligosaccharides was cumulative in brain, lymph node and pancreas (Fig. 2; Jolly *et al.*, 1980 a). In the liver, amounts remained constant while in the kidney, they fell over the first few weeks of life and then remained constant. The liver has minor parenchymal lesions and is presumably able to cope with storage material either by exocytosis into bile canaliculi or space of Disse or by residual enzyme activity. In regard to the latter, it is noteworthy that in mannosidosis the bovine liver retains approximately 15 - 20% of acidic α-mannosidase activity which is believed attributable to the mutant enzyme (Burditt *et al.*, 1978).

The pattern of storage in the kidney can be explained on the basis of cumulative storage of oligosaccharides during fetal life. Thereafter there is loss into urine associated with necrosis or degeneration of tubular cells, this exceeding the amount of new material formed. A stage is reached when the amount lost is balanced by that newly formed and/or stored within tubular cells. The amount of storage material excreted in urine per day approximates the amount stored in one kidney. Preliminary results from one calf indicate that the predominant source of mannose-containing oligosaccharides in urine is the blood stream (Daniel and Jolly unpublished). This implies that a considerable percentage of such material is formed intracellularly and excreted or otherwise lost from cells because extra-cellular catabolism of glycoproteins by α-mannosidase is unlikely.

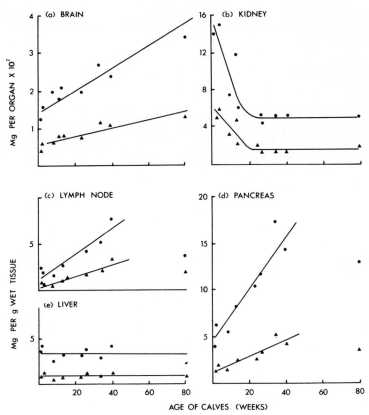

Fig. 2. Patterns of storage of oligosaccharides relative to age in various organs of calves with mannosidosis. Oligosaccharides are expressed as neutral sugar ● and hexosamine ▲ either in whole organ (a and b) or per g of wet tissue (c, d, e). (Reprinted from Jolly *et al.*, 1980 a with permission of the editor of Aust J Exp Biol Med Sc).

The expectations and limitations of two approaches to specific therapy have been explored in the bovine mannosidosis model. In the first, the effect of a natural transplant of lymphoid and perhaps other cell types on the course of mannosidosis was studied in a calf born co-twin to a normal calf of opposite sex. When twins occur in cattle there may be fusion of the placentas allowing mixture of blood. As this occurs prior to immunological

competence, blood cell lines from one individual may develop
in the other. In the case of twins of opposite sex this can
be confirmed by demonstrating both male and female karyotypes
in peripheral blood lymphocytes. In the present case, the
male mannosidosis calf had 77% female peripheral lymphocytes.
This transplant, occurring as it did under the most favourable
of circumstances, had a significant beneficial effect on
visceral organs such as exocrine pancreas, lymph nodes and
liver. There was some reduction in storage material in
the brain but nevertheless the calf developed severe
neurological signs typical of mannosidosis. It was concluded
that such tissue transplants were unlikely to significantly
influence the course of the neurological disturbances in
this type of disease (Jolly *et al.*, 1976).

In the second experiment, three affected calves were
fed high levels of zinc sulphate over a period of up to
3 months (Jolly *et al.*, 1980 b). The rationale for this
approach arose from the knowledge that α-mannosidase requires
zinc ions for optimum activity. Preliminary experiments had
established that zinc ions increased *in vitro* activity and
heat stability of the mutant acidic α-mannosidase, although
not to normal levels. It was reasoned that the deficiency
of α-mannosidase activity might be due to a reduced amount
of mutant enzyme resulting from its instability. If such
were the case, it might be possible to stabilise it *in vivo*
by additional zinc ions. A slower rate of decay could then
contribute significantly to the amount of residual enzyme
present as well as increase substrate binding. When zinc
sulphate was fed to calves, a proportion of the zinc was
stored in the liver, kidney and pancreas but not in lymph
nodes or brain. In those organs in which it was stored,
there was a very modest increase in activity attributed
to the mutant enzyme. Concurrently there was a minor
depletion of storage oligosaccharides. In contrast, organs
in which zinc was not stored showed no indication of
increased enzyme activity or decreased storage. The absence
of increased enzyme activity in brain, the relatively small
increase in organs in which zinc was stored and the inherent
toxicity, particularly to the pancreas, indicated that zinc
therapy was unlikely to be efficacious in human patients.

OVINE CEROID-LIPOFUSCINOSIS

The ceroid-lipofuscinoses are a heterogeneous group of

inherited diseases of man and animals characterised by the storage of fluorescent lipopigment within neurons and a variety of other cells (Zeman, 1976; Koppang, 1973; Jolly *et al.*, 1980 c). Although generalised in nature, secondary degenerative lesions leading to clinical disease are limited to the nervous system. The age of onset varies with the precise syndrome as do the presenting signs and course of the disease. In general though, there is blindness, behavioural abnormalities, loss of intellect, motor dysfunction and premature death.

The ovine disease is inherited in an autosomal recessive manner. Affected lambs become blind at approximately 12 months of age and usually die by 20 months (Jolly *et al.*, 1980 c). The electroretinogram of affected lambs is indicative of degeneration of rod visual receptor cells, a feature which is confirmed by microscopy. At autopsy the only gross lesion of note is a moderate atrophy of the cerebrum. Microscopically there is a loss of neurons in the cerebral cortex. Remaining neurons, astrocytes and microglial cells contain varying numbers of granules which are non-staining or slightly eosinophilic in conventional hemotoxylin and eosin stained sections. However the granules stain with Sudan black, slightly with Schiff reagent but more strongly when preceded by oxidation with periodic acid (i.e. they are PAS+ve) and they are slightly acid fast. Under blue light they show a yellow/green fluorescence in unstained deparaffinised sections, but this is more intense in frozen sections. Similar lipopigment is found within a wide variety of cells in other parts of the body. Ultrastructurally, storage bodies vary in shape from round to oval to irregular, sometimes lobulated electron-dense structures. Many appear granular but a common denominator amongst nearly all is the presence of a variety of membranous arrays that conform to those usually described as fingerprint bodies, curvilinear bodies, or crystaloids in the analogous human diseases. Those in cells of organs such as liver and pancreas are predominantly of the curvilinear type. Because of this and the fact that cells of these organs have a shorter life span than those in the central nervous system, it is postulated that these bodies are younger than those in the brain. As such, we believe that their structure and chemical composition might more accurately reflect the basic biochemical anomaly. For this reason we are concentrating on chemical and physical analyses of storage bodies isolated from liver as well as

from brain by the techniques of Siakotos and Koppang (1973).
They have a density between 1.16 and 1.22. Preliminary
observations on chloroform : methanol (2:1) extracts showed
the heterogeneous nature of both stored lipid and fluorescent
components. Silica gel TLC (ether:n-hexane:acetic acid,
20:80:1) of liver storage body neutral lipids showed several
quantitative differences from the total liver composition.
Very much smaller amounts of retinyls and triglycerides are
present in storage bodies compared to highly elevated levels
of a number of compounds that stain as alcohols. The predominant phospholipids noted on silica gel TLC (chloroform:
methanol:acetic acid: water, 50:25:4:2) were phosphatidylethanolamine, phosphatidylinositol and sphingomyelin. A
fluorescent band remained at the origin. Fluorescence in all
fractions varies with the freshness of preparation.

Phosphatidylethanolamine extracted from cerebral grey
matter showed a 25% diminution in the fatty acid 22:6 $\omega 3$
and minor changes in others. No differences have been seen
in fatty acid profiles of this phospholipid in the livers
of affected sheep.

DISCUSSION

Bovine mannosidosis is an example of a classical type
lysosomal storage disease associated with deficient activity
of a single acid hydrolase. Its study has led to control
of bovine mannosidosis in a particular population of cattle
through heterozygote detection. Such control was possible
because breeding is regulated and heterozygotes can be
culled from bull breeding herds. This is the first time
a genetic disease has been so controlled and the mutant
gene virtually eliminated from a specific population by a
heterozygote screening program. In contrast, the Tay Sachs
screening programs in Jewish populations assist in control
of the disease, but do nothing to reduce the gene frequency.
Experience gained in developing and applying this control
program has led to knowledge which may be applicable to
heterozygote screening in humans (Jolly and Desnick, 1979).
Of importance were the observations that (i) plasma is more
suitable than serum for assay as there may be variable
release of lysosomal enzymes from platelets during the
clotting process; (ii) plasma α-mannosidase activity levels
increase with age until maturity; (iii) plasma α-mannosidase
activity levels are greatly influenced by environmental

factors; (iv) when using leucocytes for enzyme assays, purified preparations of polymorph neutrophils or lymphocytes are preferable to mixed preparations; (v) leucocyte preparations are less influenced by environmental factors than plasma; (vi) that before a reference parameter (e.g. protein or reference enzyme) is chosen it should be shown to be highly correlated with the test enzyme; (vii) that the distribution of normal values in a population seldom conforms to a normal curve and as such, definition of its shape in terms of standard deviations is inappropriate.

The study of bovine mannosidosis has also contributed to an understanding of some of the expectations and limitations of specific therapy. Neither a natural *in utero* transplant of lymphocytes or zinc therapy significantly altered the course of mannosidosis. In the former experiment however, there was a relatively good response in visceral organs which is encouraging in regard to possible therapy of diseases such as Gaucher disease which have predominantly visceral lesions.

In contrast to the above inherited disease, an induced mannosidosis caused by ingestion of plants of *Swainsona* spp. occurs naturally in grazing animals or experimentally in laboratory animals. Such plants contain an indolizidine - 1, 2, 8, triol named Swainsonine that inhibits acidic α-mannosidase activity and allows accumulation of secondary lysosomes of mannose-rich oligosaccharides (Dorling *et al.*, 1978; Colgate *et al.*, 1979). The lesions and clinical signs are reversible if the plant or purified alkaloid is removed from the diet. This induced mannosidosis is also a useful model for studying some aspects of neurological dysfunction in inherited forms of mannosidosis.

The pathogenesis of the ceroid-lipofuscinoses remains an enigma. The fact that no dominant storage chemical species has been found, or was found in our material, implies that they may not belong to the classical group of lysosomal storage diseases characterised by a single acid-hydrolase deficiency with accumulation of its substrate. The hypothesis that storage of fluorescent lipopigment reflected lysosomal storage of ceroid or lipofuscin-like pigment as a result of peroxidation of unsaturated fatty acids of lipids (Zeman, 1976) is not universally supported. This hypothesis received considerable support when Armstrong *et al.*, (1974) reported a deficiency of p-phenylene-diamine specific peroxidase in leucocytes of patients but it was later suggested that the abnormality may be an epiphenomenon rather than reflecting the primary biochemical anomaly (Zeman, 1976). This peroxidase deficiency was also recorded in the English Setter canine model (Patel *et al.*, 1974). Peroxidative damage with the formation of ceroid could also occur as a consequence of lipid storage as occurs in some other specific storage diseases such as sphingomyelinosis (Brady, 1978). Although this is essentially due to a deficiency of sphingomyelinase and the dominant storage species is sphingomyelin (ceramide-phosphatidylcholine), other lipids and glycolipids are stored coincidently. The unsaturated fatty acids of these presumably undergo peroxidative damage with the formation of ceroid. The presence of ceroid in the ceroid-lipofuscinses may therefore not necessarily be of aetiological significance. Nevertheless production of free radicals during the course of peroxidative damage could conceivably contribute to the secondary degenerative changes in brain and retina.

The formation of "ceroid-lipofuscin" might also be explained by the finding of very abnormal polyunsaturated fatty acid profiles in phospholipids from brain of patients with infantile form of the disease (Svennerholm *et al.*, 1976). On the basis of these abnormalities it was suggested that the primary disturbance in this syndrome might be in the metabolism of 20:4 (ω6) fatty acid due to a defect in enzyme systems that desaturate and elongate fatty acids of the linoleic series. It was proposed that this form of ceroid-lipofuscinosis be termed "polyunsaturated fatty acid lipidosis". A different and less severely abnormal poly-unsaturated fatty acid profile was found in phosphatidylserine from grey matter of an adult patient with a pigment variant of ceroid-lipofuscinosis (Jervis and Pullakart, 1978). In our ovine model there is a 25% decrease in 22.6 ω3 fatty acid in phosphatidylethanolamine from cerebral cortex and minor differences in other fatty acids. The significance of this is not understood but as the fatty acid profiles of phospholipids from livers of the same affected sheep were normal, the lipid storage phenomenon is unlikely to reflect a general polyunsaturated fatty acid lipidosis as proposed for the infantile syndrome.

Wolfe *et al.* (1981) have found high levels of dolichols as well as retinoid complexes in storage material from a case of late infantile ceroid-lipofuscinoses and note that both types of compound are involved as intermediates in glycosylation of proteins. They suggest that their storage in this disease might reflect an inability to effectively recycle these compounds and postulate the possibility of a deficiency of a polyprenol esterase.

Alternate mechanisms of storage in the ceroid-lipofuscinoses are suggested by recent studies on chloroquine toxicosis and mucolipidosis II (Gonzalez-Noriega *et al.*, (1980) which extend those of many others. The former disease causes secondary interference with the normal lysosomal apparatus. The latter disease reflects an anomaly in the processing of lysosomal enzymes leading to a multiple enzyme deficiency. Lysosomal enzymes are synthesised in rough endoplasmic reticulum and then undergo glycosylation. Delivery to lysosomes depends on intracellular receptors which bind to newly synthesised enzymes bearing phospho-mannosyl recognition markers. The receptor-bound enzymes collect in vesicles (primary lysosomes) that bud off Golgi or endoplasmic reticulum and deliver the hydrolases to secondary lysosomes. There, the enzyme and receptor dissociate with recycling of receptor. Some enzyme may also be secreted but is recaptured by receptors in the cell membrane, internalised by pinocytosis and delivered to lysosomes.

In mucolipidosis II, newly synthesised enzymes fail to develop their markers. This is due to a deficiency in N-acetylglycosaminyl-UDP transferase which transfers phosphate to the mannose-rich oligosaccharide side chains of enzyme glycoproteins (Hasilk *et al.*, 1981). As a consequence, lysosomal enzymes tend to be secreted rather than delivered to lysosomes. The extracellular enzymes are likewise not recaptured as they lack the marker to bind to normal receptor in the plasma membrane. It is noteworthy that not all lysosomal enzymes are so affected. This implies that there may be variations of the marker-receptor complex for different lysosomal enzymes and the possibility of a family of diseases of similar pathogenesis. In addition, mutations affecting the phospho-mannosyl receptor or receptors for other possible markers, as well as mutations affecting activating proteins, are other possibilities to be kept in mind.

Chloroquine is lysomytropic and in lysosomes complexes with lipids. Lysosomal pH rises above that which favours dissociation of phospho-mannosyl markers from receptors. Failure to recycle receptors favours secretion of newly synthesised enzymes rather than delivery to lysosomes. The storage of heterogeneous lipid in the form of granular and membranous material probably reflects a combination of raised pH, induced enzyme deficiency and indigestibility of drug-lipid complexes. It is possible that the primary metabolic lesions in the ceroid-lipoguscinoses result in metabolites that initiate storage in a manner more or less similar to chloroquine or other cationic amphiphilic drugs.

The canine and ovine models of the ceroid-lipofuscinoses are of particular value in the study of these diseases as they allow invasive and sacrificial experiments in non-terminal cases. If unsaturated fatty acids or other unsaturated compounds are involved in the primary biochemical defect, they are liable to undergo post-mortem change in human derived material. We also suggest that preoccupation with nervous tissue that has governed much research may have tended to obscure the true nature of these diseases. This is because of additional physical and chemical changes that could be expected with this type of pigment in nervous tissue, as well as the severe secondary degenerative changes that occur, with consequent qualitative and quantitative changes in brain lipids. Analyses of storage material from liver and pancreas, where the turnover of parenchymal cells is such that intracellular pigment is likely to be of a younger and more even age, may more accurately reflect the basic biochemical anomaly.

REFERENCES

Armstrong D, Dimmitt S, Van Wormer DE (1974). Studies in Batten disease: Peroxidase deficiency in granulocytes. Arch Neurol 30:430

Brady RO (1978). Sphingomyelin lipidosis: Niemann-Pick disease. In Stanbury, JB, Fredrickson DS (eds): "The metabolic basis of inherited disease",New York: McGraw-Hill Book Co. p 718.

Burditt LJ, Phillips NC, Robinson D, Winchester BG,Jolly RD (1978). Characterisation of the mutant α-mannosidase in bovine mannosidosis. Biochem J 175:1013.

Colgate SM, Dorling PR, Huxtable CR (1979). A spectroscopic investigation of Swainsonine an α-mannosidase inhibitor isolated from *Swainsona canescens*, Aust J Chem 32:2257.

Dorling PR, Huxtable CR, Vogel P (1978). Lysosomal storage in *Swainsona* spp toxicosis: An induced mannosidosis. Neuropathol and Appl Neurobiol 4:285.

Gonzalez-Noriega A, Grub JH, Talkad V, Sly WS (1980). Chloroquine inhibits lysosomal enzyme pinocytosis and enhances lysosomal enzyme secretion by impaired receptor recycling. J Cell Biol 85:839.

Gordon JL (1975). Blood platelet lysosomes and their contribution to the pathophysiological role of platelets. In Dingle JT, Dean RT (eds): "Lysosomes in Biology and Pathology," Amsterdam: North Holland, Vol 4 p 1.

Hasilik A, Waheed A, Von Figura K (1981). Enzymatic phosphorylation of lysosomal enzymes in the presence of UDP-acetylglucosamine. Absence of the activity in I-cell fibroblasts. Biochem Biophys Res Comm 98:761.

Healy PJ, Nicholls PJ, Butrej P (1978). A granulocyte test for detection of cattle heterozygous for mannosidosis. Clin Chim Acta 88:429.

Hocking JD, Jolly RD, Batt RD (1972). Deficiency of α-mannosidase in Angus cattle. Biochem J 128:69.

Jervis GA, Pullakat RK (1978). Pigment variant of lipofuscinosis. Neurology 28:500

Jolly RD (1971). Pathology of the central nervous system in pseudolipidosis Angus calves. J Pathol 103:113.

Jolly RD (1975). Mannosidosis of Angus cattle: A prototype disease control program for some genetic diseases. In Cornelius CF, Brandley CA (eds): "Advances in Veterinary Science and Comparative Medicine," New York: Academic Press, Vol 19 p 1.

Jolly RD (1978 a). Annotation: Lysosomal storage diseases. J Neuropathol Appl Neurol 4:419.

Jolly RD (1978 b). Mannosidosis and its control in Angus and Murray Grey cattle. NZ Vet J 26:194.

Jolly RD, Desnick RJ (1979). Inborn errors of lysosomal catabolism - Principles of heterozygote detection. Am J Med Genet 4:393.

Jolly RD, Thompson KG (1978). The pathology of bovine mannosidosis. Vet Pathol 15:141.

Jolly RD, Digby JG, Rammell CG (1974 a). A mass screening programme of Angus cattle for the mannosidosis genotype - A prototype programme for control of inherited diseases in animals. NZ Vet J 22:218.

Jolly RD, Janmaat A, Van der Water NS (1977). Heterozygote detection: A comparative study using neutrophils, lymphocytes and two reference parameters in the bovine mannosidosis model. Biochem Med 18:402.

Jolly RD, Janmaat A, West DM, Morrison I (1980 c). Ovine ceroid-lipofuscinosis. Neuropathol and Appl Neurobiol 6:195.

Jolly RD, Slack PM, Winter PJ, Murphy CE (1980 a).
Mannosidosis: Patterns of storage and urinary excretion
of oligosaccharides in the bovine model. Aust J Exp
Biol Med Sci 58:421.

Jolly RD, Thompson KG, Murphy CE, Manktelow BW, Bruere AN,
Winchester BG (1976). Enzyme replacement therapy:
An experiment of nature in a chimeric mannosidosis
calf. Pediat Res 10:219.

Jolly RD, Thompson KG, Tse CA (1974 c). Evaluation of a
screening programme for identification of mannosidosis
heterozygotes: Factors affecting normal plasma
α-mannosidase levels. NZ Vet J 22:185.

Jolly RD, Thompson KG, Tse CA, Munford RE, Merrall M (1974 b).
Identification of mannosidosis heterozygotes - Factors
affecting normal plasma α-mannosidase levels. NZ Vet J
22:155.

Jolly RD, Tse CA, Greenway RM (1973). Plasma α-mannosidase
as a means of detecting mannosidosis heterozygotes.
NZ Vet J 21:64.

Jolly RD, Van de Water NS, Janmaat A, Slack PM, McKenzie RG
(1980 b). Zinc therapy in the bovine mannosidosis model.
In Desnick RJ (ed): "Enzyme Therapy in Genetic Disease:
2. Birth Defects: Original Article Series," New York
Alan R Liss Inc, Vol 16 (1) p 305.

Koppang N (1973). Canine ceroid-lipofuscinosis - A model for
human neuronal ceroid-lipofuscinosis and aging.
Mechanisms of Ageing and Development 2:421.

Lundblad A, Nilsson B, Norden N, Svensson S, Öckerman PA,
Jolly RD (1975). A urinary pentasaccharide in bovine
mannosidosis. Eur J Biochem 59:601.

Matsuura F, Nunez HA, Grabowski A, Sweeley CC (1981).
Structural studies of urinary oligosaccharides from
patients with mannosidosis. Arch Biochem Biophys
207:337.

Öckerman PA (1967). A generalised storage disorder resembling
Hurler's syndrome. Lancet 2:239.

Patel V, Koppang N, Patel B, Zeman W (1974). p-Phenylene-
diamine mediated peroxidase deficiency in English
setters with neuronal ceroid-lipofuscinoses. Lab Invest
30:366.

Phillips NC, Winchester BG, Jolly RD (1977). A serological
investigation into the acidic α-D-mannosidase in normal
Angus cattle and a calf with mannosidosis. Biochem
J 163:269.

Siakotos AN, Koppang N (1973). Procedures for the isolation
of lipopigments from brain, heart and liver, and their
properties: A review. Mechanisms of Ageing and Development
2:177.
Svennerholm L (1976). Polyunsaturated fatty acid lipidosis:
A new nosological entity. In Volk BW, Schneck L (eds):
"Current Trends in Sphingolipidoses and Allied Disorders,"
New York: Plenum Publishing Corp, p 389.
Thompson KG, Jolly RD, Winchester BG (1976). Mannosidosis:
Use of reference enzymes in heterozygote detection.
Biochem Med 15:233.
Wolfe LS, Ng Ying Kin NMK, Baker RR (1981). Batten diseases
and related disorders: New findings on the chemistry
of the storage material. In Callahan JW, Lowden JA
(eds): "Lysosomes and Lysosomal Storage Diseases,"
New York: Raven Press, p 315.
Yamashita K, Tachibana Y, Mihara K, Okada S, Yabuuchi H,
Kobata A (1980). Urinary oligosaccharides of
mannosidosis. J Biol Chem 255:5126.
Zeman W (1976). The neuronal ceroid-lipofuscinoses. In
Zimmerman HM (ed): "Progress in Neuropathology,"
New York: Grune & Stratton, Vol 3 p 1360.

DR. RATTAZZI: Dr. Jolly, what is the level of lysosomal enzymes in the plasma of the ceroid-lipofuscinosis
sheep? Wouldn't you expect something similar to what is
found in I-cell disease patients?

DR. JOLLY: We have not screened our sheep for this at
this stage. We have been working for three years, but basically it has been building up the model, learning techniques
of early diagnosis and describing the pathology. We are now
getting on to analyzing the storage bodies, and we have not
really looked at lysosomal enzymes, but it is something that
should be done.

DR. RATTAZZI: That would be a quick check of whether
your hypothesis is correct.

DR. JOLLY: Yes.

DR. PERRYMAN: What dosage of zinc was used in cows to
correct the α-mannosidase deficiency?

DR JOLLY: I could not tell you offhand. I think we
were giving something to the order of 1 or more grams of
zinc sulphate a day, but it varied throughout the experiment
depending on plasma levels. We did not have many calves,
and we thought we were not going to do an experiment where
we did not give enough, so we erred on the high side. There
was a lot of work being done on zinc toxicity in sheep in
New Zealand at the time, and we were able to extrapolate a
little bit about how much we should give, but it was a
rather hefty dose.

DR. PERRYMAN: I raised the question because workers in
Denmark have used oral zinc sulfate therapy to correct zinc
deficiency in cattle. They used 1/2 gram per day and obtained results without apparent toxicity.

DR. JOLLY: Yes I know, but we kept the dose high on
purpose.

DR. DESNICK: Have you had an opportunity to compare
the pathology of bovine α-mannosidosis with that of the recently described caprine model of β-mannosidosis? Do they
have common pathologic findings?

DR. JOLLY: There are differences, as I am sure Dr. M.
Jones will point out. The common factor, of course, is the
presence of highly vacuolated cells, but there are differences in terms of myelination and things like that which she
will talk about, and these have to be explained. I know she
has some ideas, and I won't steal her thunder by making suggestions.

DR. M. JONES: You mentioned that the urinary oligosaccharides are mainly derived from plasma in α-mannosidosis.
Has that been documented in both the bovine and the human

forms?

DR. JOLLY: It has not been documented. There are some differences, I believe. Our work is based on one calf that had not been kept in a metabolism cage. It was just a calf that became available and before we euthanatized it, we took pre- and post-renal blood. As such the experiment has to be repeated.

DR. BALAZS: As you alluded, Dr. Jolly, several structurally unrelated lyophilic drugs, both cationic and anionic charged are able to produce lysosomal storage disease; for example, certain anorectic agents, hypocholesteremic agents and you mentioned chloroquine. With the exception of chloroquine, however, none of these produce any clinical syndrome; no clinical or pathologic consequence has been recognized. Lysosomal changes develop also in man; it has been described even in the peripheral leukocyte. Apart from these signs, there is no consequence, with the exception of chloroquine. Even in chloroquine I am not sure that any of the toxicities are attributed to the abnormal lysosomal storage.

DR. JOLLY: My knowledge of this group of drug-induced storage diseases is relatively small and confined to my reading and talking in association with my own research with ceroid-lipofuscinosis, but I do understand that some of these other drugs have been incriminated in clinical syndromes, particularly in the eye. I know there is an ophthalmologist in New Zealand working on such a drug.

DR. PERRYMAN: You mentioned your surprise that the heterozygotes have less than half the normal level of the enzyme. What is the experience for other heterozygote screening programs that involve enzyme quantitation? Do the heterozygotes have half the normal value or less than half?

DR. JOLLY: I could not answer that.

DR. PERRYMAN: Parents of children with severe combined immunodeficiency and adenosine deaminase deficiency have less than half of normal quantities of the enzyme, suggesting that the gene dosage phenomenon is not totally quantitative.

DR. JOLLY: Yes. There must be someone here, perhaps Dr. Desnick, who could say what happens in Tay-Sachs. What is the relationship there, Dr. Desnick?

DR. DESNICK: There is about half normal activity in Tay-Sachs carriers. But one must recognize that all biological parameters are going to be distributed along a Gaussian curve. So there will always be problems of discrimination for a small group of inconclusive values as carriers or noncarriers. Therefore, more sensitive backup

tests are used in Tay-Sachs screening programs. In most
cases, you usually find half normal activity as the average
for obligate heterozygotes. However, you could find higher
or lower mean values, depending on whether the mutant and
normal gene products form hybrid molecules and whether the
mutant hybrid molecules are active. In other words, if the
enzyme is a dimer, trimer, or tetramer, it may hybridize
with one, two, or three mutant proteins, depending on the
subunit structure, and one or more of those hybrid molecules
may be active, giving an activity value other than half-
normal.

DR. DODDS: In the inherited bleeding disorders we find
less than 50 percent of normal activity levels in obligate
heterozygotes, usually between 25 and 35 or 40 percent; but
this may be an artifact of the measurements used.

DR. O'BRIEN: In the ADA system that you brought up,
there are at least two other genes, other than the structural gene, that participate in the generation of the adenosine deaminase you see in human tissues. I am curious to
know if your results may not be related to defects in genes
other than structural genes. Have the defects in the children that have this disease been mapped to one or the other
of these gene classes? Do you know, Dr. Desnick?

DR. DESNICK: Yes, the ADA deaminase structural gene.
It is not the binding protein.

DR. RATTAZZI: Dr. Jolly, given the number of heterozygote animals you have had access to, have you been able to
detect any trace of storage, either morphologically or biochemically, in these heterozygote animals? We always assume
that heterozygotes are normal individuals, and there is no
way to try to find out in humans, but you can in your animals. Have you done that?

DR. JOLLY: Of course, we should have done it, but we
haven't. It is the old story of priorities.

DR. WOOD: I wondered if the variation over the year of
your enzyme activity in the herd data you showed was perhaps
due to the differences in zinc nutrition at different times
of the year, and I wondered if you had ever had an opportunity to measure enzyme activity in perhaps a zinc-deficient
animal to see if it is α-mannosidase deficient?

DR. JOLLY: First, find your zinc deficient animal.
No, I don't think that is the answer. I think it is more
related to nutrition. Cattle tend to undergo a lot of nutritional stress in the winter months. They tend to be
below their requirements. At different times of the year
they are producing a calf or milking. I think if you chase

your cattle into the yard before you bleed them, this may affect them. There are all sorts of possibilities, and it is a field which we wanted to look at once because I am sure it is important, but again, priorities.

DR. SNYDER: We have begun screening bovine α-mannosidase activity in Western Canada for breeding stock prior to export. I wonder if you might comment on the experience in Tay-Sachs screening where gestational hormones influenced the serum activity, and secondly, whether there are any heterozygotes available in North America to give us confidence that what we are doing is appropriate. Thirdly, do you look at animals when they arrive at your borders?

DR. JOLLY: First of all, I don't think that the estrogens or pregnancy have an effect on our tests directly as in Tay-Sachs. We did look at this many years ago, and I cannot quite remember the details. Remember though that we are able to look at age and sex and matched groups; so they will all be much the same anyway. There are cases of mannosidosis that have been found in America. Drs. H. Leipold and J. Smith at Kansas State University have screened quite a large number of cattle, and although they found mannosidosis in two or three herds, the gene frequency overall appears low in this country. The cattle don't come out from Canada to New Zealand but we import semen. We will have the progeny tested before they are registered. I think you have problems in testing unless you are going to get going on a fairly large scale.

DR. HIGAKI: We have been interested in neuronal ceroid-lipofuscinosis in the dog. What is your opinion as to the primary defect in the dog? Is it the same in the sheep as in the dog?

DR. JOLLY: In humans there are at least three major syndromes with various subtypes or variants. There are a number of different defects. One would imagine that when they are sorted out they will be something like, say, the gangliosidoses where you have a family of diseases. So, I presume they are related to that extent. We don't know, but one presumes and works on that philosophy, and as such the sheep and the dogs belong to the same family, but may not necessarily be exactly the same. This is a common group of diseases. You walk into any good veterinary laboratory, and you will find cases of ceroid-lipofuscinosis in this or that breed of dogs. It occurs in chihuahuas, and that is one animal model I will not develop. We have had two cases in sheepdogs in New Zealand. What we would like to do is get heterozygous sheepdogs or chihuahuas and cross them with the

English setter and see whether we get the disease with the two different types bred together. Also it would indicate the same gene was involved.

Animal Models of Inherited Metabolic Diseases, pages 165–176
© 1982 Alan R. Liss, Inc., 150 Fifth Avenue, New York, NY 10011

CAPRINE β-MANNOSIDOSIS[1]

Margaret Z. Jones,[†] James G. Cunningham,[‡] Albert W.
Dade,[‖] Glyn Dawson,[§] Roger A. Laine,[⟨] Christine S.F.
Williams,[†] David M. Alessi,[†] Ulreh V. Mostosky,[⟨⟨] and
Joseph R. Vorro.[*]

[†]Departments of Pathology, [⟨⟨]Small Animal Surgery and
Medicine, [‡]Physiology, and [*]Anatomy, Michigan State
University, E. Lansing, MI 48824. [‖]Department of
Pathology, Tuskegee Institute, Tuskegee Institute, AL
36088. [§]Department of Biochemistry, University of
Chicago, Chicago, IL 60637. [⟨]Department of Biochem-
istry, University of Kentucky, Lexington, KY 40536.

Inherited disorders of glycoprotein catabolism are associated with marked neurological dysfunction in man and other species. α-Mannosidosis, for example, is associated with neurological deficits, storage, and excretion of oligosaccharides with
terminal α-linked mannose residues and deficiency of α-D-mannosi-
dase activity (Autio, Norden, Öckerman, Riekkinen, Rapola,
Louhimo 1973; Burditt, Chotai, Hirani, Nugent, Winchester,
Blakemore 1980; Desnick, Sharp, Grabowski, Brunning, Quie, Sung,
Gorlin, Ikonne 1976; Jolly 1971; Jolly, Thompson 1978; Kjellman,
Gamstorp, Brun, Öckerman, Palmgren 1969; Leipold, Smith, Jolly,
Eldridge 1979; Öckerman 1967; Öckerman 1967; Phillips, Robinson,
Winchester, Jolly 1974; Sung, Hayano, Desnick 1977; Whittem,
Walker 1957). Diseases associated with deficiencies of most of
the exoglycosidases responsible for sequentially degrading the
glycoprotein oligosaccharides have been described (Autio, Norden,
Öckerman, Riekkinen, Rapola, Louhimo 1973; Baker, Lindsey,
McKhann, Farrell 1971; Burditt, Chotai, Hirani, Nugent, Win-
chester, Blakemore 1980; Cantz, Gehler, Spranger 1976; Cork,
Munnell, Lorenz, Murphy, Baker, Rattazzi 1977; Dawson 1979;

[1]This work was supported in part by Biomedical Research Sup-
port Grants RR-05772 and RR-05623, by Grant NS16886 to M.Z.J.,
Grants GM23902 and AM25101 to R.A.L., HD06426 and HD09402 to
G.D..

Durand, Borrone, Della Cella 1969; Öckerman 1967; Okada, O'Brien 1968; Palo, Riekkinen, Arstila, Autio, Kivimäki 1972; Phillips, Robinson, Winchester, Jolly 1974; Sandhoff, Harzer, Wassle, Jatzkewitz 1971). Despite extensive searches, a deficiency of β-mannosidase activity has been detected only in the caprine species. In this report, the clinical, pathological, genetic, and biochemical characteristics of β-mannosidosis, a fatal neurological disease in goats associated with the accumulation of tissue oligosaccharides and deficiency of β-D-mannosidase, are described.

A normal Nubian doe, accidentally bred by her own 9-month-old offspring, gave birth to non-identical triplets. The female appeared normal, but the two males were unable to rise at birth and remained in a lateral recumbant position. Abnormal facial characteristics included a dome-shaped skull, narrowed palpebral fissures and an elongate muzzle. A coarse intention tremor and pendular nystagmus were noted. Severe muscle atrophy affected the shoulder and rear limbs. Pastern joints were hyperextended and carpal joints were contracted. However, the limbs moved in response to stimulation and the less severely affected male was able to turn over and to bear weight on the front legs when partially supported. Neither the doe nor any goat on the Michigan farm had shown evidence of a similar disease, and the locale is free of known neurotoxins (Dorling, Huxtable, Vogel 1978). Subsequent offspring included: a clinically normal female (5); affected (8), and unaffected (9) twin males; an unaffected, stillborn female (10); an affected twin female (11) and unaffected twin male (12); and unaffected quadruplets (20, 21, 22, 23) (Fig. 1A).

The sire (24) was outbred to unrelated grade Saanen females and then bred back to his female offspring, producing two more affected goats; a female (38) with an unaffected female twin (39); and male (40) with unaffected male (41) and female (42) triplets (Fig. 1B).

Physical and neurological examinations, diagnostic and laboratory studies of all affected and age-sex-matched clinically normal kids were compared. The depressed nasal bridge and dome-shaped skull were more pronounced in affected males than females. Both showed the same degree of elongation and narrowing of the muzzle with a tendency for the lower jaw to protrude. The small, narrowed palpebral fissures, immobile upper eyelid, prolapsed nictitating membrane, and small pupils were associated with a pendular nystagmus. The latter abated

after about 3 weeks of age. The contractures of the carpal
joints varied with respect to degree at birth, were associated
with hypermobility, and rapidly progressed (Fig. 2A, B).

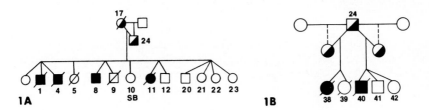

Fig. 1. ⊘ obligate carrier female; ◨ obligate carrier male;
● affected female; ■ affected male; ○ unaffected female;
□ unaffected male; 1 proband; SB stillborn; slash indicates
necropsy.
A. When a Nubian doe was bred to her own first born offspring,
three males and one female of thirteen progeny were affected with
β-mannosidosis, suggesting an autosomal recessive mode of inheritance. B. Two additional affected animals were produced by
father-daughter matings.

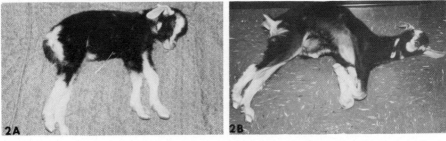

Fig. 2. A. Affected male (40) shows the dome-shaped skull, depressed nasal bridge, elongate muzzle and narrow, small palpebral fissures. Mild carpal contractures are associated with
hyperextended pastern joints at the time of birth. B. At
twelve weeks of age, carpal contractures have progressed and
these joints are fixed at a 45° angle. Hindlimb pastern joint
hyperflexion persists. Note the marked pectus carinatum.

The intention tremor was marked at birth but abated in the
two animals surviving beyond 3 weeks. The affected kids were
alert and demonstrated most expected newborn behaviors, including grooming, sucking, bleating, urination, defecation and responsiveness to handling. Vision and olfaction appeared to be
intact, but deafness was present. Affected kids used their con-

tracted forelimbs and hindlimbs to propel and right themselves
to a limited degree (righting was possible from one side only).
Seizure-like activity was observed three times in affected female (38). The affected male (40) developed a marked pectus
carinatum and, concomitantly, a loud systolic murmur.

Significant laboratory studies included an elevated serum
acid phosphatase in the one affected animal evaluated. Serum
electrolytes, calcium, phosphorus, and creatinine were within
normal limits. Peripheral blood smears showed no obvious abnormalities.

There were no significant radiographic lesions. Computer-
ized axial tomography revealed ventricular dilatation in the
one affected animal examined when compared to an age-sex-matched
control. Electroencephalograms of three affected kids were not
significantly different from those of 7 clinically normal kids.
Electroretinograms in two affected kids were unremarkable.
Electromyographic abnormalities included spontaneous potentials
resembling positive sharp waves and fibrillation potentials in
three affected kids but not in 5 clinically normal kids. Elec-
trocardiograms showed right ventricular hypertrophy and right
axis deviation in the affected male (40). Affected animals
were kept alive only by meticulous, intensive care provided by
experienced personnel.

The affected male triplets (1 and 4) were sacrificed at 1
and 3 weeks of age, respectively. The affected male (8) died
almost immediately after birth. The affected twin female (11)
was sacrificed at 1 day of age. The affected twin female (38)
was sacrificed at 4 weeks of age, when her unaffected twin died.
The affected triplet male (40) died at 16 weeks of age.

Autopsy examination revealed few gross lesions other than
those noted. Right and left ventricular hypertrophy in kid (40)
was unassociated with valvular thickening, but a jet lesion was
present on the left atrium above the mitral valve. The weights
of the heart, liver, spleen, and kidneys in this animal exceeded
those of weight-matched control animals by 2-3 times each. Examination of the brain of all six affected animals revealed
ventricular dilatation and striking paucity of cerebral hemisphere and cerebellar myelin (Fig. 3).

Microscopic examination revealed fine to coarse vacuolation in neurons (Fig. 4), autonomic ganglion cells, Schwann
cells, oligodendroglia, fibroblasts, endothelial and perithelial

cells, reticuloendothelial cells of lymph nodes, bone marrow,
and liver, in renal tubular and glomerular epithelial, thyroid
follicular and pancreatic acinar cells, in chondrocytes, and
other cell types.

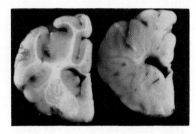

Fig. 3. Myelin paucity in cerebral hemisphere of affected goat
(11) brain (right) is associated
with ventricular dilatation, compared with well myelinated age-
sex-matched control sample at 1
day of age.

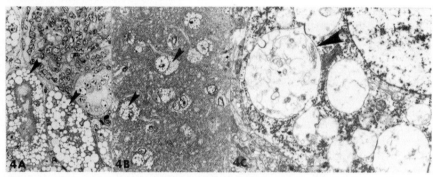

Fig. 4. A. Proximal tubular epithelium of the kidney shows
marked vacuolation (➤). B. Parietal cortex neurons are vacuolated (➤). C. Parietal cortex neuronal vacuoles (➤) are
membrane-bound.

At the ultrastructural level, membrane-bound vacuoles were
often associated with the concave face of the Golgi apparatus
and were sometimes continuous with the endoplasmic reticulum
(Fig. 4C). Vacuolar contents included membranous fragments and
floccular material on a lucent background. Axonal lesions,
like those in α-mannosidosis (Jolly 1971; Jolly, Thompson 1978;
Whittem, Walker 1957) and in the caprine neurological disease
described by Hartley and Blakemore (Hartley, Blakemore 1973)
included marked expansion near the soma of Purkinje cells and
at distances from other neuronal cell bodies. The numerous
eosinophilic, PAS-positive axonal spheroids in the white matter
were sometimes associated with calcification. Rarely, giant
filamentous axonal expansions were identified near neuronal

cell bodies. At the ultrastructural level, the axonal spheroids consisted of collections of amorphous or membranous dense
bodies and mitochondria. Myelin was only rarely preserved
over these axonal expansions. Peripheral nerve axons were not
remarkable and myelin was preserved despite the marked vacuolation of Schwann cell cytoplasm. Skeletal muscle fibers contained no vacuoles. Except for the marked central nervous
system myelin paucity and oligodendroglial lysosomal storage
vacuoles, lesions closely resembled those described by Hartley
and Blakemore (Hartley, Blakemore 1973) as well as those which
have been reported in α-mannosidosis.

    Brain lipids from (4), the affected 3-week-old male trip-
let, were analyzed according to methods previously described
(Jones, Sweeley, Yang 1972), but revealed no specific abnormalities other than those associated with hypomyelination. Following the demonstration of increased amounts of mannose and
N-Acetylglucosamine (GlcNAc) in the urine of an affected goat
(Jones, Cunningham, Dade, Alessi 1979; Jones, Dawson 1981)
water extracts of 0.1g of brain and kidney from (4) and an age-
sex-matched control animal were separated by thin layer chromatography (Holmes, O'Brien 1979; Humbel, Collart 1975) and
clearly showed the abnormal accumulation of both trisaccharide
and disaccharide (Fig. 5). Liver, peripheral nerve, and urine
also contained these accumulated oligosaccharides. Gas chromatographic (GC) analysis of the urinary, kidney, and brain-
derived trimethylsilyl-methylglycosides (Vance, Sweeley 1967)
showed the trisaccharide to primarily consist of mannose and
GlcNAc residues.

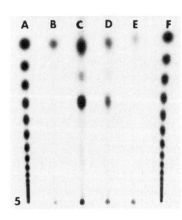

Fig. 5. Thin layer chromatogram:
Water extracts from 0.1 g kidney and
brain were concentrated and taken to
0.2 ml. Ten μl of extract from control kidney (B), β-mannosidosis kidney (C), β-mannosidosis brain (D) and
control brain (E), were applied to an
Analtech 20 x 20 cm thin layer plate
along with glucose oligomer standards
(A, F). After development with
butanol/acetic acid/water, 3/3/2, the
accumulated trisaccharide and disaccharide are in the tetra-, tri-, and
disaccharide regions.

Brain and kidney oligosaccharides were separated by Bio-

Gel P-2 chromatography and hexoses were quantified (DuBois, Gilles, Hamilton, Rebers, Smith 1956). Structures were determined by combined GC-mass spectrometry of permethylated acetates (Hakamori 1964; Stellner, Saito, Hakomori 1973). Man(β1-4)GlcNAc(β1-4)GlcNAc and Man(β1-4)GlcNAc were present in brain (Jones, Laine 1981) and kidney (Matsuura, Laine, Jones 1981) in a ratio of approximately 4:1. The amount of oligosaccharide accumulating in the brain was similar to that reported in α-mannosidosis and fucosidosis, but the massive accumulation in kidney was unexpected (Table 1).

Activity of tissue lysosomal hydrolases was determined with synthetic substrates p-nitrophenyl- and 4-methylumbelliferyl-β-D-mannopyranoside (Dawson, Tsay 1977; VanHoof, Hers 1968). A complete deficiency of β-mannosidase activity was found in both brain (4 and 11) and kidney (4) as shown in Table 2.

TABLE 1

	Trisaccharide Man(β1-4)GlcNAc(β1-4)GlcNAc	Disaccharide Man(β1-4)GlcNAc
BRAIN	2.2	0.5[a]
KIDNEY	7.6	1.6

TABLE 1. Tissue Oligosaccharides. Values are expressed as μmol mannose/g wet tissue from one affected animal (4). Age-sex-matched control animal tissues contained neither oligosaccharide.
[a]Calculated from ratio of trisaccharide to disaccharide.

TABLE 2

BRAIN	Affected (n=2)	Heterozygote (n=1)	Control (n=4)
β-mannosidase	0	2.0	8.7
α-mannosidase	208	30.0	28.2
KIDNEY	(n=1)	(n=1)	(n=3)
β-mannosidase	0	9	14
α-mannosidase	50	39	31

TABLE 2. Enzyme activity in brain and kidney of affected, carrier and clinically normal age-matched control goats. Values are expressed as nmol of p-nitrophenol liberated/mg protein/h.

The obligate heterozygote (17) showed intermediate (50% of normal) activity confirming the inherited nature of the disorder. In affected animals, deficiency of tissue β-mannosidase activity was associated with marked elevation of α-mannosidase and α-fucosidase activities while other lysosomal hydrolase activities were either normal or above normal (Jones, Dawson 1981). In contrast, liver β-mannosidase activity from affected goat (4) was 50% of control values. Goat liver β-mannosidase activity measured at pH 5.0 was more than 10 times that in brain and 5 times that in kidney and contained a large amount of neutral β-mannosidase activity. Overlap of this neutral - mannosidase activity, analogous to the situation with α-mannosidase activity in α-mannosidosis liver (Autio, Norden, Öckerman, Riekkinen, Rapola, Louhimo 1973; Tsay, Dawson 1975) and - glucosidase activity in Gaucher liver and spleen (Peters, Coyle, Glew 1976), is believed to be the reason for the failure to demonstrate a complete β-mannosidase deficiency in affected goat liver. Mixing studies revealed no evidence for the presence of an inhibitor (Jones, Dawson 1981).

This investigation strongly suggests that caprine β-mannosidosis is inherited as an autosomal recessive trait. Data in support of this hypothesis include the observations that (i) both the parents were phenotypically normal, (ii) the sire and dam were consanguinous, (iii) both male and female offspring were affected, (iv) the ratio of diseased to phenotypically normal goats was consistent with that expected for autosomal recessive inheritance, (v) lesions were observed in all six clinically affected animals, (vi) an obligate heterozygote showed intermediate levels of tissue β-mannosidase activity when compared to values in control and affected animals.

Thus, the neonatal caprine disease originally observed in New South Wales (Hartley, Blakemore 1973) and arising independently in Michigan goats appears, by our data, to represent the only characterized example of β-mannosidosis. Caprine β-mannosidosis differs from α-mannosidosis in several important respects. Expression of such a severe neurological disorder at the time of birth is not typical of α-mannosidosis nor of other caprine diseases (Cork, Hadlow, Crawford, Gorham, Piper 1974). Caprine β-mannosidosis is associated with dysmorphic facial features and joint contractures. The human and feline forms of α-mannosidosis show different skeletal abnormalities. The genetically determined deficiency of β-mannosidase is predictably related to the accumulation of products of glycoprotein catabolism with β-mannoside residues as observed in this study.

The presence of a trisaccharide with an uncleaved chito-biosyl linkage may be species specific or may represent an associated perturbation in the glycoprotein catabolic pathway. The pattern of accumulated and excreted oligosaccharides is different in α-mannosidosis and also varies among species (Burditt, Chotai, Hirani, Nugent 1980). Thus, when the human counterpart of caprine β-mannosidosis is discovered, the disaccharide Man(β1-4)GlcNAc may prove to be the major accumulated oligosaccharide. The characteristics of the caprine prototype are expected to assist with the identification of β-mannosidosis in man and other species.

ACKNOWLEDGMENTS

We are especially grateful to Jan Kelley, Holly Jensen, James Malachowski, Ronald VanderHeyden, Judith Dean, and the Brenner family for their contributions to this research. We thank Doctors Robert W. Leader, George A. Padgett, Charles C. Sweeley, Kathryn L. Lovell and Frances Kennedy for helpful consultations. We thank Doctors James Potchen and Kathryn Hart for providing the CT scans and interpretations.

Autio S, Norden NE, Öckerman P-A, Riekkinen P, Rapola J, Lou-himo T (1973). Mannosidosis: Clinical, fine-structural and biochemical findings in three cases. Acta Paediat Scand 62: 555-565.
Baker HJ, Lindsey R, McKhann GM, Farrell DF (1971). Neuronal GM_1 gangliosidosis in a Siamese cat with β-galactosidase deficiency. Science 174:838-839.
Burditt LJ, Chotai K, Hirani S, Nugent PG, Winchester BG, Blake-more WF (1980). Biochemical studies on a case of feline mannosidosis. Biochem J 189:467-473.
Cantz M, Gehler J, Spranger J (1974). Mucolipidosis I: In-creased sialic acid content and deficiency of an α-N-acetyl-neuraminidase in cultured fibroblasts. Biochem Biophys Res Commun 74:732-738.
Cork LC, Hadlow WJ, Crawford TB, Gorham JR, Piper RC (1974). Infectious leukoencephalomyelitis of young goats. J Infect Dis 129:134-141.
Cork LC, Munnell JF, Lorenz MD, Murphy JV, Baker JH, Rattazzi MC (1977). GM_2 ganglioside lysosomal storage disease in cats with β-hexosaminidase deficiency. Science 196:1014-1017.
Dawson, G (1979). Glycoprotein storage diseases and the muco-polysaccharidoses. In Margolis RU, Margolis RK (eds): "Complex Carbohydrates of Nervous Tissue," New York:

Academic Press, pp 347-375.

Dawson G, Tsay G (1977). Substrate specificity of human α-L-fucosidase. Arch Biochem Biophys 184:12-23.

Desnick RJ, Sharp HL, Grabowski GA, Brunning RD, Quie PG, Sung JH, Gorlin RJ, Ikonne JU (1976). Mannosidosis: Clinical, morphologic, immunologic, and biochemical studies. Pediat Res 10:985-996.

Dorling PR, Huxtable CR, Vogel P (1978). Lysosomal storage in Swainsona spp. toxicosis: An induced mannosidosis. Neuropath Appl Neurobiol 4:285-295.

DuBois M, Gilles KA, Hamilton JK, Rebers PA, Smith F (1956). Colorimetric method for determination of sugars and related substances. Anal Chem 28:350-356.

Durand P, Borrone C, Della Cella G (1969). Fucosidosis. J Pediat 75:665-674.

Hakamori S (1964). A rapid permethylation of glycolipid and polysaccharide catalyzed by methylsulfinyl carbanion in dimethyl sulfoxide. J Biochem (Tokyo) 55:205-208.

Hartley WJ, Blakemore WF (1973). Neurovisceral storage and dysmyelinogenesis in neonatal goats. Acta Neuropath 25:325-333.

Holmes EW, O'Brien JS (1979). Separation of glycoprotein-derived oligosaccharides by thin-layer chromatography. Anal Biochem 93:167-170.

Humbel R, Collart M (1975). Oligosaccharides in urine of patients with glycoprotein storage diseases. Clin Chim Acta 60:143-145.

Jolly RD (1971). The pathology of the central nervous system in pseudolipidosis of Angus calves. J Pathol 103:113-121.

Jolly RD, Thompson KG (1978). The pathology of bovine mannosidosis. Vet Pathol 15:141-152.

Jones MZ, Cunningham JG, Dade AW, Alessi DM (1979). Caprine neurovisceral storage disorder resembling mannosidosis Soc Neurosci Abstr 5:513.

Jones MZ, Dawson G (1981). Caprine β-mannosidosis: Inherited deficiency of β-D-mannosidase. J Biol Chem 256:5185-5188.

Jones MZ, Laine RA (1981). Caprine oligosaccharide storage disorder: Accumulation of β-Mannosyl(1-4)β-N-Acetylglucosaminyl(1-4)β-N-Acetylglucosamine in brain. J Biol Chem 256:5181-5184.

Jones MZ, Sweeley C, Yang M (1972). Lipid composition of the cerebellum and spinal cord in postnatal cycasin-treated Swiss albino mice: Preliminary observations. Fed Proc 31:1512-1516.

Kjellman B, Gamstorp I, Brun A, Ockerman P-A, Palmgren B

(1969). Mannosidosis: A clinical and histopathologic study. J Pediat 75:366-373.

Leipold HW, Smith JE, Jolly RD, Eldridge FE (1979). Mannosidosis of Angus calves. JAVMA 175:457-459.

Matsuura F, Laine RA, Jones MZ (1981). Oligosaccharides accumulated in the kidney of a goat with β-mannosidosis: Mass spectrometry of intact permethylated derivatives. Arch Biochem Biophys 211:485-493.

Öckerman P-A (1967). Deficiency of β-galactosidase and α-mannosidase: Primary enzyme defects in gargoylism and a new generalized disease? Acta Paediat Scand 177(Suppl):35-36.

Öckerman P-A (1967). A generalized storage disorder resembling Hurler's syndrome. Lancet 2:239-241.

Okada S, O'Brien JS (1968). Generalized gangliosidosis: β-galactosidase deficiency. Science 160:1002-1004.

Palo J, Riekkinen P, Arstila AU, Autio S, Kivimäki T (1972). Aspartylglucosaminuria II: Biochemical studies on brain, liver, kidney, and spleen. Acta Neuropathol 20:217-224.

Peters SP, Coyle P, Glew RH (1976). Differentiation of β-glucocerebrosidase from β-glucosidase in human tissues using sodium taurocholate. Arch Biochem Biophys 175:569-582.

Phillips NC, Robinson D, Winchester BG, Jolly RD (1974). Mannosidosis in Angus cattle: The enzymic defect. Biochem J 137:363-371.

Sandhoff K, Harzer K, Wässle W, Jatzkewitz H (1971). Enzyme alterations and lipid storage in three variants of Tay-Sachs disease. J Neurochem 18:2469-2489.

Stellner K, Saito H, Hakomori S-I (1973), Determination of aminosugar linkages in glycolipids by methylation. Arch Biochem Biophys 155:464-472.

Sung JH, Hayano M, Desnick RJ (1977). Mannosidosis: Pathology of the nervous system. J Neuropathol Exp Neurol 36: 807-820.

Tsay GC, Dawson G (1975). Glycopeptide storage in fibroblasts from patients with inborn errors of glycoprotein and glycosphingolipid catabolism. Biochem Biophys Res Commun 63:807-814.

Vance DE, Sweeley CC (1967). Quantitative determination of the neutral glycosyl ceramides in human blood. J Lipid Res 8: 621-630.

VanHoof F, Hers HG (1968). The abnormalities of lysosomal enzymes in mucopolysaccharidoses. Eur J Biochem 7:34-44.

Whittem JH, Walker D (1957). "Neuronopathy" and "pseudolipidosis" in Aberdeen-Angus calves. J Pathol Bact 74:281-288.

DR. WOOD: Do you have a hypothesis to explain the myelin deficiency?

DR. M. JONES: Myelin deficiency is a complex problem. The peripheral nervous system and the spinal cord appear to be normally myelinated. It is the later developing myelin that is abnormal. Since this is an oligosaccharide storage disease, and there may be some implications with respect to cell-cell recognition, one could postulate that there is an axonal/oligodendroglial problem in terms of cell surface recognition. Since the oligodendroglial cells store oligosaccharides, their membranes could be modified; the axons likewise could be modified in such a way that either recognition or maintenance of myelin is not possible at a later stage of development. Abnormal axons are present which may preclude normal development or maintenance of myelin.

So an interaction of enzyme deficiency, the amount of accumulated material and the time of the myelination may be important factors in this condition, and there may be other possible explanations.

DR. JOLLY: What is your explanation for the two N-acetylglucosamine residues in the storage product?

DR. M. JONES: As Dr. Jolly just pointed out, one of the interesting things about the problem is the two N-acetylglucosamine residues in the major accumulated material. Such a chitobiosyl residue also has been found in the oligosaccharides in canine GM_1 gangliosidosis by Werner and O'Brien. In the bovine α-mannosidosis, there are three N-acetylglucosamine residues in one of the accumulated products. The hypotheses that are present to explain this include the following: There may be new, perhaps species specific, N-linked glycoproteins which have multiple N-acetylglucosamine residues linked to the protein. Another possibility is that the elevated α-mannosidase and α-fucosidase catabolize the oligosaccharide chain quite rapidly and exceed the possiblity for the endoglycosidase to cleave the chitobiosyl linkage. The endoglycosidase may not work on a molecule as small as a trisaccharide. It may be effective only on a much longer molecule with certain constituent terminal residues. The latter alternative appears most attractive as a hypothesis.

Animal Models of Inherited Metabolic Diseases, pages 177–201
© **1982 Alan R. Liss, Inc., 150 Fifth Avenue, New York, NY 10011**

ANIMAL MODELS OF MUCOPOLYSACCHARIDOSIS

Haskins, M.E., Jezyk, P.F., Desnick, R.J.,
McGovern, M.M., Vine, D.T., Patterson, D.F.
Sections of Pathology & Medical Genetics,
School of Veterinary Medicine & Genetics Center,
University of Pennsylvania, Phila., PA 19104,
Division of Medical Genetics, Mt. Sinai School of
Medicine, New York, New York 10029.

In man, the genetic mucopolysaccharidoses (MPS) are
a group of well recognized syndromes resulting from defects
in glycosaminoglycan (GAG) degradation. Each syndrome has
a characteristic combination of clinical signs, urinary
GAG excretion, and a specific lysosomal enzyme deficiency
(Dorfman and Matalon, 1976, McKusick et al, 1978, Neufeld
et al, 1975).

Two animal models of mucopolysaccharidoses have been
described in the cat and in both the enzyme deficiency is
known (Jezyk et al, 1977, Haskins et al, 1979, 1979a).
A third mucopolysaccharide storage disease in a dog is
presently being studied. These models allow investigations
into the pathogenesis, and an evaluation of therapeutic
regimens in these lysosomal storage diseases.

MUCOPOLYSACCHARIDOSIS VI (Maroteaux-Lamy Syndrome)

Human MPS VI, first described in 1963, is characterized
by growth retardation, facial abnormalities that include
apparent hypertelorism, a depressed bridge of the nose,
full cheeks, and relatively broad jaws; corneal opacity,
hepatosplenomegaly, normal or near normal intelligence, and
dysostosis multiplex (Maroteaux and Lamy, 1965, McKusick,
1972, Spranger et al, 1970). Alder-Reilly bodies are
prominent in peripheral granulocytic leukocytes (Hansen,
1972, Spranger et al, 1970). Urinary GAGs are considerably elevated with the predominant urinary GAG being
dermatan sulfate (Pennock, 1976, Taniguchi et al, 1975).

The enzyme which is deficient in this disease, identified as arylsulfatase B (ASB), has been shown to be an N-acetyl-galactosamine-6-sulfate sulfatase, which is required for complete degradation of chondroitin-4-sulfate and dermatan sulfate (Fluharty et al, 1974, 1975, Matalon et al, 1974, O'Brien et al, 1974, Shapira et al, 1975, Stumpf and Austin, 1972). MPS VI is inherited as an autosomal recessive trait.

Feline MPS VI - Clinical Manifestations

Naturally occurring MPS VI in the cat has so far been recognized only in animals of Siamese ancestry. Affected cats have flat, broad facies with an apparent hypertelorism and depressed bridge of the nose (Fig. 1).

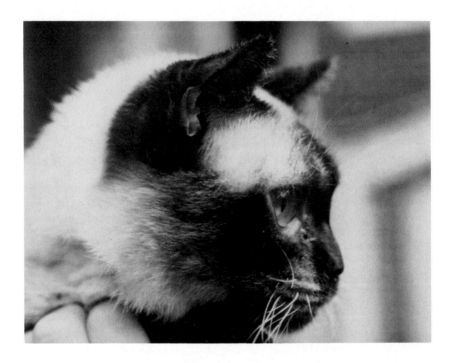

Fig. 1   The facies of a Siamese cat with
          mucopolysaccharidosis VI. Note the
          flattened face and small ears.

The animals also are of a small body size, with relatively small ears and short tail compared to age, sex-matched, unaffected family members. The facial dysmorphia is readily identifiable in the Siamese cat, which normally has a somewhat elongated face. Breeding experiments have subsequently produced the disease in non-Siamese hybrids by outcrossing to non-Siamese cats and backcrossing to Siamese carriers. The facial dysmorphia is somewhat less pronounced in these hybrids, but is recognizable. Affected animals also have a diffuse bilateral corneal clouding resulting from fine granular opacities present at all levels of the corneal stroma; retinal atrophy and corneal vascularization were observed individually in two affected cats. At 18 months of age, one animal developed cutaneous nodules, 4-10 mm in diameter, over her face and head. These nodules were not pruritic, gradually regressed, and were not apparent six weeks later.

The radiographic osseous changes are most severe in the oldest affected cats. In those animals, the spine is severely affected, with fusions and multiple proliferative lesions of the cervical, thoracic, and lumbar regions. The odontoid process is hypoplastic, the pelvis has shallow irregular acetabulae, and the femoral heads are flattened and bilaterally subluxated with a valgus deformity of the femoral neck. All long bones have severe epiphyseal dysplasia with multiple exostoses and irregular articular surfaces. Short tubular bones are similarly affected. A variable degree of generalized osteoporosis is present radiographically, as well as an increased opacity (sclerosis) at the vertebral end-plates and articular facets. Skeletal lesions in younger animals are less severe, particularly long bone epiphyseal changes. Radiographic observations of skeletal abnormalities over time indicates the progressive nature of the disease.

Progressive locomotor difficulty is observed and generally reflects the degree of skeletal change. However, in several animals a profound posterior paresis with depressed pain perception and increased extensor tone has been observed. To date, all but one of these animals have been male, with the onset of this clinical sign occurring at about 7 months of age. Myelograms indicate an obstruction to the flow of radio-opaque dye at the area of the thoraco-lumbar junction. This is the only evidence of neurologic dysfunction we have observed in affected animals. Although mentation is difficult to assess in domestic animals, there have been no indications in any of these cats of any deficit comparable to what is defined in man as mental retardation.

On examination of peripheral blood smears stained with toluidine blue, 90-100% of polymorphonuclear leukocytes contain excessive coarse granulations in the cytoplasm. Abnormal granulations in lymphocytes have not been recognized by light microscopy.

Spot tests (Berry and Spinanger, 1960) on urine from all clinically affected animals are positive for glycosamino-glycans while spot tests on urine from all clinically normal animals, including obligate heterozygotes, are negative. The electrophoretic patterns obtained on cetylpiridinium chloride precipitated GAG show that the primary GAG excreted by affected cats co-migrates with dermatan sulfate. Variable amounts of chondroitin sulfate and a trace of heparan sulfate are also present. Normal cat urine contains primarily chondroitin sulfate with a small amount of dermatan sulfate and a trace of heparan sulfate.

The incorporation of $^{35}SO_4$ into mucopolysaccharides of cultured fibroblasts grown from skin biopsies from normal cats and an affected animal, indicates an intra-cellular accumulation of $^{35}SO_4$ in affected cats consistent with defective degradation of GAG (Fratantoni et al, 1968).

Pathology

The gross pathology of animals affected with MPS VI includes thickened atrio-ventricular heart valves and chordae tendinae, bony proliferations at the epiphyses and, in animals with posterior paresis, bony overgrowth into the spinal canal producing indentations along the spinal cord just anterior to the nerve roots (Fig. 2) (Haskins et al, 1980). Moderate cerebral ventricular dilatation has been noted in several animals. Hepato-splenomegaly is not a feature of this disease in the cat.

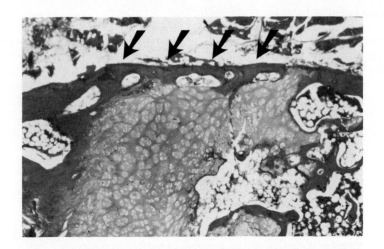

Fig. 2   Light micrograph of the cervical spine of a
          five year old female cat. Note the bony bridge
          (arrows) between the vertebral bodies. The
          intervertebral tissue is primarily cartilage.
          (H & E X 10)

     Reports of the histologic and ultrastructural pathology
of MPS VI in man have been limited to descriptions of the
eye, liver, skin and heart valves (Kenyon et al, 1972,
Lagunoff et al, 1962, Quigley and Kenyon, 1974,
Spranger, 1972, Tondeur and Neufeld, 1975, Van Hoof and
Hers, 1972). In contrast to most of the other mucopolysaccharidoses, human patients with MPS VI are of
normal and near normal intelligence and therefore,
examination of the histologic and ultrastructural features
of the central nervous system (CNS) is of interest.
Reports of the CNS pathology in human cases of MPS VI,
however, have been limited to discussions of hydrocephalus or myelopathy secondary to C1-C2 subluxations
and/or cervical cord compression associated with thickening of the cervical dura (Goldberg et al, 1970, McKusick,
1972, Peterson et al, 1975, Van Hoof and Hers, 1972).
The first histologic and ultrastructural descriptions of
the CNS, as well as the spleen, bone marrow and skeleton
in MPS VI, have been made in the feline model.

The histologic pathology of MPS VI in the cat is characterized by cytoplasmic vacuolations in fibroblasts of the atrio-ventricular heart valves, the eye and skin; smooth muscle cells of the spleen and aorta, bone marrow granulocytes, keratocytes, pigment epithelium, and perithelial cells (Haskins et al, 1980). Fusion of cervical vertebrae is evidenced by bony bridges between vertebral bodies and complete disruption of the inter-vertebral discs (Fig. 3). The degree of neuronal pathology within compressed areas of the spinal cord has not been adequate to explain the degree of clinical dysfunction.

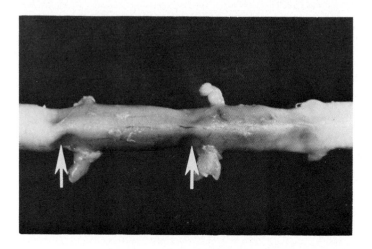

Fig. 3   Photograph of the thoraco-lumbar spinal cord of a 10 month old cat with posterior paresis. Note the discoloration of the cord and the depressions (arrows) just caudal to the nerve roots.

By electron microscopy, membrane-bound cytoplasmic inclusions are present within those tissues containing cytoplasmic granulations by light microscopy (Fig. 4).

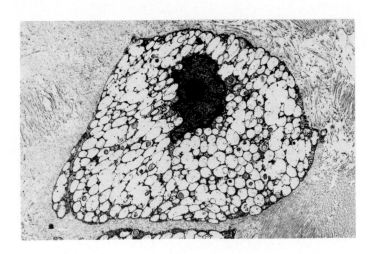

Fig. 4   Electron micrograph of a cartilage cell
          from the proximal tibia. The cytoplasm
          is packed with membrane-bound cytoplasmic
          inclusions (Uranyl acetate-lead citrate
          X 1900).

These inclusions vary from empty to granular to lamellar and have been observed within hepatocytes (Fig. 5), as small granular inclusions not readily visible at the light microscopic level. The only storage observed within the central nervous system is within the meninges, and perithelial cells of the vascular system.

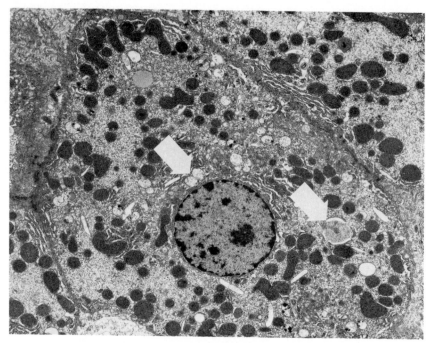

Fig. 5   Electron micrograph of a hepatocyte which
contains numerous membrane bound granular
inclusions (arrows), (Uranyl acetate-lead
citrate X 1900).

Enzymology

   Arylsulfatase B activity in white blood cells and
cultured fibroblasts is markedly reduced in affected
individuals and is, as expected, approximately 50% of
normal in obligate heterozygotes (McGovern et al, 1981).
Hepatic ASB from normal and MPS VI cats has been purified
and the physical and kinetic properties described (Vine
et al, 1981). Partially purified residual arylsulfatase B
has a significantly greater Km value, a more negative charge,
and is markedly less stable to thermo-, cryo-, and pH-
inactivation than the normal feline enzyme. In addition,
the enzyme in affected cats is approximately half the
molecular weight of the normal feline enzyme, which has

been shown to be a homodimer. These results suggest that
the mutation in the structural gene for feline ASB alters
the gene product in such a way that it is unable to form
and/or maintain its normal dimeric subunit configuration,
resulting in altered catalytic properties. Subunit re-
association with increases in specific activity by thiol
reducing agents has been demonstrated in vitro and in vivo,
which provides one approach to therapy in the feline
disease (Desnick et al, 1981). It should be noted that
ASB isolated from human tissues (and that of other species)
has been presumed to be a monomer of molecular weight about
half that of the normal cat homodimer. In view of this, it
is unlikely that the molecular pathology of feline MPS VI
is identical to that of human MPS VI. However, this should
not limit the usefulness of the model, since the objective
of devising and evaluating enzyme replacement strategies
is the same in either case. Family studies of spontaneously
occurring MPS VI in Siamese cat families, as well as breeding experiments within the established colony at the
University of Pennsylvania, School of Veterinary Medicine,
indicates MPS VI is transmitted as an autosomal recessive
trait (Fig. 6).

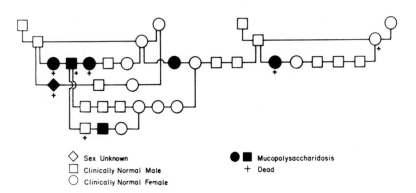

◇ Sex Unknown   ● ■ Mucopolysaccharidosis
□ Clinically Normal Male   + Dead
○ Clinically Normal Female

Fig. 6   The pedigree of a family of cats with mucopolysaccharidosis VI. Note that most of the
breedings are incestuous and that an affected
male cat has successfully reproduced.

Spontaneous cases have been diagnosed in cats from the mid-Atlantic states, Oklahoma and Oregon and, as all of these cases have occurred in non-registered Siamese families, it appears that the gene for MPS VI is widespread throughout the Siamese feline population within the United States. We have, by outcrossing and backcrossing to affected and carrier Siamese cats been able to produce affected animals that do not have the Siamese coat color pattern. Thus, there is no evidence indicating a close linkage between the locus for the Siamese dilution gene and the locus for ASB.

MUCOPOLYSACCHARIDOSIS I

In man, MPS I is presently sub-divided into three separate clinical syndromes, each having deficient alpha-L-iduronidase activity (McKusick et al, 1978) and each apparently resulting from different combinations of at least two mutant alleles at the same gene locus (Fortuin and Kleijer, 1980, McKusick et al, 1972). The Hurler syndrome (MPS I H), the most severe form, is characterized by corneal clouding, facial dysmorphia, severe dyostosis multiplex, mental retardation, and. death usually before age 10. In the least severe form (Scheie syndrome, MPS I S) patients have corneal clouding, joint involvement, normal intelligence, and possibly normal life span. A form, which has been considered to be a Hurler/Scheie compound heterozygote (MPS I H/S), has an intermediate phenotype. In all three syndromes, Alder-Reilly bodies are present in peripheral blood lymphocytes, GAGs excreted in excess in the urine are dermatan and heparan sulfates, and alpha-L-iduronidase activity is deficient, as measured in cell lysates. There is evidence that the residual enzyme kinetics of MPS I H patients differs from that of MPS I S patients, indicating a difference in enzyme structure (Hopwood and Muller, 1979). This finding supports the hypothesis that at least two different mutations within the same enzyme are responsible for these separate clinical syndromes. The possibility that at least some of the individuals classified as MPS I H/S are not compound heterozygotes but represent a third mutant allele at this locus cannot be excluded. All 3 forms of MPS I are inherited as an autosomal recessive trait.

The major pathologic variation between the three
MPS I syndromes in man appears to be in the degree of
lysosomal storage within CNS neurons, with MPS I H having
widespread neuronal storage, MPS I S having none and
MPS I H/S being intermediate in the numbers and distribution of neurons affected (Aleu et al, 1965, Dekaban and
Constantopoulos, 1977, Lagunoff et al, 1962, Loeb et al,
1968, Martin et al, 1978). However, at present the
number of reports of CNS pathology in MPS I S and MPS I
H/S patients are few.

Feline MPS I - Clinical Manifestations

Feline MPS I was first reported in a one year old
male white domestic short-haired cat (Haskins et al,
1979a). A colony of carriers and affected animals has
been established by out-crossing the mother of the
initial affected cat, identifying carriers of MPS I
through enzyme assay, and mating carriers to produce
affected individuals. All affected animals have large
heads with short ears, wide spaced eyes and a broad nose.
Dwarfing is not seen; in fact these cats, particularly
the males, are larger than normal, sex-matched relatives
of the same age. Typical facial dysmorphia is present
at weaning, but because of the normal facial variability
of domestic short-haired cats, it is not as striking as
that seen in Siamese cats with MPS VI. All affected
cats have diffuse, bilateral, fine granular corneal
clouding. Leucocytes and peripheral blood smears do
not contain prominent metachromatic granules, as are
usually seen in children with this disease. Affected
animals can be identified at weaning (six weeks) by a
spot test for excessive urinary glycosaminoglycans
(Berry and Spinanger, 1960); the GAGs excreted in
excess are dermatan and heparan sulfates. A grade
IV/V holosystolic heart murmur, compatible with mitral
insufficiency, has been detected in three animals under
one year of age and chest radiographs gave evidence
of left atrial enlargement.

The radiographic features of the skeletal disease
in the cat include bilateral hip subluxation, fusions
of cervical vertebrae, and pectus excavatum. The degree
of skeletal involvement, particularly long bone
epiphyseal dysplasia, is not as prominent as is seen
in cats with mucopolysaccharidosis VI.

Accumulation of $^{35}SO_4$ by cultured fibroblasts has been shown to be abnormal; the pattern being consistent with defective degradation of glycosaminoglycans.

The oldest cats evaluated, at two years of age, are alert but have hindlimb gait abnormalities. They appear painful when they walk or when the joints of these limbs are manipulated. There have been no indications in any of the affected cats of central nervous system deficits comparable either to mental retardation in man or to those abnormalities seen in other storage diseases described in the cat such as GM_1 and GM_2 gangliosidoses, sphingomyelinosis, and mannosidosis (Baker et al, 1971, Cork et al, 1977, Chrisp et al, 1970, Wenger et al, 1980, Burditt, 1980). Cats affected with MPS I live long enough to reach sexual maturity and both a male and a female have been bred successfully.

Pathology

Gross pathologic changes have included mild hepato-splenomegaly and thickening of mitral valve leaflets in chordae tendinae (Haskins et al, 1981). By light microscopy, neurons were swollen with vacuolated cyto-plasm (Fig. 7) in several areas of the central nervous system including the middle layers of the cerebral cortex. By electron microscopy, membrane bound inclusions containing zebra-bodies (Fig. 8) were present in neurons; granular inclusions were present in periph-eral granulocytes, hepatocytes (Fig. 9), smooth muscle cells of the spleen, keratocytes and in fibroblastic elements of liver, kidney, and mitral valve. The presence of storage within central nervous system neurons without obvious clinical signs of neurologic dysfunction raises questions concerning the relationship between the presence of storage within neurons and dysfunction.

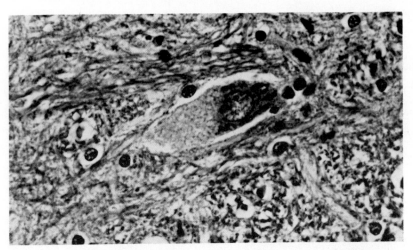

Fig. 7   Light micrograph of a sensory neuron from the dorsal horn of the spinal cord having vesicular cytoplasm (H & E, X 1680).

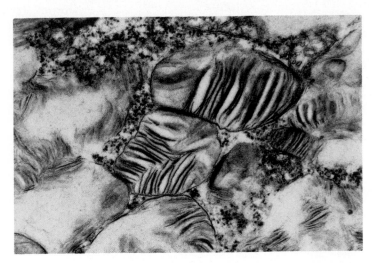

Fig. 8   An electron micrograph of the vesicular area of a dorsal horn neuron illustrating "zebra" bodies (lead citrate, uranyl acetate, X 3150).

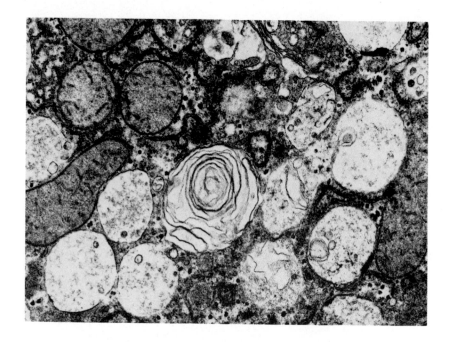

Fig. 9   Electron micrograph of an hepatocyte with
          membrane bound cytoplasmic inclusions
          (Uranyl acetate-lead citrate, X 4800).

Enzymology

        Alpha-L-iduronidase activity in peripheral blood
granulocytes and cultured fibroblasts of affected cats
is less than 1% of normal, and obligate heterozygotes have
alpha-L-iduronidase activities intermediate between those
of normal and affected cats. This disease is transmitted
as an autosomal recessive trait and because all of the
affected animals now present within the breeding colony
at the University of Pennsylvania, School of Veterinary
Medicine were derived from a single carrier, they are
homozygous for the mutant allele which is identical by
descent (Fig. 10). Thus, while the clinical and pathologic phenotype of feline MPS I is best described as being
intermediate between MPS IH and MPS IS in man resembling
the putative compound heterozygote, this cannot be the

case in these cats, indicating that the existence of a compound heterozygote is not necessary to explain an intermediate phenotype in this syndrome.

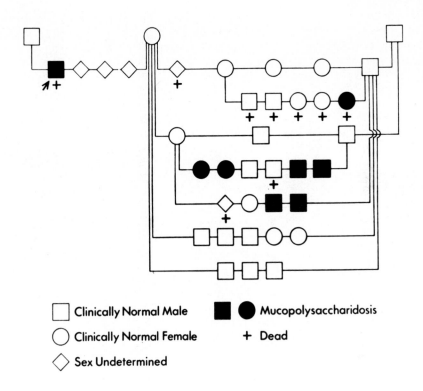

Clinically Normal Male   ■ ● **Mucopolysaccharidosis**

Clinically Normal Female   **+ Dead**

Sex Undetermined

Fig. 10   The pedigree of domestic short-haired cats with mucopolysaccharidosis I. Subsequent to the diagramming of this pedigree both male and female affected cats have been bred successfully.

MUCOPOLYSACCHARIDOSIS IN A DOG

We have recently investigated a dog with clinical signs of mucopolysaccharidosis, referred to us by Dr. Niels Pedersen of the Veterinary School, University of California at Davis. This male, mixed-breed dog was first observed to be weak, particularly in the rear legs, at 8 weeks of age and became progressively worse. When presented to us at age 8 months the animal had a large head in proportion to his body with a shortened maxilla and protruding mandible. The animal's tongue usually protruded beyond the labial margins and he had peg-shaped, wide-spaced teeth. Both corneas contained diffuse fine stromal granularities with areas of edema and what were considered to be cholesterol deposits. Both the axial and appendicular skeletons appeared deformed. The spine seemed short and the rib-cage was compressed in a dorso-ventral direction (anterior-posterior in man). The long bones appeared shortened and curved and most joints were extremely lax and were easily subluxated and crepitant. Joint capsules were swollen and seemed fluid-filled on palpation. Both patellae were luxated medially. The animal was incapable of standing or fully supporting weight on his limbs, being particularly weak in the hind limbs. He was bright and alert, and had apparently normal pain perception in all areas. Function of all cranial nerves was evaluated as within normal limits, and segmental reflexes appeared normal, within the limits imposed by severe skeletal disease. Many of the muscles of locomotion were atrophied. Cardiovascular examination revealed no abnormalities.

In peripheral blood smears stained with toluidine blue, most lymphocytes and granulocytes contained metachromatic cytoplasmic granules. The urinary spot test for GAGs was positive and electrophoresis of precipitated GAG co-migrated with chondroitin and keratan sulfates.

At 13 months of age the animal had radiographic evidence of extensive skeletal disease including bilateral femoral head luxation (Fig. 11) and degeneration, extensive degenerations of carpal and tarsal bones, lytic lesions in the epiphyseal regions of most long bones, and cervical vertebral dysplasia and platyspondyly (Fig. 12). These lesions became progressively worse with time.

The animal had an active libido and was mated by artificial insemination to three bitches, one of which conceived.

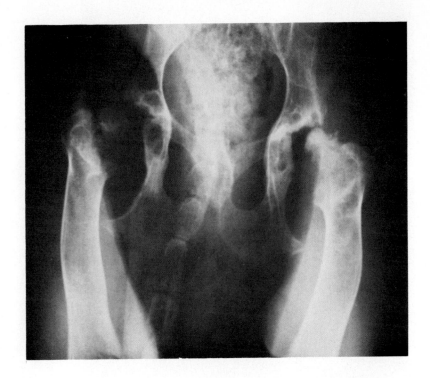

Fig. 11   Ventro-dorsal radiograph of the hips of a
           dog with mucopolysaccharidosis. Note the
           bilateral hip luxation and irregular femoral
           head destruction.

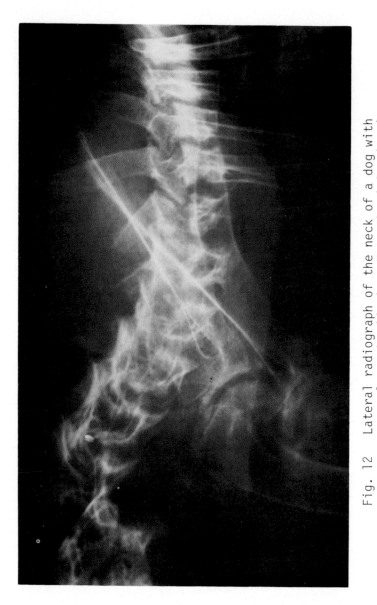

Fig. 12 Lateral radiograph of the neck of a dog with mucopolysaccharidosis. Note the deformity in size and shape of the vertebral bodies and irregular articular surfaces in the scapulo-humeral joints.

Electron microscopic examination of conjunctiva and peripheral white blood cells revealed the presence of multiple, membrane-bound, granular cytoplasmic vacuoles within conjunctival fibroblasts, polymorphonuclear leucocytes and lymphocytes (Fig. 13).

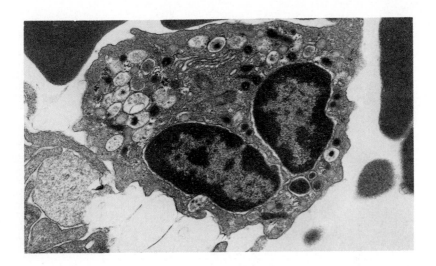

Fig. 13   Electron micrograph of a peripheral blood polymorphonuclear leucocyte with granular cytoplasmic vacuoles (Uranyl acetate-lead citrate, X 1900).

The animal died suddenly from apparent gastric dilatation with ascites, hydrothorax, and pulmonary congestion. There was generalized hepatomegaly, the atrio-ventricular heart valves were thickened, and a generalized polyarthropathy with villous proliferation of synovial membranes was observed in the joints of the appendicular skeleton.

Studies are presently underway to define the enzymatic defect in tissues from this animal. $^{35}SO_4$ incorporation studies on cultured skin fibroblasts and electron microscopy of other major visceral organs are also in progress.

Based upon the clinical and radiographic signs, and the excretion of excessive amounts of keratan sulfate in the urine, a tentative diagnosis of mucopolysaccharidosis IV or Morquio's syndrome has been made.

ACKNOWLEDGEMENTS

This work was supported by NIH grant AM 25759 and Genetics Center Grant GM 20138, March of Dimes Birth Defects Foundation Grant 1-578. M. M. McGovern is the recipient of an NIH predoctoral fellowship in genetics (IT 32 HDO 7105).

REFERENCES

Aleu FP, Terry RD, Zellweger H (1965). Electron microscopy of two cerebral biopsies in gargoylism. J Neuropath Exp Neurol 24:304.

Baker HJ, Lindsey JR, McKhann GM, Farrell DF (1971). Neuronal G_{M1} gangliosidosis in a siamese cat with β-galactosidase deficiency. Science 174:838.

Berry HK, Spinanger J (1960). A paper spot test useful in study of Hurler's syndrome. J Lab Clin Med 55:136.

Burditt LJ, Chotai K, Hirani S, Nugent PG, Winchester, BG (1980). Biochemical studies on a case of feline mannosidosis. Biochem J 189:467.

Chrisp CE, Ringler DH, Abrams GD, Radin NS, Brenkert A (1970). Lipid storage disease in a siamese cat. J Am Vet Med Assoc 156:616.

Cork LC, Munnell JF, Lorenz MD, Murphy JV, Baker HJ, Rattazzi MC (1977). G_{M2} ganglioside lysosomal storage disease in cats with β-hexosaminidase deficiency. Science 196:1014.

Dekaban AS, Constantopoulos G (1977). Mucopolysaccharidosis types I, II, IIIA and V: Pathological and biochemical abnormalities in the neural and mesenchymal elements of the brain. Acta Neuropathol (Berl) 39:1.

Desnick RJ, McGovern MM, Haskins ME, Patterson DF, Vine DT (1981). Characterization of the residual arylsulfatase B activity in feline mucopolysaccharidosis VI. Implications for enzyme manipulation therapy. In Desnick RJ (ed): "Advances in the Treatment of Inborn Errors of Metabolism," in press.

Dorfman A, Matalon R (1976). The mucopolysaccharidoses: A review. Proc Natl Acad Sci USA 73:630.

Fluharty AL, Stebens RL, Fung D, Peak S, Kihara, H (1975). Uridine diphospho-N-acetylgalactosamine-4-sulfate sulfohydrolase activity of human arylsulfatase B and its deficiency in the Maroteaux-Lamy syndrome. Biochem Biophys Res Commun 64:955.

Fluharty AL, Stevens RL, Sanders DL, Kihara H (1974). Arylsulfatase B deficiency in Maroteaux-Lamy syndrome cultured fibroblasts. Biochem Biophys Res Commun 59:455.

Fortuin JJH, Kleijer WJ (1980). Hybridization studies of fibroblasts from Hurler, Scheie, and Hurler/Scheie compound patients: Support for the hypothesis of allelic mutants. Hum Genet 53:155.

Fratantoni JC, Hall CW, Neufeld EF (1968). Hurler and
    Hunter Syndromes: Mutual correction of the defect in
    cultured fibroblasts. Science 162:470.
Goldberg MF, Scott CI, McKusick V (1970). Hydrocephalus
    and papilledema in the Maroteaux-Lamy syndrome (Muco-
    polysaccharidosis, Type VI). Am J Ophthalmol 69:969.
Hansen G (1972). Hematologic studies in mucopolysaccha-
    ridoses and mucolipidoses. Birth defects original
    article series. Vol. VIII:115.
Haskins ME, Jezyk PF, Patterson DF (1979). Mucopoly-
    saccharidosis VI in three families of cats with
    arylsulfatase B deficiency: Leukocyte studies and
    carrier identification. Ped Res 13:1203.
Haskins ME, Jezyk PF, Desnick RJ, McDonough SK,
    Patterson DF (1979a). Alpha-L-iduronidase deficiency
    in a cat. A model of mucopolysaccharidosis I.
    Ped Res 13:1294.
Haskins ME, Aguirre GD, Jezyk PF, Patterson DF (1980).
    The pathology of feline arylsulfatase B deficient
    mucopolysaccharidosis. Am J Pathol 101:657.
Haskins ME, Jezyk PF, Desnick RJ, Patterson DF (1981).
    Animal model of human disease. Mucopolysaccharidosis I
    (Hurler, Scheie, Hurler/Scheie Syndrome).
    Comp Pathol Bulletin VIII:3.
Hopwood JJ, Muller V (1979). Biochemical discrimination
    of Hurler and Scheie syndromes. Clin Sci 57:265.
Jezyk PF, Haskins ME, Patterson DF, Mellman WJ,
    Greenstein M (1977). Mucopolysaccharidosis in a
    cat with arylsulfatase B deficiency: A model of
    Maroteaux-Lamy syndrome. Science 198:834.
Kenyon KR, Quigley HA, Hussels IE, Wyllie RG (1972). The
    systemic mucopolysaccharidoses: Ultrastructure and histo-
    chemical studies of conjunctiva and skin.
    Am J Ophthalmol 73:811.
Lagunoff D, Ross R, Benditt EP (1962). Histochemical and
    electron microscopic study in a case of Hurler's disease.
    Am J Pathol 41:273.
Loeb H, Jonniaux G, Resibois A, Cremer N, Dodion J,
    Tondeur M, Gregoire PE, Richard J, Cieters P (1968).
    Biochemical and ultrastructural studies in Hurler's
    syndrome. J Pediat 73:860.
Maroteaux P, Leveque B, Marie J and Lamy M (1963). Une
    nouvelle dyostose avec elimination urinaire de
    chondroitine sulfate B. Presse Med 71:1849.

Martin JJ, Centerick C, Leroy JG, Neetens A (1975). Pathology in MPS IH/IS, Comparison with allelic and non-allelic mucopolysaccharidoses (MPS-OSES). Proceedings of the VIII International Congress of Neuropathology:655.

Matalon R, Arbogast B, Dorfman A (1974). Deficiency of chondroitin sulfate N-acetylgalactosamine-4-sulfate sulfatase in Maroteaux-Lamy syndrome. Biochem Biophys Res Commun 61:1450.

McGovern MM, Vine DT, Haskins ME, Desnick RJ (1981). An improved method for heterozygote identification in feline and human mucopolysaccharidosis VI, arylsulfatase B deficiency. Enzyme 26:206.

McKusick VA (1972). The mucopolysaccharidoses. In "Heritable Disorders of Connective Tissue," St. Louis MO:C. V. Mosby, p.521.

McKusick VA, Neufeld EF, Kelly TE (1978). The mucopolysaccharide storage diseases. In Stanbury JB, Wyngaarden JB, Fredrickson DS (eds): "The Metabolic Basis of Inherited Disease," New York:McGraw Hill, p.1282.

Neufeld EF, Lim TW, Shapiro LJ (1975). Inherited disorders of lysosomal metabolism. Ann Rev Biochem 44:357.

O'Brien JF, Cantz M, Spranger J (1974). Maroteaux-Lamy disease (MPS VI), subtype A: deficiency of a N-acetyl-galactosamine-4-sulfatase. Biochem Biophys Res Commun 60:1170.

Pennock CA (1976). A review and selection of simple laboratory methods used for the study of glycosamino-glycan excretion and the diagnosis of the mucopoly-saccharidoses. J Clin Pathol 29:111.

Peterson DI, Bacchus H, Seaich L, Kelly TE (1975). Myelopathy associated with Maroteaux-Lamy syndrome. Arch Neurol 32:127-129.

Quigley HA, Kenyon KR (1974). Ultrastructural and histo-chemical studies of a newly recognized form of systemic mucopolysaccharidosis (Maroteaux-Lamy syndrome, mild phenotype). Am J Ophthalmol 77:809.

Shapira E, DeGregorie RR, Matalon R, Nadler HL (1975). Reduced arylsulfatase B activity of the mutant enzyme protein in Maroteaux-Lamy syndrome. Biochem Biophys Res Commun 62:448.

Spranger JW, Koch F, McKusick VA, Natzschka J, Wiedmann, HR, Zellweger H (1970). Mucopolysaccharidosis VI (Maroteaux-Lamy's disease). Helv Paediatr Acta 25:337.

Spranger JW (1972). "The Systemic Mucopolysaccharidoses. Ergebnisse der Luneren Midizin und Kinderheilkunde." New York:Springer-Verlag, p.165.

Stumpf DA, Austin JH (1972). Sulfatase B deficiency in
the Maroteaux-Lamy syndrome (MPS VI). Trans Am Neurol
Assoc 97:29.

Taniguchi N, Koizumi S, Masake K, Kobayashi Y (1975).
Diagnosis of genetic mucopolysaccharidosis: electrophoretic and enzymatic characterization of urinary
glycosaminoglycans. Biochem Med 14:241.

Tondeur M, Neufeld EF (1975). The mucopolysaccharidoses,
biochemistry and ultrastructure. In Good RA, Day SB,
Yunis JJ (eds): "Molecular Pathology," Springfield, Ill:
p.600.

Van Hoof F, Hers HG (1972). "The Mucopolysaccharidoses as
Lysosomal Diseases, Sphingolipids, Sphingolipidoses
and Allied Disorders." New York:Plenum Press, p.211.

Vine DT, McGovern MM, Haskins ME, Desnick RJ (1981).
Feline mucopolysaccharidosis VI: Purification on
characterization of the residual arylsulfatase B
activity. Am J Hum Genet (in press).

Wenger DA, Sattler M, Kudoh T, Snyder SP, Kingston RS
(1980). Niemann-Pick disease: A genetic model in
siamese cats. Science 208:1471.

DR. CORK: Were you able to do any muscle biopsies in your dog with MPS, and if so, what were the results? I ask because the protrusion of the tongue and the flaring of the rib cage may represent muscle weakness.

DR. HASKINS: We did not do a muscle biopsy. We do have muscle from the post mortem. There was a large amount of muscle wasting which we had assumed was secondary to disuse atrophy because of the skeletal disease and the inability to move. The areas that were wasted were the areas that one would expect because of disuse atrophy.

DR. CORK: Were you able to get EMG's?

DR. HASKINS: No, we did not do EMG's on the dog.

DR. RATTAZZI: With regard to your MPS I animal, I don't quite understand. Are you postulating that this is really a kind of compound heterozygote? If it were so, an analysis of the pedigree would show it.

DR. HASKINS: Right. A compound heterozygote is not possible. The animal is homozygous by descent for its mutant allele. What we are saying is that it is possible to have an intermediate phenotype without having a genetic compound which perhaps will help delineate the human situation.

DR. DESNICK: We have developed a very sensitive α-L-iduronidase assay. When we assay human Hurler disease tissues, no activity is detected in a number of patients. However, when we assay the same tissues in the Hurler cat, we find about 10 percent residual activity. Perhaps the presence of residual activity is consistent with the intermediate phenotype, analogous to the human Hurler-Scheie compound. Maybe the study of the feline model will support the concept that the human Hurler-Scheie disease is due to homozygosity for a different allele, rather than a compound of the Hurler and Scheie alleles.

Animal Models of Inherited Metabolic Diseases, pages 203-212
© **1982 Alan R. Liss, Inc., 150 Fifth Avenue, New York, NY 10011**

FELINE GANGLIOSIDOSES AS MODELS OF HUMAN LYSOSOMAL STORAGE
DISEASES

Henry J. Baker, D.V.M.[1], Steven U. Walkley, D.V.M., Ph.D.[2],
Mario C. Rattazzi, M.D.[3], Harvey S. Singer, M.D.[4],
Harold L. Watson, M.S.[1], and Philip A. Wood, D.V.M, M.S.[1]

[1]University of Alabama in Birmingham, Birmingham, AL 35294
[2]Albert Einstein College of Medicine, Bronx, NY 10461
[3]Children's Hospital of Buffalo, Buffalo, NY 14222
[4]Johns Hopkins Hospital, Baltimore, MD 21205

This year marks the centennial of Waren Tay's original
description of ophthalmological and other clinical stigmata
of the form of human Gm_2 gangliosidosis that now bears his
name, Tay-Sachs disease (Tay 1881). Today, the gangliosidoses
are recognized as a family of clinically and/or biochemically
distinct entities that represent a subset of inherited
diseases of lysosomal function (Table 1).

Although much has been learned about lysosomal storage
diseases through study of human patients, many fundamental,
complex questions remain which can be answered only by the
use of well characterized experimental models. Reports of
lysosomal diseases affecting various animals are numerous
(see Jolly this volume). However, careful analysis of this
apparent plethora of animal models reveals that very few
colonies of animals with these mutations have been developed
for experimental use. Animal models of the gangliosidoses
rank among the most advanced experimental systems for research
on the lysosomal storage diseases (Table 1) (Baker 1979). Of
these, feline Gm_1 and Gm_2 gangliosidosis provide a number of
important advantages for research use which have been exploited for the past decade (Baker 1979). The clinical,
genetic, pathological and biochemical characteristics of these
models are well documented (Table 2) (Baker 1979; Cork 1979).

This paper will review some important contributions being
made currently by feline models of the gangliosidoses in
research on the pathogenesis and therapy of lysosomal storage
diseases.

Table 1. Ganglioside Storage Diseases in Man and Animals

Storage product	Human disease	Animal analog[1]
Gm_1 ganglioside	Generalized gangliosidosis, type 1, Norman–Landing disease Juvenile Gm_1 gangliosidosis, type 2, Derry's disease Adult (chronic) Gm_1 gangliosidosis	Gm_1 gangliosidosis Bovine–Friesan cattle Canine–Beagle/mixed breed dogs Feline–Siamese, Korat and other breeds of cats
Gm_2 ganglioside	Gm_2 gangliosidosis, type 1, Tay–Sachs disease Gm_2 gangliosidosis, type 2, Sandhoff's disease Juvenile Gm_2 gangliosidosis, type 3, Bernheimer–Seitelberger disease Adult (chronic) Gm_2 gangliosidosis	Gm_2 gangliosidosis Canine–German Shorthair Pointer dogs Feline–Mixed breed cats Porcine–Yorkshire swine

[1] Arrangement in table does not imply analogy between animal disease and clinical subtype of human disease. Only feline Gm_2 gangliosidosis is known to be a biochemical analog of human Sandhoff's subtype.

Table 2. Feline Gangliosidoses

	Gm_1	Gm_2
Breed	Siamese, Korat, other	Mixed
Signs	Progressive tremors, motor disability, and others	Same
Onset	3–4 mo.	1–2 mo.
Progression	Slow	Rapid
Death	10–12 mo.	Less than 6 mo.
Appearance	Normal	Dwarf, corneal-opacity (rare)
Inheritance	Autosomal recessive	Same
Histopathology	Vacuolation neurons and liver	Same
Ultrastructure	Neurons–lamellar bodies Hepatocytes–flocculent	Same Same
Neuronal storage	Gm_1 ganglioside	Gm_2 ganglioside
Hepatic storage	Glycopeptides	Glycolipids
Enzyme defect	B–galactosidase	B–hexosaminidases A and B
Analog	Derry's disease	Sandhoff's disease

PATHOGENESIS OF GANGLIOSIDOSES

Conspicuous evidence of cellular pathology due to lysosomal disease includes: bizarre morphological alterations,
massive changes in biochemical characteristics, and relent-
lessly progressive loss of nervous system function. Ironi-
cally, in spite of such spectacular changes, the precise
cellular events underlying cellular dysfunction (particularly
of neurons) remains entirely unknown. The traditional "cytotoxicity" hypothesis which suggests that hypertrophied
lysosomes simply compress other organelles, is unsupported by
experimental evidence. Our studies using the feline gangliosidoses provide provocative new evidence indicating that
altered membrane structure and function may be a major factor
contributing to neuronal dysfunction.

Using Golgi stains to outline entire neurons from human
patients with gangliosidosis, Purpura and Suzuki (1976)
revealed bizarre distortions of neurons. Comprehensive
studies of the feline gangliosidoses confirmed and extended
these observations to include the following. (1) A variety
of significant structural alterations have been observed, such
as: prominent expansions (meganeurites) between the soma and
initial axonal segment, inappropriate proliferation of

secondary neurites, aberrant synaptogenesis, somatic swelling, and abnormal somatic processes. (2) Neurons from different brain regions vary in their morphological expression of disease. (3) Neuronal loss is not obvious until very late in the clinical course of disease. (4) Electrogenic properties and retrograde axonal transport appear to be unaffected. (Purpura 1978; Purpura 1980; Walkley 1980; Walkley 1981).

Preliminary assessment of neurotransmitter function by Singer et al (1981) using cats with advanced neurobehavioral disease due to Gm_1 gangliosidosis revealed the following. (1) Activities of neurotransmitter synthesizing enzymes in diseased cats were not different from normal sibling controls, supporting morphological observations that neuronal loss is not a significant factor. (2) Endogenous neurotransmitters approximated those of controls. (3) Significant reduction was found in high affinity uptake of glutamate, gama amino-butyric acid (GABA) and norepinephrine in cerebral cortex and cerebellum of diseased cats. This finding suggests that regulation of major excitatory and inhibitory neurotransmitters is defective.

Unpublished observations by Wood et al (1981) on the biophysical properties of synaptosomal membrane using lipid fluorescent probes indicate reduced fluidity of neuronal membrane from cats with Gm_1 gangliosidosis, probably due to altered lipid composition.

Neurons are distinguished by a uniquely high proportion of gangliosides in the lipid composition of plasma membranes, particularly at synapses (Svennerholm 1980). While the prominence of gangliosides in neuronal membrane structure infers a principal role in neuronal function, specific mechanisms are just beginning to be revealed. These early findings suggest a unifying role for gangliosides in membrane mediated cell surface regulatory events such as: (1) receptors for various bioactive compounds including neurotrans-mitters (Svennerholm 1980), (2) transduction of membrane associated regulatory systems (Brady 1978; Yamakowa 1978), and ion transfer (Leon 1981).

An attractive hypothesis explaining neuronal dysfunction in the gangliosidoses begins to emerge from this fragmentary evidence. Obstructed ganglioside catabolism undoubtedly has significant influence on the lipid composition of neuronal membranes. Major alteration in membrane content of any specific lipid (e.g., excess Gm_1 ganglioside) could cause a profound distortion in the relative distribution of other lipid and protein constituents. Derangement of neuronal membrane structure might be manifested morphologically (e.g., neurite proliferation) and functionally (e.g., reduced neuro-transmitter uptake).

The feline gangliosidoses will continue to play a key role in understanding the pathogenesis of neuronal dysfunction in lysosomal storage diseases, and perhaps as important, in understanding normal structure and function of the normal nervous system.

THERAPY OF LYSOSOMAL STORAGE DISEASES

Definition of specific enzyme defects in lysosomal storage diseases has provided the opportunity to prevent birth of diseased children by heterozygote detection and therapeutic abortion based on prenatal diagnosis. However, treatment of these devastating diseases remains limited to palliative measures. The thrust of current research is directed toward corrective strategies, particularly enzyme replacement. The rationale for this approach is based on the concept that exogenous enzyme would be assimilated by diseased cells, transported to hypertrophied lysosomes and degrade accumu-lated substrate. Substantial evidence derived from studies using cultured cells from children and cats with gangliosi-dosis confirm the validity of this concept including the following. (1) Assimilation of lysosomal enzymes is con-trolled by cell surface receptors. (2) Enzyme activity approximating normal (or higher) can be achieved in enzyme deficient cells by endocytosis of exogenous enzyme with appropriate recognition markers or by use of carriers. (3) Assimilated enzyme is lysosomotrophic. (4) Half-life of assimilated enzyme approximates 7-10 days. (5) Accumulated substrate is effectively hydrolized. (Reynolds and Baker 1978; Brooks 1980; Brooks 1981).

Using cats with Gm_2 gangliosidosis, Rattazzi et al (1981) have made remarkable progress in demonstrating the feasibility of enzyme replacement therapy *in vivo* (see Rattazzi this volume). Key findings to date include the following. (1) The circulating half-life of exogenous enzyme can be pro-longed by selective blockade of reticuloendothelial cells using competitive inhibition of cell surface recognition sites. (2) The blood-brain barrier, which normally excludes lysosomal enzymes, can be disrupted temporarily, permitting entry of exogenous enzyme to brain without apparent deleterious effects on neurobehavioral function (Figure 1). (3) The activity of (exogenous) hexosaminidases can be restored in mutant cat brain to that found in normal cats. (4) Clearance of the principal hepatocellular storage product, globoside, from liver is nearly complete in cats with Gm_2 gangliosidosis 72 hours after administration of exogenous hexosaminidase purified from human placenta (Rattazzi 1980).

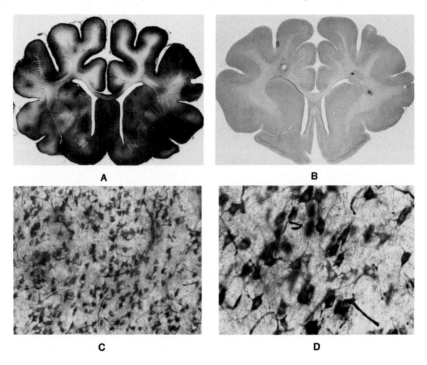

Fig. 1. Coronal brain sections of cats subjected to temporary disruption of the blood-brain barrier (BBB) by the method of Rattazzi and given horseradish peroxidase (HRP) as an enzyme marker (A), or sham operated and given HRP(B). Sections were cut frozen, developed with diaminobenzidine tetrahydrochloride to demonstrate HRP, and counter stained with cresyl violet. A high concentration of HRP was found in gray matter of cats subjected to BBB disruption, while no HRP was found in brain parenchyma of sham operated cats. Histological sections (C,D) of brain shown in (A) demonstrates extensive assimilation of HRP in cortical neurons.

Full validation of this promising therapeutic approach for clinical application must await conclusive evidence pertaining to the following questions. (1) What are the long term consequences of temporary blood-brain barrier disruption and perfusion of brain with exogenous enzyme? (2) Are cells of the central nervous system capable of endocytosis? (3) Is exogenous enzyme capable of catabolizing long standing accumulation of complex, highly organized glycolipids? (4) Are neurons with significant structural and functional distortions capable of revival? (5) What is the prognosis for long term maintenance of normal nervous system function after temporary correction of disrupted lysosomal catabolism?

It appears that all of the principal technical measures are at last in hand to fully explore these remaining questions, and the feline gangliosidoses provide nearly ideal models for these studies that are crucial for continued progress toward therapy of lysosomal diseases.

ACKNOWLEDGEMENTS

This work was supported in part by NIH Grants NS-10967, RR07003, and NS-13677.

REFERENCES

Baker HJ, Reynolds GD, Walkley SU, Cox, NR, Baker, GH (1979). The gangliosidoses. Comparative features and research applications. Vet Path 16:635.

Brady RO, Fishman PH (1978). Gangliosides as biotransducers of membrane mediated information. In Silverstein SC (ed): Life Sciences Research Reports vol 2 "Transport of Macromolecules in Cellular Systems", New York: G Fisher, p 69.

Brooks SE, Hoffman LM, Adachi M, Amsterdam D, Schneck L (1980). Enzyme replacement treatment for Tay-Sachs disease brain cells in culture utilizing conconovalin-A mediated hexosaminidase-A uptake: Biochemical and morphological evidence of Gm_2 mobilization. Acta Neuropath (Berl) 50:9.

Brooks SE, Hoffman LM, Amsterdam D, Adachi M, Schneck L (1981). Long term intracellular retention of hexosaminidase-A by Tay-Sachs disease brain and lung cells *in vitro*. J Neurosci Res 6:381.

Cork LC, Munnell JF, Baker HJ, Rattazzi MC (1979). A comparative pathological study of feline and human Gm_2 gangliosidosis. In Zimmerman H (ed): "Progress in Neuropathology", New York: Raven Press, p 161.

Leon A, Facci L, Toffano G, Sonnino S, Tettamanti G, (1981). Activation of Na+, K+ ATPase by nanomolar concentrations of Gm_1 ganglioside. J Neurochem 37:350.

Purpura DP, Suzuki K (1976). Distortion of neuronal geometry and formation of aberrant synapses in neuronal storage diseases. Brain Res 116:1.

Purpura DP, Baker HJ (1978). Meganeurites and other aberrant processes of neurons in feline Gm_1 gangliosidosis: A Golgi study. Brain Res 143:13.

Purpura DP, Highstein SM, Karabelas AB, Walkley SU (1980). Intracellular recording and HRP staining of cortical neurons in feline ganglioside storage disease. Brain Res 181:446.

Rattazzi MC, Appel AM, Baker HJ (1980). Enzyme replacement in feline Gm_2 gangliosidosis: Reduction of glycolipid storage in visceral organs. Am J Human Genetics 32:51.

Rattazzi MC, Appel AM, Baker HJ, Nester J (1981). Towards enzyme replacement in Gm_2 gangliosidosis: Inhibition of hepatic uptake and induction of CNS uptake of human β-hexosaminidase in the cat. In Callahan J, Lowder JA (eds): "Lysosomes and Lysosomal Storage Diseases", New York: Raven Press, p 405.

Reynolds GD, Baker HJ (1978). Enzyme replacement using liposome carriers in feline Gm_1 gangliosidosis fibro-blasts. Nature 275:754.

Singer HS, Coyle JT, Weaver DL, Kawamura N, Baker HJ (1981). Neurotransmitter chemistry in feline Gm_1 gangliosidosis: A model for human ganglioside storage disease. Ann Neurol In press.

Svennerholm L (1980). Gangliosides and synaptic transmission. In Svennerholm L, Mandel P, Dreyfus H, Urban PF (eds): "Structure and Function of Gangliosides", New York: Plenum Press, p 533.

Tay W (1881). Symmetrical changes in the region of the yellow spot in each eye of an infant. Trans Ophth Soc 1:155.

Walkley SU, Baker HJ, Purpura DP (1980). Morphological changes in feline gangliosidosis: A Golgi study. In Rose FC, Behon PO (eds): "Animal Models of Neurological Diseases", London: Pitmans Medical, p 419.

Walkley SU, Wurzelmann S, Purpura, DP (1981). Ultrastructure of neurites and meganeurites of cortical pyramidal neurons in feline gangliosidosis as revealed by the combined Golgi-EM technique. Brain Res 211:393.

Wood PA, McBride M, Christian ST, Baker HJ (1981). Fluorescent probe analysis of synaptosomal membrane from cats with Gm_1 gangliosidosis. In preparation.

Yamakawa T, Nagai Y (1978). Glycolipids at the cell surface and their biological functions. Trends Biochem Sci 3:128.

DR. RATTAZZI: I would like to add to Dr. Baker's comments. We now have evidence that the exogenous enzyme induces degradation of substrate in visceral organs, not only as far as globoside in liver, but also, GM_2 ganglioside in liver, GM_2 ganglioside in bone, and globoside in kidney and spleen. Unfortunately our initial finding is that a similar amount of exogenous enzyme delivered to the brain does not result in the same effect as we see in visceral organs. So, as Dr. Baker said, there are a lot of things that we have to explore before a catabolic effect can be achieved at the neuronal level.

DR. SCARPELLI: Dr. Baker, it is now reasonably well established that lipid peroxidation causes significant alteration in membrane lipid moieties and these in turn may contribute to changes in membrane permeability. Is the hyperoxic effect reversible, and if so, how quickly do the permeability characteristics return to normal?

DR. BAKER: Unfortunately, we don't know the basic mechanism of the barrier opening, either due to oxygen administration or hypertonic solutions or any number of other ways that have been demonstrated to open the barrier. As far as the Rattazzi method is concerned, it is a temporary opening, probably not lasting more than about 30 minutes. It does not cause clinically apparent disease in normal cats although there is some question about the histological lesions that might result.

DR. SCARPELLI: Have you tried the effects of antioxidants in your experimental system?

DR. BAKER: No.

DR. RATTAZZI: Relative to your question, Dr. Scarpelli, blood brain barrier permeability can be induced not only with oxygen but also with air, and with nitrogen and with CO_2. So, lipid peroxidation doesn't seem to be involved. There is a hypothesis that formation of histamine by the enzyme histidine decarboxylase (which seems to be activated by the shearing stress of the gas bubbles against the endothelial cells) may be involved, but there are no direct data bearing on this.

Animal Models of Inherited Metabolic Diseases, pages 213-220
© **1982 Alan R. Liss, Inc., 150 Fifth Avenue, New York, NY 10011**

ENZYME REPLACEMENT IN FELINE GM$_2$ GANGLIOSIDOSIS:
CATABOLIC EFFECTS OF HUMAN β-HEXOSAMINIDASE A

M.C. Rattazzi[1], A.M. Appel[1], H.J. Baker[2]

[1]Dept. Pediatrics, Children's Hospital,
SUNY, Buffalo, NY; [2]Dept. Comparative
Medicine, U. Alabama, Birmingham, AL

STORAGE DISEASES: NEED FOR A THERAPEUTIC APPROACH

Human lysosomal storage diseases result from
genetic defects of lysosomal hydrolases and impaired
catabolism of biological compounds, which accumulate in the cellular vacuolar-lysosomal apparatus
leading to impairment of cell functions. Although
individually rare, storage diseases collectively
account for a significant portion of neurodegenerative disorders of infancy. Most of them are very
severe and lead to early death, but clinical
variants are known with later onset and protracted
course. In couples genetically at risk it is
possible to prevent the birth of a diseased infant
by enzymatic prenatal diagnosis and selective
abortion. With the exception of Tay-Sachs disease
in the Ashkenazic Jewish population, in which their
frequency is high, and their identification by
screening programs is feasible, couples at risk
are identified in most instances only after the
birth of an affected child. Thus, therapy of
storage diseases would be useful in those cases
which escape, or are not amenable to, prevention
by screening programs; and in cases in which the
prenatal diagnosis-selective abortion approach is
not acceptable.

PRINCIPLE AND PROBLEMS OF ENZYME REPLACEMENT

Therapy of lysosomal storage diseases is possible, at least in principle. Enzyme-deficient cells, exposed to exogenous, normal enzyme, should endocytose it; the fusion processes which characterize the vacuolar-lysosomal system should bring the exogenous enzyme in contact with the stored material, resulting in its catabolism (De Duve, 1964). The principle of enzyme replacement therapy (ERT) has received support from several experiments in cell culture systems; its application to patients, however, has not yielded clear evidence of biochemical or clinical effectiveness (Tager et al., 1980; Desnick and Grabowski, 1981).

Therapeutic trials in patients, though clinically unrewarding, have identified the main methodologic problems of ERT. Most important is that of delivering exogenous enzymes across biochemical or anatomical barriers to organs or tissues which are the main site of pathology. On the one hand, most lysosomal enzymes are glycoproteins, and the structure of their carbohydrate moiety determines their organ disposition, by virtue of glycosyl residue-specific mechanisms on different cells. Thus, mannosyl- and N-acetylglucosaminyl-specific endocytosis by non-parenchymal liver cells (Stahl et al., 1976), or galactosyl-specific endocytosis by hepatocytes (Furbish et al., 1981) result in preferential hepatic uptake. On the other hand, the existence of a blood-brain barrier (BBB) to proteins (Rapoport, 1976) prevents delivery of exogenous enzymes to the CNS for the treatment of storage diseases with prominent neurologic involvement. Not less important is the practical problem of assessing the biochemical effect of exogenous enzymes in the patients' organs, a prerequisite for any rational therapeutic approach.

Well characterized animal models of human storage diseases, such as the cat with genetic β-hexosaminidase deficiency and Gm_2 gangliosidosis (Cork et al., 1977,1979) offer the opportunity to experiment with methodologies aimed at solving these problems, and to assess in vivo the effectiveness of various ERT strategies, at the biochemical and at the clinical level.

APPROACHES TO ENZYME REPLACEMENT IN THE CAT

Visceral Organs

In earlier experiments, we showed that β-hexosaminidase from human placenta is cleared very rapidly from the cat circulation, mainly by a hepatic mechanism recognizing mannosyl and N-acetylglucosaminyl residues (Rattazzi et al., 1979,1980). Preferential hepatic uptake of enzyme can be depressed competitively by preinjection of mannosyl-rich, S. cerevisiae mannans; uptake by other organs and tissues, however, is inhibited to a lower degree (Rattazzi et al., 1981). In this way, injection of high doses of purified β-hexosaminidase in affected animals can result in levels of exogenous enzyme activity approaching those found in normal animals, as exemplified in Table 1.

Table 1: Human placental Hex A (as % of normal activity) in tissues of 2 kittens with Gm_2 gangliosidosis

	A7*	A10**		A7	A10
Liver	108.4	351.5	Adrenals	81.6	146.0
Spleen	70.8	29.9	Gonads	50.7	44.0
Kidney	63.7	26.3	Sk. muscle	66.7	83.3
Lung	84.4	35.6	Lymph node	16.1	159.4
Bone	18.9	56.9	Sm. intestine	6.5	57.8
Pancreas	39.6	44.9			

*Mannans: 150 mg/kg bw; Hex A:7 x 10^7 U; perfusion: 1 lt saline @ 10 min
**Mannans: 75 mg/kg bw; Hex A:1.5 x 10^8 U; perfusion: 1 lt saline @ 24 hrs

In addition to CNS storage of Gm_2 ganglioside, affected cats have glycolipid storage in liver and most extrahepatic tissues (Cork et al., 1977,1979). Thus, in Hex A-injected kittens we could assess not only whether exogenous enzyme can catabolize stored substrates; but also whether this can happen in liver and extrahepatic sites when the main hepatic uptake mechanism is inhibited. In a series of affected kittens injected with various doses of enzyme and sacrificed at different times, we analyzed neutral lipids from saponified Folch extract lower phase, and gangliosides from Folch upper phase, by high efficiency TLC, and densitometry of iodine vapor- and resorcinol-stained plates, respectively. In the liver of the animals which received high doses and were sacrificed at 24-72 hrs from injection (A10,A4) the levels of GL4 globoside were drastically reduced, approaching the levels found in normal animals; similarly, Gm_2 ganglioside levels were significantly ($p < .01$) reduced in affected, enzyme-injected animals, as exemplified in Table 2.

Table 2: Liver GL4 globoside and Gm_2 ganglioside (as % of age-matched values in untreated, affected animals) in Hex A-injected, affected kittens

	A2	A3	A4	A5	A6	A10
GL4*	51.0	66.2	17.6	72.3	49.3	12.4
Gm_2**	30.1	31.8	18.1	43.1	17.6	12.1

*Ratio GL4 globoside/sphingomyelin (=internal reference)
**Ratio Gm_2 ganglioside/Gm_3 ganglioside (=substrate/product).

A similar, but somewhat less drastic effect (as expected from the lower exogenous enzyme activity) was evident in spleen, kidney, and bone extracts, as exemplified in Table 3.

Table 3:   GL4 globoside* and Gm_2 ganglioside* in some extrahepatic tissues of Hex A-injected, affected kittens**

	A3	A4	A5	A6	A8	A10
GL4,spleen	---	46.5	35.4	67.4	68.1	24.5
kidney	61.1	78.5	---	92.7	---	17.3
bone	94.3	43.5	---	66.3	18.4	40.7
Gm_2,bone	26.9	31.3	38.8	47.1	35.2	36.1

*see notes to Table 2
**expressed as % of age-matched values in untreated affected animals

These data represent the first clear demonstration of a catabolic effect of exogenous lysosomal enzyme in vivo at organ level; they also show that it is possible to circumvent the specific hepatic uptake and still retain significant catabolic activity in hepatic and extrahepatic tissues. Histologic studies are needed, however, to determine whether different cell types are preferentially depleted of stored substrates.

Central Nervous System

In experimental animals cerebral air embolism induces transient BBB permeability to proteins (Lee and Olszewski, 1957). Our current approach consists in unilateral intracarotid (IC) injection of a small bolus (<1 ml) of oxygen, rather than air as in earlier experiments (Rattazzi et al., 1981), and is compatible with survival in >90% of the animals, without gross neurologic complications. If oxygen embolism is followed by IC injection of β-hexosaminidase (with mannan preinjection), significant levels of exogenous enzyme are found in the animals' CNS, persisting for at least 72 hrs, as exemplified in Table 4.

Table 4: Human placental Hex A (as % of normal activity) in CNS of affected kittens subjected to cerebral oxygen embolism

	A4	A6	A8	A9	A10
Cortex					
-ipsilateral	14.6	54.2	84.5	174.6	100.1
-controlateral	5.4	45.5	82.2	167.9	53.1

A4: 5×10^7 U Hex A IV; perfusion @ 72 hrs
A6: 5×10^7 U Hex A IC; perf. @ 12 hrs
A8: 7×10^7 U Hex A IV + 4×10^7 U IC; perf. @ 7 hrs
A9,A10: 1.5×10^8 U Hex A IC; perf. @ 4 & 24 hrs, resp

Analysis of gangliosides from the cortex of 9 enzyme-injected, affected kittens did not show a decrease in Gm_2 ganglioside comparable to what we have found in visceral tissues. However, in animals in which a high CNS activity of Hex A and a longer survival were obtained, there was a significant increase in Gm_3 ganglioside (the expected product of Hex A activity on Gm_2 ganglioside). For example, in kittens A4, A5, A8, A10 the glycolipid was 186%, 159%, 188% and 205%, respectively, of the age-matched values from untreated affected animals. This, however, corresponds to only ~5-7% of the Gm_2 ganglioside stored in these animals' cortex. These data are encouraging, as they suggest that exogenous Hex A did degrade Gm_2 ganglioside in the CNS, but it is not known whether this was a consequence of neuronal uptake of the enzyme. The low endocytic activity of perikarya and dendrites; the time factor in retrograde axonal transport of proteins endocytosed at the axon terminal (Broadwell and Brightman, 1979); and the unclear carbohydrate specificity of neuronal uptake (Kusiak et al., 1979) are some of the problems that have to be considered in order to obtain a more significant catabolic effect.

CONCLUSIONS

Our experiments demonstrate clearly the usefulness of a well-characterized animal model in assessing the biochemical effect of ERT methodologies. This essential first step must be followed by a careful assessment of their clinical effectiveness. Given our poor understanding of the causal and temporal relationships between lysosomal enzyme defect, storage, and impaired cellular function, even a biochemically effective ERT approach may not be therapeutically significant, or may result in a partial cure, for instance just prolonging the survival of a severely neurologically affected patient. This makes important that ERT methodologies be thoroughly tested in animal models before they are applied to patients.

ACKNOWLEDGMENTS

The work in Dr. Rattazzi's laboratory was supported in part by grants NS-13677 and RR-05493-17 from the NIH; by March of Dimes grant 1-646; and by MCHS project 417. Dr. Baker's support was from NIH grant NS-10967. We thank Jane A Melisz for excellent technical assistance.

REFERENCES

Broadwell RD, Brightman MW (1979). Cytochemistry of undamaged neurons transporting exogenous protein in vivo. J Comp Neurol 185:31.
Cork LC, Munnell JF, Baker HJ, Rattazzi MC (1979). A comparative study of feline and human Gm$_2$ gangliosidosis. In Zimmerman HM (ed): "Progress in Neuropathology," New York: Raven Press, 4:161.
Cork LC, Munnell JF, Lorenz MD, Murphy JW, Baker HJ, Rattazzi MC (1977). Gm$_2$ ganglioside storage disease in cats with β-hexosaminidase deficiency. Science 196:1014.
De Duve C (1964). From cytases to lysosomes. Fed Proc 23:1045.
Desnick RJ, Grabowski GA (1981). Advances in the treatment of inherited metabolic diseases. In Harris H, Hirschhorn K (eds): "Advances in Human Genetics," New York: Plenum Press, 11:281.

Furbish FC, Steer CS, Krett NL, Barranger JA (1981).
  Uptake and distribution of placental glucocerebro-
  sidase in rat hepatic cells and effects of
  sequential deglycosylation. Biochim Biophys Acta
  673:425.
Kusiak JW, Toney JH, Quirk JM, Brady RO (1979).
  Specific binding of ^{125}I-labeled β-hexosaminidase A
  to rat brain synaptosomes. Proc Natl Acad Sci
  USA 76:982.
Lee JC, Olszewski J (1959). Effect of air embolism
  on permeability of cerebral blood vessels.
  Neurology 9:619.
Rapoport SI (1976). "Blood-Brain Barrier in Physio-
  logy and Medicine." New York: Raven Press.
Rattazzi MC, Appel AM, Baker HJ, Nester J (1981).
  Toward enzyme replacement in Gm$_2$ gangliosidosis:
  Inhibition of hepatic uptake and induction of CNS
  uptake of human β-hexosaminidase in the cat. In
  Callahan JW, Lowden AJ (eds): "Lysosomes and Lyso-
  somal Storage Diseases," New York: Raven Press,
  p. 405.
Rattazzi MC, Lanse SB, McCullough RA, Nester JA,
  Jacobs EA (1980). Towards enzyme replacement in
  Gm$_2$ gangliosidosis: Organ disposition and induced
  central nervous system uptake of human β-hexos-
  aminidase in the cat. In Desnick RJ (ed): "Enzyme
  Therapy in Genetic Diseases:2," New York: Alan R.
  Liss for the March of Dimes-Birth Defects Foun-
  dation. Birth Defects: Original Article Series,
  XVI (1):179.
Rattazzi MC, McCullough RA, Downing CJ, Kung M-P
  (1979). Toward enzyme therapy in Gm$_2$ ganglio-
  sidosis: β-hexosaminidase infusion in normal
  cats. Pediatr Res 13:916.
Stahl PD, Six H, Rodman J, Schlesinger P, Tulsiani
  DR, Touster O (1976). Evidence for specific recog-
  nition sites mediating clearance of lysosomal
  enzymes in vivo. Proc Natl Acad Sci USA 73:4045.
Tager JM, Hamers MN, Schram AW, Van den Berg FA,
  Rietra PJ, Loonen C, Koster JF, Slee R (1980).
  An appraisal of human trials in enzyme replace-
  ment therapy of genetic diseases. In Desnick RJ
  (ed): "Enzyme Therapy in Genetic Diseases:2,"
  New York: Alan R. Liss for the March of Dimes-
  Birth Defects Foundation. Birth Defects: Original
  Article Series XVI (1):343.

Animal Models of Inherited Metabolic Diseases, pages 221-225
© **1982 Alan R. Liss, Inc., 150 Fifth Avenue, New York, NY 10011**

LIVER NEURAMINIDASE DEFICIENCY INHERITED AS A SINGLE GENE
ON MOUSE CHROMOSOME 17

James E. Womack, Denise L.S. Yan, and Michel
Potier
Veterinary Pathology, Texas A&M University,
College Station, Texas and Hospital St. Justine,
University of Montreal, Montreal, Quebec

Electrophoretic variation of liver acid phosphatase
(Lalley and Shows, 1977), α-mannosidase (Dizik and Elliot,
1978), arylsulfatase-B (Daniel et al., 1981), and α-glucosidase (Peters and Swallow, 1979) has been reported in strain
SM/J mice. Genes for posttranslational modification were
suggested in each study by the conversion of the SM/J enzyme
to a form electrophoretically indistinguishable from that of
other inbred strains after incubation with bacterial neuraminidase. A single gene on chromosome 17 was found to be
responsible for the processing of each hydrolase. The occurrence of four independent mutations in strain SM/J, each
affecting the processing of a different liver enzyme, and
each linked to chromosome 17 markers, is highly unlikely.
A more plausable explanation of these data is a unique
SM/J allele at a single locus with pleiotropic effects on
the posttranslational processing of multiple hydrolases.

Changes in electrophoretic mobility after incubation
with neuraminidase suggest that SM/J enzymes are hypersial-
ylated. Thus, a single gene responsible for alteration of
at least four enzymes might code for a sialytransferase, in
which case SM/J has a hyperactive allele, or a neuraminidase,
in which SM/J is defective. The second hypothesis became
testable with the synthesis of 4-methylumbelliferyl-α-D-N-
acetylneuraminate, an artificial substrate of neuraminidase
(Potier et al., 1979a).

Specific activity of liver neuraminidase was tested in
20 inbred strains of mice, in SM/J x C57BL/6J F_1 hybrids,
and in the congenic strain B10.SM(70NS)/Sn. The assay

methods are described by Potier *et al.*, (1979b) and the results of this experiment are summarized in Table 1.

Table 1. Specific activity of liver neuraminidase, expressed as micromoles of 4-methylumbelliferone released per hour per gram of protein in 20 inbred strains of mice, one F_1 hybrid, and one congenic strain. Two assay were conducted per mouse.

Strain	Number of Mice tested	Activity
MOL/Wo	6	4.2 ± 0.9
C57BR/cdJ	4	4.1 ± 1.0
SWR/J	4	4.1 ± 1.1
KK/Wo	6	4.0 ± 1.1
CE/J	4	3.8 ± 1.0
SJL/J	4	3.7 ± 1.0
C57BL/6J	17	3.5 ± 0.2
C57L/J	4	3.5 ± 0.8
DBA/2J	4	3.5 ± 0.9
SK/Cam	6	3.5 ± 1.1
A/J	4	3.4 ± 0.9
C57BL/10J	4	3.4 ± 0.6
BALB/cJ	4	3.3 ± 0.9
P/J	4	3.3 ± 0.6
AKR/J	4	3.2 ± 0.7
RF/J	4	3.2 ± 0.7
C3H/HeJ	4	3.2 ± 0.8
PL/J	4	3.0 ± 0.6
CBA/J	4	3.0 ± 0.8
(SM/J x C57BL/6J)F_1	19	1.7 ± 0.3*
B10.SM(70NS)Sn	4	0.6 ± 0.3**
SM/J	15	0.6 ± 0.1**

*Significantly different from all other means at $P \leq .01$.
**Significantly different from all other means at $P < .01$ but not different from each other.

Strain SM/J is deficient in liver neuraminidase relative to other inbred strains. F_1 hybrids between SM/J and C57BL/6J are of intermediate activity. A backcross of F_1 animals to SM/J produces two phenotypic classes, low and intermediate, and the F_2 generation of this cross demonstrates the three phenotypic classes expected in the segregation of a single autosomal locus with co-dominant expression (Womack *et al.*, 1981). We have designated this locus neuraminidase-1 (*Neu-1*).

Strain SM/J has about 15 percent of the activity of most other strains. An extremely labile component that comprises about 85 percent of the C57BL/6J activity is absent in SM/J (Potier et al., 1979b).

Low activity in the congenic strain B10.SM(70NS)/Sn (Table 1) suggests that the gene for liver neuraminidase activity is on chromosome 17. This strain was constructed by backcrossing the H-2 locus of strain SM/J onto strain C57BL/10Sn and then inbreeding. The Neu-1 gene of SM/J, presumably near H-2, was incorporated into the congenic strain along with the SM/J H-2 haplotype. Backcrosses and intercrosses support either identity or extremely close linkage of Neu-1 with Apl and Map-2. No recombinants have occurred between these three loci in 52 F_2 and 51 backcross offspring (Womack et al., 1981)

We propose that Neu-1, Apl, and Map-2 are one and the same gene. Variation in liver arylsulfatase-B and α-glucosidase are likely pleiotropic manifestations of this gene as well. A model in which neuraminidase deficiency accounts for genetic variation in multiple enzymes has several requirements: (1) the strain distributions of neuraminidase activity and alleles at the other loci must be identical, (2) neuraminidase activity must be inherited as a single gene on the same chromosome to which variation of the other enzymes has been mapped, and (3) there should be no genetic recombination between neuraminidase activity and the other variants in segregating crosses. These conditions appear to be met.

A number of inherited human diseases including mucolipidoses I, II, and III (Cantz et al., 1977; Kelly and Graetz, 1977; Spranger et al., 1977; Thomas et al., 1976; Strecker et al., 1976) and cherry-red spot myoclonus syndrome with or without dementia (Wenger et al., 1978; O'Brien, 1977), are associated with neuraminidase deficiency. While it is yet unclear how neuraminidase deficiency in healthy SM/J mice relates to these diseases, the Neu-1 locus will likely be useful for defining the role of neuraminidase in enzyme processing. Also, the SM/J mouse is a potentially valuable model for enzyme replacement therapy. Successful delivery and subsequent function of the missing enzyme should result in conversion of electrophoretic patterns of acid phosphatase, α-mannosidase, arylsulfatase-B, and α-glucosidase to to that of the lesser sialylated forms of most mouse strains.

Supported by grants from the March of Dimes Birth Defects Foundation and the Medical Research Council of Canada.

References:
Cantz M, Gehler J, Spranger J (1977). Mucolipidosis I: increased sialic acid content and deficiency of α-N-acetylneuraminidase in cultured fibroblasts. Biochem Biophys Res Commun 74:732.

Daniel WL, Womack JE, Henthorn PS (1981). Murine liver arylsulfatase B processing influenced by region on chromosome 17. Biochem Genet 19:211.

Dizik M, Elliot RW (1978). A second gene affecting the sialylation of lysosomal α-mannosidase in mouse liver. Biochem Genet 16:247.

Kelly TE, Graetz G (1977). Isolated acid neuraminidase deficiency: a distinct lysosomal storage disease. Amer J Med Genet 1:31.

Lalley PA, Shows TB (1977). Lysosomal acid phosphatase deficiency: liver specific variant in the mouse. Genetics 87:305.

O'Brien JS (1977). Neuraminidase deficiency in the cherry-red spot-myolconus syndrome. Biochem Biophys Res Commun 79:1136.

Peters J, Swallow DM (1979). Private communication. Mouse News Lett 60:46.

Potier M, Mameli L, Belisle M, Dallaire L, Melancon, SB (1979a). Fluorometric assay of neuraminidase with a sodium (4-methylumbelliferyl-α-D-N-acetylneuraminate) substrate Anal Biochem 94:287.

Potier M, Yan DLS, Womack JE (1979b). Neuraminidase deficiency in the mouse. FEBS Lett 108:345.

Spranger, J, Gehler J, Cantz M (1977). Mucolipidosis I-A sialidosis. Am J Med Genet 1:21.

Strecker G, Michalski JC, Montreuil J, Farraux JP (1976). Defect in neuraminidase associated with mucolipidosis II (I-cell disease), Biomed Exp 25:238.

Thomas GH, Tiller GE Jr, Reynolds LW, Miller CS, Brace JW (1977). Increased levels of sialic acid associated with a sialidase deficiency in I cell disease (mucolipidosis II) fibroblasts. Biochem Biophys Res Commun 71:188.

Wegner DA, Tarby TJ, Wharton C (1978). Macular cherry-red spots and myoclonus with dementia: co-existent neuraminidase and β-galactosidase deficiencies. Biochem Biophys Res Commun 82:589.

Womack JE, Yan DLS, Potier M (1981). Gene for neuraminidase activity on mouse chromosome 17 near H-2: pleiotropic effects on multiple hydrolases. Science 212:63.

SECTION IV.
INBORN ERRORS OF CONNECTIVE AND EPIDERMAL TISSUES

Animal Models of Inherited Metabolic Diseases, pages 229-244
© 1982 Alan R. Liss, Inc., 150 Fifth Avenue, New York, NY 10011

ANIMAL MODELS OF COLLAGEN DISEASE

G. A. Hegreberg

Department of Veterinary Microbiology and Pathology
Washington State University
Pullman, WA 99164

INTRODUCTION

Inherited collagen disorders are a family of genetic
entities in which changes in the structural and functional
integrity of the tissues result from a primary collagen
defect, especially involving collagen formation and maturation. These inherited disorders should not be confused with
a group of chronic degenerative disorders, also termed
collagen diseases, but which are accompanied by fibrinoid
degeneration of apparently properly formed and matured
collagen (Klemperer, Pollack, and Baehr, 1942). Included in
this group of chronic degenerative diseases are systemic
lupus erythematosus, dermatomyositis, and periarteritis
nodosa.

Inherited collagen disorders were originally recognized
using clinical, genetic, and morphologic criteria; however,
biochemical alterations have been identified in some members
of this group, and these biochemical changes have provided a
more finite basis for the identification and subclassifica-
tion of these diseases. Although the primary alteration may
involve either the biosynthesis or degradation of collagen,
defects in the biosynthetic formation or maturation of collagen are thus far the most commonly recognized sites of the
molecular defects.

A number of inherited collagen disorders have been identified in people, including the following:

Ehlers-Danlos syndromes (ED-S), including types I
   through VII
Marfan's syndrome
Osteogenesis imperfecta, including congenita and
   tarda forms
Cutis laxa
Menke's kinky hair syndrome
Of the above collagen disorders, only a few types of the
Ehlers-Danlos syndrome have been well defined in animals
(Table I).

This discussion will concentrate on a brief discussion
of collagen metabolism and on comparisons of the ED-S of
people and animals. A great portion of both the understanding and research direction of inherited collagen disorders is
based on recent findings which have defined a number of
important molecular events in collagen biosynthesis. Several
excellent reviews are available which discuss this subject
thoroughly (Bornstein, 1974; Nimni, 1974; Uitto and
Lichtenstein, 1976; Piez, 1976; Pinnell, 1978). The following
is a brief review of these processes.

The biosynthesis of each collagen polypeptide chain is a
multi-step process involving, in part, a classical series of
transcriptional and translational steps (Bornstein, 1974).
Collagen is rather unique in several respects, especially
relating to composition of the primary structure and to posttranslational modifications. Collagen has an unusually high
content of glycine, proline, and lysine and is also characterized by the presence of two amino acids, hydroxyproline
and hydroxylysine.

Collagen is synthesized in a precursor form (procollagen)
and this precursor is characterized by both amino and carboxy
end extensions (Bellamy and Bornstein, 1971; Jimenez, Dehm,
and Prockop, 1971; Martin, Byers, and Piez, 1975). The
extensions differ considerably in their amino acid composition from the parent helical portion of the polypeptide and
are enzymatically cleaved extracellularly prior to assembly
of the collagen molecules into fibrils. The function of the
extensions is believed to involve the stabilization of three
polypeptide chains in order to form the triple helical molecule and the proper movement and alignment of the collagen
molecule both intra- and extracellularly.

Table 1. Summary of ED-S Types in People and Animals

ED-S Type	Species	Inheritance	Clinical Signs	Biochemical Defect
I-III	Human beings, dogs, cats, mink	Autosomal dominant	Type I - skin fragility, skin and joint hyperextensibility, skin laxity Type II - similar to type I, however manifestations are milder Type III - joint hypermobility, minimal skin fragility and hyperextensibility	Unknown
IV	Human beings	Autosomal recessive	Thin, easily bruised skin, rupture of large blood vessels and bowel	Altered metabolism of type III collagen
V	Human beings	Sex-linked recessive	Skin fragility and bruisability, hyperextensibility of skin and joints, cardiac valvular defects, short stature	Lysyl oxidase deficiency?
V	Mice	Sex-linked recessive	Fragile skin, aortic aneurysms, bone abnormalities	Lysyl oxidase deficiency
VI	Human beings	Autosomal recessive	Thin, hyperextensible, easily bruised skin; corneal collagen weakness; long, slender digits; kyphoscoliosis	Lysyl hydroxylase deficiency
VII	Human beings	Autosomal dominant	Skin hyperelasticity but not fragility; severe joint laxity and dislocation; short stature	Structural mutation of pro-alpha$_2$ collagen
VII	Cattle, sheep, cat	Autosomal recessive (cattle and sheep)	Severe skin fragility	Procollagen N-protease deficiency

The synthesis of the precursor polypeptide chain is
followed by a series of reactions which modify the polypeptide chain both intracellularly (including glycosylation and
hydroxylation of certain prolyl and lysyl residues in the
polypeptide chain) and a series of modifications which occur
exterior to the cell (conversion of procollagen to collagen),
oxidation of the epsilon amino group of certain lysyl and
hydroxylysyl residues, and intra- and intermolecular cross-
link formation. These post-translational polypeptide modifications are essential for the maturation of collagen.

It is recognized that collagen in different parts of the
body has different chemical compositions, and at least 4
different molecular species of collagen are now recognized.
Type I collagen predominates in the skin, tendon, dentin,
and bone. This molecule is composed of 2 identical polypeptide chains termed $alpha_1$ (I) and a similar but distinct
polypeptide termed $alpha_2$ (I) (Click and Bornstein, 1970).
Type II collagen is found primarily in cartilage, and the
molecule consists of three identical polypeptides termed
$alpha_1$ (II) (Miller and Lunde, 1973). Type III collagen has
been isolated from fetal skin and blood vessels and in other
tissues which are rich in type I collagen (Chung and Miller,
1974). The type III collagen molecule is solely composed of
the $alpha_1$ (III) monomeric unit. Type IV collagen is found
primarily in basement membrane. Variations in the hydroxylysine, cysteine, and carbohydrate content are among the
differences which distinguish the various types of collagen.

EHLERS-DANLOS SYNDROME, TYPES I, II, AND III

People

In the early 1900's, Ehlers and Danlos independently
recognized a syndrome in people characterized by a triad of
cardinal clinical signs, including skin fragility and hyperextensibility, and joint hyperextensibility. Skin fragility
was considered to be the most distinctive clinical manifestation of this syndrome. In many cases, the collagen defect
appeared to be restricted to the skin; however, some ED-S
patients exhibit connective tissue defects in other organ
systems, including the ocular, cardiovascular, respiratory,
gastrointestinal, and central and peripheral nervous systems.
Ehlers and Danlos recognized a familial pattern of transmission of the syndrome, and the mode of inheritance of the
classical form of the disease was later shown to be autosomal
dominant.

Three similar but distinct forms of the ED-S in people, all inherited as autosomal dominant traits, are now recognized, and they have been designated types I, II, and III (Pinnell, 1978; Bornstein and Byers, 1980). Type I, also referred to as the gravis form, is accompanied by the most severe connective tissue changes, including very fragile and hyperextensible skin; thin, poorly contracted scars; and prominent joint hypermobility. Hernias, varicose veins, prolapse of mitral valves, vascular fragility, and other weaknesses related to the connective tissue weakness may be observed as clinical manifestations.

Type II (mitis) is accompanied by many of the same clinical changes observed in type I ED-S, but these changes are less severe than the type I clinical changes. The skin fragility and thin, poorly contracted scars found in type I ED-S are not a prominent feature of the type II ED-S. Type III ED-S, also termed familial benign joint hypermobility, is accompanied primarily by joint hypermobility with minimal skin fragility or hyperextensibility.

The major dermal changes observed in the ED-S include quantitative change in the amount of collagen, and occasionally elastin, and alterations in the appearance of collagen and elastin. Normally, the syncytium of highly cross-linked collagen bundles limits the movement of fibrous connective tissue. The hyperextensibility and decreased tensile strength of the skin in the ED-S was first explained on the basis of altered collagen arrangement in which freely movable collagen bundles, lacking proper cross-linking, could slide across each other.

Recent studies have demonstrated ultrastructural changes in dermal collagen fibrils from cases of ED-S type I (Vogel et al, 1979). In cross-section, the collagen fibrils from these patients varied in diameter with the presence of unusually large-diametered fibrils. The contours of many fibrils were irregular and lobular in appearance. In longitudinal plane, the collagen fibrils had an unraveled appearance because of the poorly integrated filamentous components of the fibril. The periodicity of the fibrils from affected individuals did not appear to be altered.

The biochemical derrangement in the ED-S, types I, II and III has not been determined, however, it is believed to involve type I collagen, because the connective tissue weakness predominates in those tissues with high concentrations of that collagen type.

Animals

A condition in dogs characterized by severe skin weakness was described independently by Arlein and Wall in 1947. The dog presented to Wall was a male 1-year-old Manchester terrier with skin laxity, especially prominent on the legs. Histopathologic changes in the skin included thinning of the epidermis, absence of adnexal glands, and thinning and sparsity of elastic fibers in the dermis. The case reported by Arlein involved a Spitz-cross 11-month-old female, presented because of a foot laceration. The skin in this affected dog was soft, putty-like, and extremely fragile.

Since these original reports, dominantly transmitted forms of the ED-S have been reported in dogs and mink (Hegreberg, et al, 1969, 1970a, 1970b) and cats (Patterson and Minor, 1977). Skin fragility, skin laxity, and skin hyperextensibility form distinguishing clinical characteristics of the condition in these species. In the disorder in dogs and mink, skin fragility was the most pronounced and consistent clinical feature. Multiple skin lacerations were observed. The skin fragility was generalized throughout the skin in the affected dogs and was of sufficient magnitude that the skin tore with minimal force. The tensile strength of the skin of affected dogs was only 4% that of nonaffected dogs of the same age, sex and breed. Numerous naturally occurring, broad, shallow scars were evidence of healed lacerations in the affected dogs. The rate of wound healing in the affected dogs and mink was not appreciably different from nonaffected animals, providing that adequate approximation of the wound edges was maintained to facilitate primary healing.

Hyperextensibility of the skin has been noted in the affected dogs and mink reported by Hegreberg and workers (1970a; 1970b). Skin laxity varied in severity among the individual affected animals, but was more pronounced in the older dogs. The skin laxity was especially noticeable about the head, legs, and rump. Clinical abnormalities noted in the affected dogs in areas other than the skin included umbilical and inguinal hernias, luxated patellas, and rectal prolapses. These clinical changes were not observed in affected mink.

An autosomal dominant mode of inheritance was defined in dogs and mink (Hegreberg et al, 1969) and cats (Patterson and Minor, 1977) with the ED-S. In the dog and mink studies, both affected and nonaffected F_1 generation offspring were produced from affected dam to affected sire matings, indicating that the disease was not recessive. Approximately 57% of the puppies and 51% of the mink kits from affected sire to nonaffected dam matings were affected. The trait was autosomal in both dogs and mink, and no significant differences were noted in the sex distribution of the disease in either the affected dogs or mink.

It appears that the gene involved in this dominant form of the ED-S of dogs was transmitted with complete penetrance. In dogs, nonaffected F_1 generation offspring from affected dam to affected sire matings did not produce affected F_2 generation offspring, indicating that the affected dam and sire were heterozygotes. When one affected canine sire was mated to several nonaffected females, approximately 50% of the offspring were affected, a 1:1 ratio which would be expected in heterozygote to nonaffected matings when the penetrance was complete. Nonaffected F_1 generation offspring (F_1 generation derived from affected to affected or affected to nonaffected matings) have never transmitted the defect to their F_2 progeny, indicating that these dogs were not carrying the ED-S gene.

Histologically, dermal collagen bundles from affected dogs and mink were fragmented and frayed, as opposed to the homogeneous and uniformly sized collagen bundles of the normal dermis (Hegreberg et al, 1970b). Collagen bundles were haphazardly arranged, some areas having a whorled appearance, and lacked the syncytoid interlacing arrangement seen in the normal dermis. Some collagen bundles were small in diameter (3 to 4 u) and appeared as fibrillar strands, whereas other collagen bundles were larger than normal, measuring up to 40 u in diameter. Optical changes were not apparent in the skin of cats affected with the ED-S (Patterson and Minor, 1977).

Ultrastructurally, the collagen fibrils from affected dogs and mink demonstrated variation in fiber diameter size and an irregular, branching appearance of the fibril in longitudinal profile. These alterations in organization of the collagen bundles were also observed in samples examined by scanning electron microscopy (SEM). The bundle size was small, and bundles lacked the tight, interwoven appearance of the collagen bundles from the normal dogs (Holbrook et al, 1978). Electron microscopic changes in the feline ED-S have been reported, and these changes included formation of large, irregular fibrils with indistinct banding pattern in the fiber centers. Also, there was a population of larger fibrils which gave a bimodal distribution to the fibril diameter size, and fibril packing was disorganized (Patterson and Minor, 1977).

Biochemical studies revealed that an increased quantity of collagen was solubilized in acetic acid from affected dogs and mink, suggesting a possible defect in formation or stabilization of intermolecular collagen cross-links (Hegreberg, Padgett, and Page, 1970). The levels of biosynthetic enzymes of collagen metabolism, including prolyl hydroxylase and lysyl oxidase from the dermis of affected mink, were not decreased in activity (Counts, Knighten, and Hegreberg, 1977).

On the basis of clinical and genetic characteristics, the dominant forms of the ED-S in dogs, mink and cats resemble most closely types I and II of the human ED-S classification, those which are accompanied by prominent skin fragility and hyperextensibility. Before more definitive comparisons can be made, it will be necessary to define the primary biochemical defect in both the human and animal forms.

EHLERS-DANLOS SYNDROME, TYPE IV
Type IV ED-S has been reported in people as a clinically and genetically heterogeneous group of disorders involving a defect in the metabolism of type III collagen. Recent reports indicate that type III procollagen is synthesized but cannot be secreted from the cell, resulting in severe dilation of the endoplasmic reticulum with the collagen precursor (Holbrook and Byers, 1981, Byers et al, 1981). This form of the ED-S has not been reported in animals.

EHLERS-DANLOS SYNDROME, TYPE V

People
Type V ED-S of people is a sex-linked recessive trait characterized by minimal to moderate skin fragility with easy bruisability, hyperextensibility of the skin and joints,

cardiac valvular defects, and short stature (Beighton, 1970). Lysyl oxidase has been reported to be deficient in type V ED-S (DiFerrante et al, 1975). This enzyme catalyzes the oxidative deamination of lysine and possibly hydroxylysine residues to form reactive aldehydes which are necessary to form intra- and inter-molecular collagen and elastin crosslinks.

Animals
    An inherited collagen disorder has been recognized in the mouse as a sex-linked trait associated with the mottled coat color (Rowe et al, 1974). The disorder is accompanied by reduced tensile strength of skin, development of aortic aneurysms, and bone abnormalities.

    Rowe and workers (1977) demonstrated that mice with this trait have biochemical changes similar to those described in the human ED-S type V. These changes include a marked increase in the extractability of collagen, an elevation in the alpha to beta chain ratio, and a decrease in the lysine-derived aldehyde content of purified skin collagen and aortic elastic tissue. The levels of lysyl oxidase activity in the skin of the mottled mouse were found to be significantly reduced.

EHLERS-DANLOS SYNDROME, TYPE VI
    Type VI ED-S is an autosomal recessive trait which is clinically accompanied by skin and bone changes including thinned, hyperextensible, easily bruised skin, weakening of the cornea of the eye resulting in ketatoconus, elongated slender fingers and toes, and malformations of the vertebral column resulting in kyphoscoliosis (Pinnell et al, 1972; Pinnell, 1978). Lysyl hydroxylase, which catalyzes the hydroxylation of lysyl residues, is deficient in the ED-S type VI (Pinnel et al, 1972; Bornstein and Byers, 1980). Hydroxylysine is an important component of collagen, contributing functionally to the collagen intermolecular crosslinks. No animal model for this human disorder has been reported.

EHLERS-DANLOS SYNDROME, TYPE VII

People
    Type VII ED-S, formerly termed arthroclasis multiplex congenita, is accompanied by severe joint hypermobility and associated congenital hip subluxations, soft, hyperelastic

skin, and short stature (Lichtenstein et al, 1973). This form of the ED-S is not accompanied by the severe skin fragility observed in some of the other forms of the ED-S. Biochemical studies revealed that there was an accumulation of type I procollagen in which the amino terminus of the procollagen alpha$_2$ chains was improperly cleaved (Steinmann et al, 1980). The persistence of procollagen in this disorder is believed to result from a structural mutation at the site of cleavage of the amino terminus of the procollagen, rather than a deficiency of or decreased activity of the enzyme responsible for cleavage of this portion of the procollagen molecule, termed procollagen N-protease.

Animals

Dermatosparaxia is an autosomal recessive disorder, initially described by Hanset and Ansay (1967) in cattle from the central and high regions of Belgium. The disorder was clinically characterized by extreme skin fragility and impaired healing of skin wounds. Although the skin has reduced tensile strength, other structures composed of fibrous connective tissue, such as blood vessels, do not appear to be appreciably altered. An apparently identical defect has been identified in Norway as an autosomal recessive trait in sheep (Fjolstad and Helle, 1974). Affected lambs have extensive skin lacerations, especially of the legs and neck. Skin tensile strength is markedly reduced, along with certain internal organs, such as the intestinal tract and blood vessels. A similar disorder has been identified in a cat and is accompanied by thin, fragile skin (Holbrook et al, 1980, Counts et al, 1980).

In all three species, the skin from the affected animals was characterized ultrastructurally by collagen bundles with an unraveled, tangled appearance of the collagen fibrils. This was opposed to the tightly and parallel aligned fibrils in the collagen bundles from nonaffected animals. In cross-section, the collagen fibrils showed a wide range of bizarre shapes, similar to hieroglyphic figures and apparently characteristic for this disorder.

Dermatosparaxia in cattle, sheep, and the cat was accompanied by an elevation of procollagen in the skin. In this respect, dermatosparaxia resembles ED-S type VII of people, however the disorder in cattle, sheep, and the cat resulted from a deficiency of procollagen N-protease rather than a structural mutation in the procollagen molecule as occurs in the human disease (Lapiere, Lenaers, and Kohn, 1971; Becker et al, 1976; Counts et al, 1980). The accumulation of procollagen in the skin is believed to be responsible for the marked decrease in tensile strength of this tissue.

ACKNOWLEDGEMENTS

This study was supported by NIH grants RR00515, AG00030, and FR5465.

REFERENCES

Arlein MS (1947). Generalized acute cutaneous asthesia in a dog. JAVMA 111:52.

Becker U, Timpl R, Helle O, Prockop DJ (1976). NH_2 terminal extensions on skin collagen from sheep with a genetic defect in conversion of procollagen into collagen. Biochemistry 15:2853.

Beighton P (1970). "The Ehlers-Danlos Syndrome." London: William Heinemann.

Bellamy G, Bornstein P (1971). Evidence for procollagen, a biosynthetic precursor of collagen. Proc Natl Acad Sci 68:1138.

Bornstein P (1974). The biosynthesis of collagen. Ann Rev Biochem 43:567.

Bornstein P, Byers P (1980). Collagen metabolism. In "Current Concepts," Kalamazoo, Mich.: Upjohn Co.

Byers PH, Holbrook KA, McGillivray B, Macleod PM, Lowry RB (1979). Clinical and ultrastructural heterogeneity of IV Ehlers-Danlos syndrome. Hum Genet 47:141.

Byers PH, Holbrook KA, Barsh GS, Smith LT, Bornstein P (1981). Altered secretion of type III procollagen in a form of type IV Ehlers-Danlos syndrome. Lab Invest 44:336.

Chung E, Miller EJ (1974). Collagen polymorphism: characterization of molecules with the chain composition $[\alpha P(III)]_3$ in human tissues. Science 183:1200.

Click EM, Bornstein P (1970). Isolation and characterization of the cyanogen bromide peptides from the α_1 and α_2 chains of human skin collagen. Biochemistry 9:4699.

Counts DF, Byers PH, Holbrook KA, Hegreberg GA (1980). Dermatosparaxis in a Himalayan cat: I. Biochemical studies of dermal collagen. J Invest Dermatol 74:96.

Counts D, Knighten P, Hegreberg GA (1977). Biochemical changes in the skin of mink with Ehlers-Danlos syndrome: Increased collagen biosynthesis in the dermis of affected mink. J Invest Dermatol 69:521.

Daniels JR, Chu GH (1975). Basement membrane collagen of renal glomerulus. J Biol Chem 250:3531.

DiFerrante N, Leachman RD, Angelini P, Donnelly PV, Francis G, Almazan A, Segni G, Franzblau C, Jordan RE (1975). Ehlers-Danlos type V (X-linked form): A lysyl oxidase deficiency. Birth Defects 11:31.

Fjolstad M, Helle O (1974). A hereditary dysplasia of collagen tissues in sheep. J Pathol 112:183.

Hanset R, Ansay M (1967). Dermatosparaxia (peau déchîrée) chez le veau: au defaut général du conjonctif, de nature héréditaire. Ann Med Vet 7:451.

Hegreberg GA, Padgett GA, Gorham JR, Henson JB (1969). A connective tissue disease of dogs and mink resembling the Ehlers-Danlos syndrome of man. II. Mode of inheritance. J Hered 60:249.

Hegreberg GA, Padgett GA, Henson JB (1970a). A heritable connective tissue disease of dogs and mink resembling the Ehlers-Danlos syndrome of man. III. Histopathologic changes of the skin. Arch Pathol 90:159.

Hegreberg GA, Padgett GA, Ott RL, Henson JB (1970b). A heritable connective tissue disease of dogs and mink resembling the Ehlers-Danlos syndrome of man. I. Skin tensile strength properties. J Invest Dermatol 54:377.

Hegreberg GA, Padgett GA, Page RC (1970c). The Ehlers-Danlos syndrome of dogs and mink. Symp Proc III. Animal Models for Biomedical Research, Nat Acad Sci, pp 80-90.

Holbrook K, Byers PH (1981). Ultrastructural characteristics of the skin in a form of the Ehlers-Danlos syndrome type IV. Lab Invest 44:342.

Holbrook KA, Byers PH, Counts DF, Hegreberg GA (1980). Dermatosparaxis in a Himalayan cat: II. Ultrastructural studies of dermal collagen. J Invest Dermatol 74:100.

Holbrook KA, Byers P, Hegreberg GA, Counts D (1978). Altered collagen fibrils in skin of animals with inherited connective tissue disorders. Anat Rec 190:424.

Jimenez SA, Dehm P, Prockop DJ (1971). Further evidence for a transport form of collagen. Its extrusion and extracellular conversion to tropocollagen in embryonic tendon. FEBS Lett 17:245.

Klemperer P, Pollack AD, Baehr G (1942). Diffuse collagen disease. Acute Disseminated lupus erythematosus and diffuse scleroderm. JAMA 119:331.

Lapiere CM, Lenaers A, Kohn LD (1971). Procollagen peptidase: An enzyme excising the coordination peptides of collagen. Proc Natl Acad Sci 68:3054.

Lichtenstein J, Kohn L, Byers P, Martin GR, McKusick VA (1973). Procollagen peptidase deficiency in a form of the Ehlers-Danlos syndrome. Trans Assoc Am Physicians 86:333.

McKusick VA (1972). "Heritable Disorders of Connective Tissue," St. Louis: CV Mosby.

Martin GR, Byers PH, Piez KA (1975). Procollagen. Adv Enzymol 42:167.

Miller EJ, Lunde LG (1973). Isolation and characterization of the cyanogen bromide peptides from the $\alpha 1(II)$ chain of bovine and human cartilage collagen. Biochemistry 12:3153.

Nimni ME (1974). Collagen: Its structure in normal and pathological connective tissues. Semin Arthritis Rheum 4:95.

Patterson DF, Minor RR (1977). Hereditary fragility and hyperextensibility of the skin of cats. A defect in collagen fibrillogenesis. Lab Invest 37:170.

Piez K (1976). Primary structure. Ranachandran GN and Reddi AH (eds.): "Biochemistry of Collagens," New York: Plenum, p 1.

Pinnell SR (1978). Disorders in collagen. In Stanbury JB, Wyngaarden JB, Fredrickson DS (eds.): "Metabolic Basis of Inherited Disease," New York: McGraw-Hill, p 1366.

Pinnell SR, Krane SM, Kenzora JE, Glimscher MJ (1972). A heritable disorder of connective tissue. N Engl J Med 286:1013.

Rowe DW, McGoodwin EB, Martin GR, Grahn D (1977). Decreased lysyl oxidase activity in the aneurysm-prone, mottled mouse. J Biol Chem 252:939.

Rowe DW, McGoodwin EB, Martin GR, Sussman MD, Grahn D, Faris B, Franzblau C (1974). A sex-linked defect in the cross-linking of collagen and elastin associated with the mottled locus in mice. J Exp Med 139:180.

Steinmann B, Tuderman L, Peltonen L, Martin G, McKusick VA, Prockop DJ (1980). Evidence for a structural mutation of procollagen type I in a patient with the Ehlers-Danlos syndrome type VII. J Biol Chem 255:8887.

Uitto J, Lichtenstein JR (1976). Defects in the bioche-
    mistry of collagen in diseases of connective tissue. J
    Invest Dermatol 66:59.
Vogel A, Holbrook KA, Steinmann B, Gitzelmann R, Byers P
    (1979). Abnormal collagen fibril structure in the
    gravis form (Type I) of Ehlers-Danlos syndrome. Lab
    Invest 40:201.
Wall RD (1947). Congenital defects of the skin. North
    Amer Vet 28:166.

DR. JOLLY: Two comments, one to Dr. Hegreberg and one to Dr. Desnick.   Firstly, dermatosparaxis also occurs in sheep in New Zealand, and secondly, α_1-antitrypsin deficiency has been described in the horse, and I believe in the turkey.

DR. DESNICK: Unfortunately the turkey model isn't a real model of α_1-antitrypsin deficiency.

DR. JOLLY: I suspected that, but it has been described in the horse.

DR. LEWIS: On the basis of the molecular defect in the various types of Ehlers-Danlos syndrome in animals, would you consider these models to be analogues or homologues of the human disease?

DR. HEGREBERG: I think that at this point we have to say that other than the lysyl oxidase deficiency in the mouse they are all analogues.   Certainly, dermatosparaxis has a different molecular mechanism, and the type I through type III of Ehlers-Danlos lack biochemical identification of the primary defect.   Thus, at this point they can only be called analogues of the human disorders.

DR. LEWIS: The other question I wanted to raise is the peculiar distribution of the lesions in the varying types of Ehlers-Danlos syndrome.   Is it entirely based on the normal anatomic distribution of the different collagen types?

DR. HEGREBERG: Yes, in part.   Certainly type IV ED-S with its marked clinical manifestations involving the blood vessels is an example, in that it involves type III collagen, a collagen rather characteristic of those tissues.

DR. J. SMITH: Have you tried to look at carriers for the dermatosparaxis by enzyme assay?

DR. HEGREBERG: Unfortunately, the cases of dermatosparaxis that we have obtained have been isolated cases, and the cat represented a case in which we could not trace the parentage.

DR. J. SMITH: Do you think it would be possible to measure the enzyme quantitatively?   When you must depend on extracts, it would seem to be difficult.

DR. HEGREBERG: The assay, although not particularly difficult to perform, is crude and probably would not be too useful for carrier detection.

DR. PATTERSON: You mentioned a couple of times the similarity between the cat dominant Ehlers-Danlos-like defect and that in the dog, and I certainly would agree.   I had not seen your scanning EM pictures before, but they are very nice.   They do look rather similar at that level.   As you know, Ron Minor and I have hypothesized that this might be a defect in collagen fibrillogenesis due to a mutation in the structural gene for one of the collagen polypeptide chains. Ron is still working on the biochemical characterization of this disease, but there is one other piece of information that we have come up with since our original paper, and I wondered if you had observed something similar. When we mate heterozygotes, if we do a large series, we find that there is a decreased litter size, and if you look at the uterus early in gestation you find about one-fourth of the sites are reabsorbing. This indicates that the homozygous state is lethal.

As you know, if you look at the distribution of collagen fibril diameters by EM in heterozygotes you find that there are two populations, one larger than the other. This fits a model in which you have one mutant gene at the relevant locus. Homozygotes presumably are making all abnormal collagen, leading to lethality.

I wondered if you had observed any evidence of embryonic death in the dominant dog model.

DR. HEGREBERG: We have suspected that this is occurring with our heterozygote-heterozygote matings of the dominantly inherited canine disorder. We do not yet have enough offspring to really substantiate this. We have not visualized and counted the number of developing embryos early in gestation.

DR. PATTERSON: In the cat, they seem to die rather early. I have been trying to remove embryonic material to get cell cultures, but so far I have not been successful.

DR. HEGREBERG: I think that is a very important observation.

DR. DESNICK: I would like to make a further comment on the mechanism of dominant defects. Among human genetic diseases, a great number are dominant, expressed in the heterozygous condition. However, we do not know much about the molecular mechanisms leading to their pathology. It is important to note that the animal models provide the opportunity to make matings to get the homoallelic defect expressed. Such matings ought to be pursued since these animals may provide important insights into the mechanisms of dominantly inherited disorders.

DR. BUSS: Do you find that one sex is favored in the incidence for any of the defects that you have described?

DR. HEGREBERG: The expression appears to be manifested in both sexes, and as far as we can tell the degree of severity of the disorder does not really have a sex predilection.

Animal Models of Inherited Metabolic Diseases, pages 245-249

BRACHYMORPHIC (bmm/bmm) CARTILAGE MATRIX DEFICIENCY
(cmd/cmd) AND DISPROPORTIONATE MICROMELIA
(Dmm/Dmm); THREE INBORN ERRORS OF CARTILAGE
BIOSYNTHESIS IN MICE

Kenneth S. Brown and Leslie Harne
Laboratory of Development Biology and
  Anomalies
National Instititute of Dental Research
Bethesda, Maryland

The synthesis of cartilage matrix underlies
skeletal form and growth in two ways.
Prechondrogenic mesenchyme cells of the limb bud
and axial skeleton condense, differentiate into
chondrocytes, and form cartilage models of the limb
bones and vertebrae by the synthesis of a
characteristic extracellular matrix. Subsequent
linear growth of these endochondral skeletal
elements occurs at the epiphyseal growth plate
through the multiplication of chondrocytes, active
synthesis of extracellular matrix and its
replacement by bone (Hall 1978, Brighton 1978).

More than 70 constitutional disorders of skeletal
development of man are known to be inherited
(McKusick 1975), but only a dozen or so are known
to be associated with specific metabolic defects;
the mucopolysaccharidoses, mucolipidoses, hypophos-
phatasias, hypophosphatemiemia, pseudohypoparathyroidism, and hypothyroidism. Most human
dwarfisms are recognized only by distintive
clinical findings such as radiographic features,
genetic pattern, whether they are detectable at
birth, in the first year, or in later childhood or
adoles-cence, and whether they have short limbs,
short trunk or normal body proportions (Smith
1976).

We have recently studied several syndromes of
chondrodystrophic dwarfism in mice which provide

Some molecular basis for understanding the clinical patterns of dwarfism. Brachymorphic (bm), an autosomal recessive dwarfism, has full adult viability and fertility but 10% risk of incisor malocclusion due to relatively short maxilla. Achondroplastia (cn), an autosomal recessive, is somewhat more severe than (bm) with reduced viability and infertility and occasional newborn lethality due to cleft palate (Lane and Dickie 1968). Cartilage matrix deficiency (cmd), is an autosomal recessive newborn lethal with cleft palate and respiratory failure secondary to trechea cartilage defect, and severe limb and tail shortening (Rittenhouse et al 1978). Disproportionate micromelia (Dmm), is an autosomal incomplete dominant (Brown et al 1981). Dmm/Dmm newborn resemble cmd/cmd and Dmm/+ are fully viable and fertile dwarfs with disproportionate shortening of the humerus and femur.

The biochemical bases for the skeletal growth disturbances in bm/bm, cmd/cmd and Dmm/Dmm are specific errors of cartilage matrix biosynthesis. No structural error was found in the collagen or proteoglycan of cn/cn matrix (Kleinman, Pennypacker and Brown 1977).

The defects of bm/bm and cmd/cmd were in proteoglycan biosynthesis and their matrix was characterized by reduced volume but normal structural strength. The defect of cmd/cmd was found to be the failure of synthesis of the core protein of the cartilage sepcific large proteoglycan (Kimata et al 1981). This resulted in a great reduction of cartilage matrix volume and disorganization of the epiphyseal growth plate (Rittenhouse et al 1978). The defect of bm/bm was generalized undersulfation of the glycosaminoglycans (Orkin, Pratt and Martin 1976) due to a generalized defect in the synthesis of PAPS, the sulfate donor (Pennypacker, Kimata and Brown 1981) which was rate limiting primarily for cartilage matrix biosynthesis particularily in the reduced proliferative zone of the growth plate (Greene, Brown and Pratt 1978).

In both these mutants type II collagen was made in reduced amounts but was normal in proportion to type I.

In Dmm/Dmm and Dmm/+ there is also a significant reduction of the growth plate in Dmm/Dmm and a shortening of the proliferative zone in Dmm/+. There is no structural abnormality of proteoglycan in these mutants and the cartilage matrix of Dmm/Dmm is relatively weak in contrast with cmd/cmd. There is a significant reduction in the ratio of type II to type I collagen in the Dmm/Dmm cartilage matrix as measured by electrophoresis and by immunofluorescence. Further, the type II collagen present appears to be localized in a pericellular distribution rather than throughout the extracellular matrix as in normal or cmd/cmd cartilage. The mouse mutant cho/cho, chondrodysplasia, shows great morphological, histological and cartilage structure similarities to Dmm/Dmm but has a different collagen abnormality (Seegmiller, Fraser and Sheldon 1971)and is not allelic to Dmm.

These observations suggest the following general conclusions:

1. Many different defects of the biosynthesis of cartilage matrix can result in dwarfism.

2. The clinical type of dwarfism may depend on the effect on cartilage matrix of the specific biochemical defect. A type II collagen defect reduces growth plate organization and matrix strength with a rhizomelic growth disturbance in Dmm/Dmm. A cartilage specific proteoglycan defect, whether of the core protein as in cmd/cmd, or of sulfation of glycosaminoglycans as in bm/bm reduces matrix volume but not matrix strength and results in a mesomelic growth disturbance.

3. When cartilage matrix biosynthesis is severely defective the clinical phenotypes are very similar regardless of the specific biochemical defect since it is growth plate function which

controls bone growth.

4. Dwarfism may result from a defect of a molecule
   specific to cartilage such as type II collagen
   in Dmm/Dmm or the core protein of the cartilage
   specific proteoglycan in cmd/cmd or it may
   result from a systemic deficiency which is only
   expressed as rate limiting for cartilage matrix
   biosynthesis as in the PAPS defect of bm/bm.

REFERENCES

Brighton CT (1978) Structure and function of the
   growth plate Clin. orthop. 136.
Brown KS, Cranley RE, Green R, Kleinman HK,
   Pennypacker JP (1981) "Disproportionate
   Micromelia (Dmm): an incomplete dominant mouse
   dwarfism with abnormal cartilage matrix. J
   Embroyol exp morph 62:165.
Green RM, Brown KS, and Pratt RM (1978)
   Autoradiographic analysis of altered
   glycosaminoglycan synthesis in the epiphyseal
   cartilage of neonatal brachymorphic mice.Anat
   Rec 191:19.
Hall BK (1978) "Developmental and Cellular
   Skeletal Biology" New York Academic Press.
Kimata K, Barrach HJ, Brown KS, Pennypacker JP
   (1981) Absence of proteoglycan core protein in
   cartilage from cmd/cmd (cartilage matrix
   deficiency) mouse. J. Biol. Chem. 256:6961.
Kleinman HK, Pennypacker JP and Brown KS (1977)
   Proteoglycan and collagen of "Achondroplastic
   (cn/cn) neonatal mouse cartilage.   Growth"
   41:171.
Lane P, Dickie MM (1968) Three recessive
   mutations producing disproportionate dwarfing
   in mice: achondroplasia, brachymorphic and
   stubby J. Hered 59:300.
McKusick VA (1975) "Mendelian Inheritance in Man"
   4th ed. Baltimore: The Johns Hopkins
   University Press p43.
Orkin RW, Pratt RM, Martin GR (1976) Undersulfated
   chondroitin sulfate in the cartilage matrix of
   brachymorphic mice   Develop. Biol. 50:82.
Pennypacker JP, Kimata K, Brown KS (1981)
   Brachymorphic mice (bm/bm): a generalized

biochemical defect expressed primarily in
cartilage   Develop. Biol. 81:280.
Rittenhouse E, Dunn LC, Cookingham J, Cala C,
    Spiegelman M, Dooher GB, Bennett D (1978)
    Cartilage matrix defeciency (cmd): a new
    autosomal recessive lethal mutation in the
    mouse   J Embryol exp Morph 43:71.
Seegmiller RE, Fraser FC,Sheldon H (1971) A new
    chondrodystrophic mutant in mice: electron
    microscopy of normal and abnormal
    chondrogenesis J. Cell Biol. 48:580.

Animal Models of Inherited Metabolic Diseases, pages 251-264
© **1982 Alan R. Liss, Inc., 150 Fifth Avenue, New York, NY 10011**

REPEATED EPILATION (ER): A SEMIDOMINANT AUTOSOMAL GENE REDUCING SYNTHESIS OF SKIN FILAGGRIN IN MICE

Kenneth S. Brown, Leslie C. Harne, Karen A. Holbrook, Beverly A. Dale

Laboratory of Developmental Biology and Anomalies, National Institute of Dental Research, Bethesda, Maryland; Departments of Biological Structure, Medicine and Periodontics, The University of Washington, Seattle, Washington.

The characteristic differentiated product of the epidermis is the keratinized anucleate keratinocyte of the superficial stratum corneum which is filled with α keratin in an amorphous protein matrix. Keratinocytes are derived from the basal germinative epidermal cells, which contain loose tonofilaments. They regularly pass superficially into the spinous layer where dense tonofilaments of keratin appear and then into the granular layer where keratohyalin synthesis and granule formation occur before their terminal cornification (Breathnach and Wolff, 1979).

The differentiation depends on multiple factors. There are interactions between epidermis and dermis, between basal cells and systemic hormones and between the cells of the epidermal layers. These all contribute to the region specific, species specific, variations of epidermis (Montagna, 1979).

The epidermis does not develop in its adult pattern until the organogenic period of embryogenesis, at around 10 days in mouse or 25 days in man. Prior to that time the embryonic periderm is formed as a single layer of nucleated, rapidly dividing, self supporting cells which continue to function well after the true epidermis is formed. They are sluffed into the amniotic fluid but may be retained until birth (Flaxman, 1979).

The epithelial defect of the heterozygote of Repeated Epilation, (Er) an autosomal incomplete dominant gene in the mouse was first seen at Oak Ridge National Laboratory as the result of gamma ray treatment of spermatogonia (Hunsicker, 1960). The homozygous lethal trait of this epidermal syndrome was first reported by Guenet, 1977. The linkage association of Er between Pgm-2 and Gpd-1 on chromosome 4 and a full description of the external features, skeletal abnormalities and microscopic anatomy of the Er/Er embryo at day 18 of gestation were given by Guenet, Salzgeber and Tassin (1979). We have described the abnormal synthesis of filaggrin, a matrix molecule characteristic of the stratum corneum and stratum granulosum of the epidermis, and the ultrastructural details of the embryonic and newborn epidermis of the heterozygous and homozygous mice (Holbrook et al., 1981; Dale et al., 1981).

Although this defect has no exact counterpart in man, it is similar to the Ichthyosiform Dermatoses, a heterogeneous group of hereditary epithelial defects of undetermined biochemical bases which include several forms of the collodion baby and the harlequin fetus. THese conditions share hypertrophic epidermis and abnormal keratinization with scaling or flaking of the cornified layer (Baden, 1979).

EXTERNAL FEATURES OF ER/ER AND ER/+

The Er/Er is lethal at birth (Fig. 1). It was accurately described by Guenet et al. (1979). Er/Er mice are often born alive, have a dark, hypoxic color and a very shiny skin. They make strenuous efforts to breathe but cannot because of occuluded nasal and oral airways and die of acute respiratory distress. They have stumpy limbs with poor or no differentiation of digits. The limbs, tail and external ears are fused or partially fused to adjacent body surfaces resulting in a pupoid, or mummy-like appearance.

The heterozygous Er/+ mice are distinguishable from +/+, on a C57BL/6J genetic background, at birth by the presence of a glove like edema of the paws and a bloody thickened tail tip. These traits are first seen clearly two days before birth. They are not clearly recognizable on the second day after birth.

The next stage at which Er/+ are clearly seen is when hair loss begins around the nose and eyes during the second postnatal week. The hair loss is almost complete by three weeks and there is repeated regrowth and loss of fur without topographic pattern or regular time pattern. The surviving adults have a characteristic shaggy sparse fur and are slightly smaller than +/+ (Fig. 2) but are completely fertile and have a normal life span. We have seen viable litters as large as 10 and up to 5 litters from a single female mated to Er/+ males.

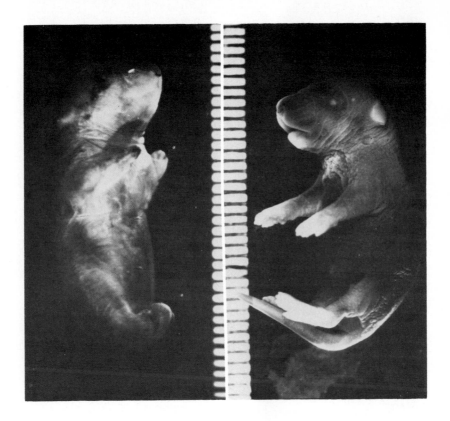

Fig. 1. Newborn Er/Er (left) and normal (right). Note fused mouth, limbs, tail and digits. Scale is mm.

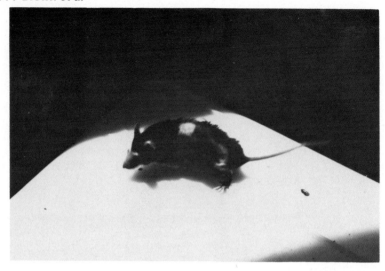

Fig. 2. Adult Er/+ mouse showing irregular fur pattern.

FETAL DEVELOPMENT OF ER/ER

An Er/Er embryo first becomes distinguishable from
its litter mates at stage 20 (Theiler, 1972) when the
first signs of front limb digits normally appear. They
are much delayed in Er/Er (Fig. 3). Prior to that time
classification is uncertain although possible at stage 19
based on abnormal shape and small size of the footplate
and shorter tail.

Truncation of limbs and tail and adhesions of approximated epithelial surfaces become clearly established by
stage 22, or day 14, and some Er/Er die at this stage
while others develop bloody amniotic fluid which is characteristic of many living Er/Er at later gestation stages.
The source of this blood has not been identified.

There are many major consequences of the epithetial
abnormality in Er/Er (Guenet et al., 1979). In the oral
cavity (Fig. 4) adhesions of tongue, and buccal and palatal mucosae prevent the closure of the secondary palate
shelves and obliterate the oral cavity so the mouse lacks
a mouth. In the distal limbs, the phalanges are shortened,

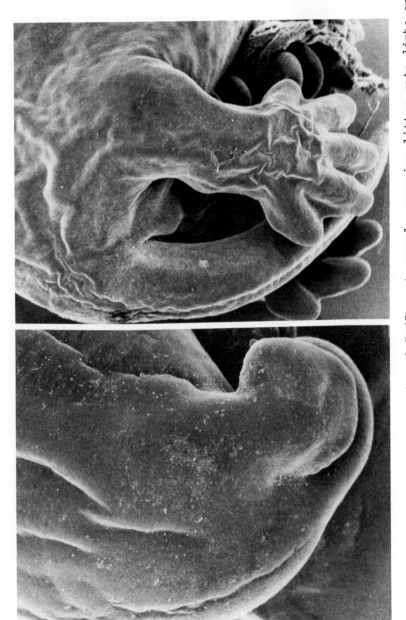

Fig. 3. Scanning electron micrographs of Er/Er and normal appearing litter mate limbs on day 13 of gestation.

fused, compressed by the skin and sometimes missing. Epithelial invagination sometimes isolates digit elements, the tail is shortened by 10 to 12 caudal vertebrae and is frequently curved and adherant to a limb or the abdominal wall. Also, the cornea and eyelids are adherant.

EPIDERMIS HISTOLOGY AND ULTRASTRUCTURE

Histology of Er/Er epidermis at birth shows hyperplasia with a highly variable abnormal organization lacking a stratum corneum. The surface of the Er/Er appeared smooth and taut compared to the puckered wrinkled pattern of normal newborns (Fig. 5). Portions of many cells were

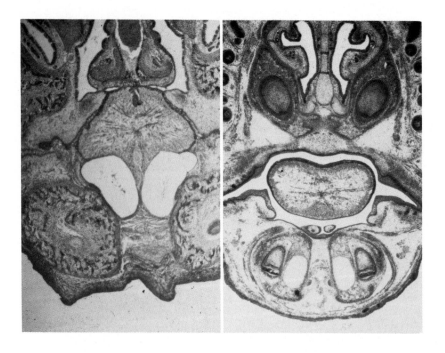

Fig. 4. Frontal section of the oral region of the newborn mouse showing adhesions of tongue, buccal and palatal mucosae in Er/Er (left). Normal (right).

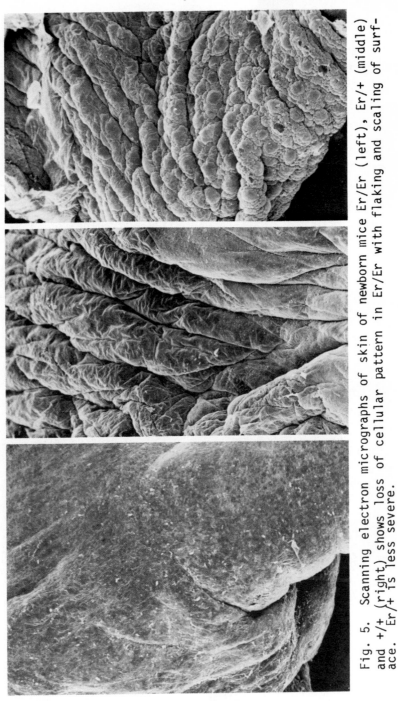

Fig. 5. Scanning electron micrographs of skin of newborn mice Er/Er (left), Er/+ (middle) and +/+ (right) shows loss of cellular pattern in Er/Er with flaking and scaling of surface. Er/+ is less severe.

loosened from the surface givng a ragged appearance. The epidermis of Er/Er was hyperplastic, yet irregular, highly inconsistent in thickness. A true cornified zone was not seen although isolated cornified areas were embedded in the epidermis surrounded by less differentiated cells (Fig. 6).

Ultrastructure had marked abnormalities in all layers of Er/Er epidermis cells. The number of desmosomes in the basal layer was reduced. The number of cells in the spinous layer was highly variable. Both the basal and spinous cells contained mitochondria with electron opaque membrane bound spheres. The granular layer was increased in thickness from 2 to 8 cells and contained a spectrum of keratohyalin granules of different sizes and shapes not related to cell position (Fig. 7). These cells were sometimes completely superfcial but were generally covered by one or more layers of nucleated, organelle containing, non-granular cells, lacking a cornified envelope. No fully cornified cells were found superficially although there were some embedded single and multiple keratinized cells of nearly normal morphology.

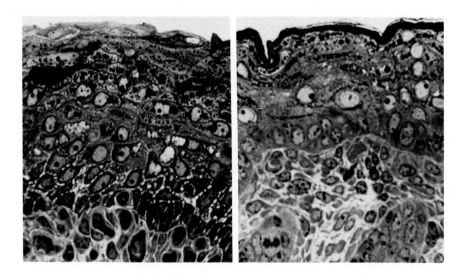

Fig. 6. Histological sections of Er/Er (left) and normal (right) newborn skin showing differences in keratinization, cellular organization and granular pattern.

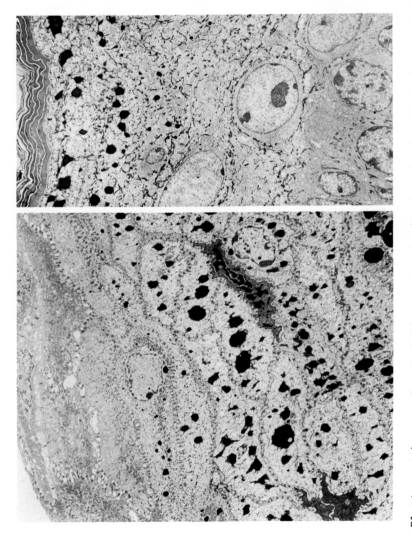

Fig. 7. Electron micrograph of Er/Er epidermis (left) showing superficial non-granular nucleated cells, irregular granules and embedded keratinized cells. Normal epidermis (right).

The Er/+ newborn mice had increased cell numbers in all superficial layers of epidermis but the granular cells had normal cytologic characteristics. The superficial cells contained a wider variety of types than normal but were often nucleated and contained a variety of organelles.

In day 13 embryos, the epidermis of Er/Er was characterized by irregular cell size, shape, and variable number of cell layers and wide separations among the deeper layers of cells which had reduced numbers of desmosomes. Increased diffuse matrix-like material was observed in the intracellular spaces of Er/Er compared to Er/+ and +/+ litter mates which were not distinguishable. The irregularity of Er/Er was seen in the periderm cells which also had reduced numbers of microvilli.

BIOCHEMISTRY

Keratin filaments embedded in a matrix are the major component of the keratinized cells of the stratum corneum. The matrix protein, called filaggrin is cationic and species specific. It is found only in keratinizing stratified epithelia and spontaneously interacts with keratin filaments to produce macrofibrils (Dale et al., 1978). A highly phosphorylated precursor of filaggrin, which does not react with keratin filaments, is stored in keratohyalin granuales of the granular layer. A profilaggrin is synthesized in the spinous or granuler layer, phosphorylated for storage in keratohyalin granules and then dephosphorylated to form the functional matrix protein (Dale et al., 1980).

In the Er/Er mouse there is a block in the normal series of post translational changes of filaggrin (Dale et al., 1981) while in Er/+ the block is incomplete resulting in a reduction in the amount of filaggrin in keratinized epithelial cells (Fig. 8).

During development there is a progression in the differentiation of the response to antibodies to filaggrin as shown by immunofluorescence. Suprabasal cells are difusely positive in all embryos of day 13 but by day 15, +/+ and Er/+ embryos show granular immunofluorescence while Er/Er does not. By day 17 the stratum corneum of +/+ and

Er/+ also becomes strongly responsive but Er/Er continues to respond like day 13.

There are also altered ratios among the keratin peptides of Er/Er epidermis and the adhesion of epithelial cells indicates alterations in the surface properties of the cells. It thus appears that filaggrin synthesis is jointly regulated with other important biochemical processes in keratinization. The control mechanism for this

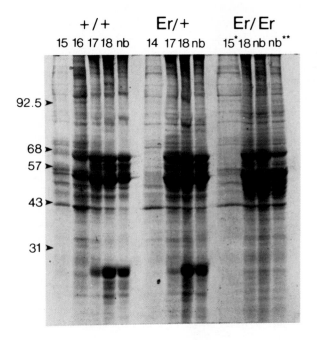

Fig. 8. Electrophoresis of epidermal extracts on 8.75% SDS-polyacrylamide gels at different days of gestation and newborn. Molecular weights (x10^{-3}) were calculated by comparison with protein standards. Note the relative increase in intensity of bands of 59 K, 53 K, 49 K and the absence of the 26.5 K band in the Er/Er extract.

regulation is unknown.

The major value of the Er/Er phenotype may be as a probe to demonstrate the previously unappreciated role of epidermal keratinization in the control of morphogenesis. It is already providing new questions and approaches for the study of the biochemistry of keratinization.

REFERENCES

Baden HP (1979). Ichthyosiform Dermatoses, Chapt. 28, In Fitzpatrick TB et al. (eds) "Dermatology in General Medicine" 2nd Ed. New York: McGraw Hill.

Breathnach As and Wolff K (1979). The structure and development of skin, Chapt. 4 in Fitzpatrick TB et al. (eds) "Dermatology in General Medicine" 2nd Ed. New York: McGraw Hill.

Dale BA, Holbrook KA, Steinert PM (1978). Assembly of stratum corneum basic protein and keratin filaments in macrofibrils. Nature 276:729.

Dale BA, Jones JCR, Goldman RD, and Brown KS (1981). Identification of flaggrin and filaggrin precursor in developing keratinocytes of normal and Er mutant mouse skin. J Cell Biol 91:35A.

Dale, BA, Lonsdale-Eccles JD, Holbrook KA (1980). Stratum corneum basic protein: An interfilamentous matrix protein of epidermal keratin. In Berstein IA, Seiji M (eds) "In Biochemistry of Normal and Abnormal Epidermal Differentiation." Tokyo: University of Tokyo Press.

Flaxman BA (1979). Control of Skin Development: Cell and Tissue Interactions Chapt. 5. In Fitzpatrick TB et al. (eds) "Dermatology in General Medicine" 2nd Ed. New York: McGraw Hill.

Guenet JL (1977). Private Communication, Mouse Newsletter 56:57.

Guenet JL, Salzbeger B, Tassin MT (1979). Repeated epilation: A genetic epidermal syndrome in mice, J Heredity 70:90.

Holbrook KA, Dale BA, Brown KS (1981). Abnormal epidermal keratinization in the repeated epilation mouse, J Cell Biol, in press.

Hunsicker PR (1960). Private communication, Mouse Newsletter 70:90.

Montagna W (1979). Comparative Anatomy and Function of Skin, Chapt. 6. In Fitzpatrick TB et al. (eds) "Dermatology in General Medicine" 2nd Ed. New York: McGraw Hill.

Theiler K (1972). "The House Mouse", Berlin: Springer-Verlag, p 87.

DR. SCARPELLI: Dr. Brown, is there any involucrin in this skin? It is a protein that forms in the fully keratinized cell at the cell surface. It is very inxoluble and serves to maintain the shape of the cell in a flattened fashion.

DR. BROWN: Involucrin is in the cornified cell envelope while the filaggrin is in the intracellular matrix. Involucrin has been found to be present in the Er/Er mouse by morphological criteria.

Animal Models of Inherited Metabolic Diseases, pages 265–267
© **1982 Alan R. Liss, Inc., 150 Fifth Avenue, New York, NY 10011**

FRAGILITAS OSSIUM (fro) : AN AUTOSOMAL RECESSIVE MUTATION
IN THE MOUSE.

Jean-Louis Guenet, D.V.M., D. Sc.
Institut Pasteur de Paris (France).

Ritta Stanescu, Pierre Maroteaux, Viktor Stanescu.
Hôpital Necker - Enfants Malades (Paris)

Osteogenesis imperfecta (brittle bones or fragilitas
ossium) is a group of heritable human syndromes characterized by osteoporosis leading to fractures and skeletal deformities. The existence of more than one genetic variety of
osteogenesis imperfecta (OI) is well documented (Mc Kusick VA
1975; Sillence, Alison, Danks 1979). Biochemical studies on
cultured fibroblasts (Penttinen, Lichtenstein, Martin, Mc Kusick VA 1975) and skin (Bauze, Smith, Francis 1975; Francis,
Smith 1975) from patients with OI support the proposed heterogeneity and suggest collagen abnormalities in some patients.
Conditions with similarities to the human syndrome have been
described in cats, dogs, lambs and zoo animals, but there is
evidence that most, if not all, of these disorders are primarily nutritional rather than genetic and are not therefore analogous to the disease in man (Scott, Mc Kusick VA.,
Mc Kusick AB 1963).

We have discovered and studied an autosomal recessive
mutation in mice with abnormalities similar to those found
in the severe form of osteogenesis imperfecta. The mutation
(fro) has been discovered in a randombred stock of mice during an experiment aimed at the detection of recessive lethal mutations, after treatment of the post meiotic germ
cells of male mice with various chemical mutagen used was an
ethyleneimine derivative : tris (1-aziridinyl phosphine-[R]
sulphide which is sold under the commercial name Thiotepa
and the target post meiotic germ cells were the spermatids.
The treated male which gave the original fro heterozygote
had received a single intraperitoneal injection of 5 micro-
grams per grams of body weight two weeks before the mating.

The affected newborns are moderately runted and had deformities in all four limbs. These two phenotypic charac- teristics were easily detectable and the limb deformities were exceptionally constant. They were characterized by a curving of the long bones. No deformities are apparent in the tail, spine or ribs. The viability of the homozygotes is greatly reduced and up to 90 percent of young fro/fro die prior to day 3. This percentage was not improved by culling the progeny size but was apparently affected by the genetic background. The fro mutations is fully penetrant. Its linkage relationships are not yet established.

Where, as occured occasionally, an affected animal survives, it remains small and deformed all its life. Bree- ding and behaviour in both sexes are normal. The life span is clearly not reduced and the condition seems to improve with age.

Six affected newborns and five controls were studied roentgenologically and histologically. The X-ray study was performed using a senograph CGR (3 sec, 19 KV). The long bones were shorter and showed important diaphyseal incur- vations. The diaphysis were wider and more translucent than in the normals, with small, irregular denser areas. The cortices were thin and irregular and several long bones showed discontinuities. The shape of the metacarpals and phalanges seemed not to be disturbed but the cortices were thin and the bones had an increased transparency. The epiphysis, the carpal and tarsal bones showed an apparently normal shape. The metaphyseal line did not show rachitic changes.

The histological study was performed on : a) speci- mens decalcified in EDTA 10 %, paraffin embedded and stai- ned with HE and with Mallory trichome; b) fresh frozen undecalcified sections stained with Azur A (pH 1.75) or with the von Kossa technique; c) undecalcified specimens, embed- ded in Spurr medium (Spurr 1969) and stained with Azur II and methylene blue.

The histological study of the bones showed : a) wide diaphysis of long bones presenting incurvations or angular deformations and thin cortices. Calluses associated with various stages of bone remodelling were found.
The number of osteoblasts did not seem to be reduced but many of them are rather flattened, osteoid rims were not

widered. Osteoclasts were not unusually conspicuous except
in some areas of bone remodelling ; b) the normal appearance of growth cartilage : normal arrangement and length
of cartilage columns, normal development of the hypertrophic zone and of provisional calcification. The vascular
invasion was regular as were the primary traveculae which
were however thinner than in controls. The metachromasis of
the growth plate was similar to that of the controls.

The type of transmission, the clinical, roentgenologi-
cal and pathologic features of this mutation, show similarities to those of the severe form of human osteogenesis
imperfecta. However, heterogeneity within this clinical
group is highly probable and biochemical studies will be
necessary to establish if the basic defect in fro/fro mice
is similar to certain human types of ostoegenesis imperfecta.

Bauze RJ, Smith R, Francis MJO (1975). A new look at
osteogenesis imperfecta. A clinical and biochemical study
of forty-two patients. J Bone Jt Surg 57 B:2.
Francis MJO, Smith R (1975). Polymeric collagen of skin
in osteogenesis imperfecta, homocystinuria and Ehlers-
Danlos, and Marfan syndromes. Birth Defects, Original
article series 11:15
Mc Kusick VA (1975). The classification of heritable
disorders of connective tissues. Birth Defect, Original
article series 11:1.
Penttinen RP, Lichtenstein JR, Martin GR, Mc Kusick VA
(1975). Abnormal collagen metabolism in cultured cells in
osteogenesis imperfecta. Proc Nat Acad Sci USA 72:586.
Scott PP, Mc Kusick VA, Mc Kusick AB (1963). The nature
of osteogenesis imperfecta in cats. J Bone Jt Surg 45A:125.
Sillence DO, Alison S, Danks DM (1979). Genetic heterogeneity in osteogenesis imperfecta. J Med Genet 16:101.
Spurr AR (1969). A low viscosity epoxy resin embedding
medium for electron microscopy. J Ultrastruct Res 26:31.

SECTION V.
INBORN ERRORS OF IMMUNE FUNCTION AND HISTOCOMPATIBILITY

Animal Models of Inherited Metabolic Diseases, pages 271–307
© **1982 Alan R. Liss, Inc., 150 Fifth Avenue, New York, NY 10011**

IMMUNODEFICIENCY DISEASE IN ANIMALS

Lance E. Perryman and Nancy S. Magnuson

Department of Veterinary Microbiology
  and Pathology
Washington State University
Pullman, Washington 99164

The importance of the immune system in prevention of and recovery from infections is graphically demonstrated by those children and animals in which there is a genetically-based deficiency of a component of the immune system (reviewed in Horowitz and Hong, 1977; Perryman, 1979). Such cases have defined the roles of various cell types in immunity and have clarified their importance in host defense.

A simplified scheme for the origin and maturation of lymphocyte subpopulations in man is presented in Figure 1. Both major lymphocyte subclasses are derived from a common stem cell precursor. Those cells destined to become T lymphocytes travel to the thymus where they undergo a series of mitotic divisions and differentiational changes before emerging as functionally mature T lymphocytes. T cells play three major roles in immune responses: 1) they may interact with B lymphocytes in the production of specific antibody, in which case they are referred to as helper T cells (T_H); 2) they may suppress immune responses and, in those cases, are classified as suppressor T lymphocytes (Ts); 3) finally, T lymphocytes are responsible for cell-mediated immunity, which is important in host defense against neoplastic cells, fungi, protozoa, intracellular bacteria, and some viral infections (reviewed in Good, 1972; Horowitz and Hong, 1977). B lymphocytes also complete a series of maturational changes in which precursor cells give rise to pre B cells and ultimately B cells. Changes occurring in these steps involve the

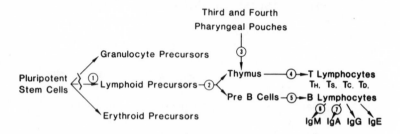

Figure 1.   Proposed sites of defects in lymphocyte
            maturation resulting in various immunodeficiency
            disorders.

acquisition of surface IgM and IgD, and the ability to
synthesize and secrete antibodies following antigenic
stimulation and cooperation with T lymphocytes and/or
macrophages. Specific antibodies play an important role in
host defense against extracellular bacteria and some viral
infections.

     Immunodeficiency disorders may involve one or both
divisions of the immune system to varying degrees (reviewed
in Horowitz and Hong, 1977). Examples of human disorders
are indicated in Figure 1. The most severe deficiency
occurs when differentiation of both myeloid and lymphoid
precursor cells is blocked (Fig. 1-1). The disorder is
termed reticular dysgenesis (immunodeficiency with hematopoietic hypoplasia) and the mode of inheritance is
unknown. Death from overwhelming infections occurs within
a few weeks of birth. Severe combined immunodeficiency
(Fig. 1-2) is a heterogeneous group of disorders
characterized by the absence of T and B lymphocytes able to
produce immunologically-specific reactions. Autosomal

recessive, sex-linked, and sporadic modes of inheritance have been described. Mechanisms and manifestations range from a virtual absence of identifiable B and T cells, to conditions where substantial numbers of cells with surface markers indicative of T and B cells can be found. In this latter group, immunoglobulin synthesis may occur, and T lymphocytes may proliferate in response to phytolectin stimulation. However, antigen-specific immune responses are not demonstrable. Another subset of children with severe combined immunodeficiency are deficient in the enzyme adenosine deaminase (ADA, EC 3.5.4.4), resulting in immunodeficiency by mechanisms which have not been totally defined (Giblett et al., 1972). Survival ranges from 6 months to about 4 years unless bone marrow transplantation or other forms of therapy restore the patients' ability to produce functional lymphocytes. The incidence of severe combined immunodeficiency is approximately 1 per 100,000 births but may be substantially higher in certain ethnic groups (Murphy et al., 1980).

Two disorders have been described in which T lymphocytes are selectively affected. The Di George syndrome (Fig. 1-3) is characterized by hypoplasia or aplasia of the third and fourth pharyngeal pouches with resulting hypoplasia or aplasia of the thymus and parathyroid glands. Affected individuals are variably deficient in their ability to manifest T cell-dependent immune responses. The Di George syndrome is not genetically determined. It is a developmental defect resulting from intrauterine insult occurring before the eighth week of gestation. Another example of a T cell deficiency (Fig. 1-4) is that associated with absence of purine nucleoside phosphorylase (PNP, EC 2.4.2.1). This autosomal recessive condition was first described in 1975 (Giblett, et al., 1975) and is associated with anemia and increased susceptibility to infections.

Disorders of B lymphocytes may involve the total B cell population or be limited to a single class of immunoglobulin-secreting cells. Boys with X-linked agammaglobulinemia (Fig. 1-5), have a virtual absence of B lymphocytes, although pre-B cells are detectable in many patients. Inability to produce significant quantities of immunoglobulin results in heightened susceptibility to certain bacterial infections. Selective deficiencies of individual immunoglobulin classes have also been described

(Fig. 1-6, 1-7). Selective IgM deficiency may occur as a primary or secondary disorder (Hobbs, 1975). Selective IgA deficiency is one of the two most common immunodeficiencies of man. Affected individuals may experience serious sinopulmonary and intestinal infections.

Common variable immunodeficiency occurs frequently in people. Because of the heterogeneity of the disorder, it cannot be readily indicated on the schematic in Figure 1. Patients experience an increased incidence of infections, and have hypogammaglobulinemia associated with variable patterns of cellular immune dysfunction. Onset of clinical signs is highly variable. The underlying mechanisms are heterogeneous, involving intrinsic B cell defects and/or excessive T lymphocyte suppressor activity (Waldmann et al., 1974; 1980).

Many other deficiencies have been described in man, and the interested reader is referred to the following

Table 1. Complement Deficiencies

Deficient component	Species	References
C1	Chicken	Hammer et al., 1981
C4	Guinea pig	Ellman and Green, 1970
	Rat	Arroyave et al., 1977
C2	Guinea pig	Bitter-Suerman et al., 1981
C3	Dog (Brittany Spaniel)	Winkelstein et al., 1981
C5	Mouse (A/HeN, AKR/N, B10.D2/ OSnN)	Doi and Cotten, 1979
C6	Rabbit	Rother et al., 1976
	Hamster	Hammer et al., 1981

reviews (Horowitz and Hong, 1977; Asherson and Webster, 1980; Seligman and Hitzing, 1980). It is interesting to note that of all the deficiencies described in man, in only a few has the metabolic basis of the disease been identified. It is now accepted that adenosine deaminase deficiency and purine nucleoside phosphorylase deficiency are responsible for the failure to produce functional lymphocytes; however the precise mechanisms have yet to be defined (reviewed in Pollara et al., 1979).

In the following sections, selected examples of immunodeficiencies in animals will be presented. Several complement deficiencies (Table 1) and leukocyte defects (Table 2) have been described in animals, and they serve as valuable models of similar diseases in man. In this review, complement and leukocyte disorders will not be detailed. Rather, the information presented will be limited to genetically-based disorders of lymphocytes, and the biochemical basis of the disease will be emphasized where possible. Reviews of additional animal immuno-deficiencies can be found in Gershwin and Merchant, 1981; and Perryman, 1979.

T LYMPHOCYTE DEFICIENCIES OF ANIMALS

Table 3 lists the currently recognized immunodefic-iencies of animals in which T lymphocytes are preferent-ially affected. Two of the disorders will be discussed to indicate the widespread use of one model and the knowledge gained concerning the metabolic basis of the second disorder.

Hairlessness and Immunodeficiency in Mice,
Rats and Guinea Pigs

Nude mice. A hairless mouse mutant with shortened life-span was discovered in 1966 (Flanagan) and subsequently shown to be athymic (Pantelouris, 1968). The value of these animals for defining the role of T lymphocytes in immune responses was immediately obvious and led to the rapid dissemination of nude mice to several laboratories. From the standpoint of widespread use and knowledge gained, the nude mouse must be viewed as the animal model of greatest impact amongst those described to date.

Table 2. Neutrophil and Macrophage Deficiencies

Disease	Defective or deficient cell population	Species	References
Canine granulocytopathy syndrome	Neutrophils	dog	Renshaw et al., 1977
Cyclic hematopoiesis	Neutrophils, monocytes	dog	Dale et al., 1972
Chediak-Higashi Syndrome (C-HS)	Neutrophils, monocytes	mouse (beige)	Lutzner et al., 1967
C-HS	Neutrophils, monocytes	mink	Padgett et al., 1964
C-HS	Neutrophils, monocytes	cattle	Padgett et al., 1964
C-HS	Neutrophils, monocytes	cat	Kramer et al., 1977
C-HS	Neutrophils, monocytes	whale	Taylor and Farrell, 1973
Macrophage defects	Macrophages	mouse	Vogel, et al., 1981

Table 3.   T Lymphocyte Deficiencies of Animals

Disorder	Reference
Hairlessness and immunodeficiency	
Nude mouse	Fogh and Giovanella (1978)
Nude rat	Festing (1981)
Hairless immunodeficient guinea pig	O'Donoghue and Reed (1981)
Lethal trait A-46 in cattle	Andresen, et al., (1970)

Hereditarily athymic-asplenic
  (Lasat) mice
	Erickson and Gershwin
	  (1981)

Hypopituitary dwarfs with immunodeficiency	
Ames dwarf mouse	Duquesnoy (1981)
Snell-Bagg dwarf mouse	Duquesnoy (1981)
Weimaraner dogs	Roth, et al. (1980)

The combination of hairlessness and thymic dysgenesis is a single gene defect in nude mice and is inherited as an autosomal recessive trait (reviewed in Hansen, 1978). The thymus normally develops from endodermal and ectodermal anlagen of the third branchial pouch and arch. Nude mouse fetuses develop a thymic rudiment visible at 14-15 days pregnancy, but the thymus is atypical in appearance and location, and does not become lymphoid. Because a thymic rudiment is present in most cases, thymic dysgenesis, rather than thymic aplasia, more accurately describes the phenomenon. The single gene defect influences development of ectodermal structures and accounts for joint occurrence of thymic dysgenesis and hairlessness, a feature which facilitates identification of immunodeficient mice from their normal littermates.

Extensive investigations of nude mice have shown them to be markedly deficient in thymic-derived lymphocytes as evidenced by very low levels of thy-bearing cells, lack of T helper cell activity with inability to produce antibodies to thymic-dependent antigens, failure to generate cytotoxic T cells, inability to reject allografts and xenografts, negligible response to T cell mitogens, (concanavalin A and phytohemagglutinin P), diminished contact sensitization reactions, and inability to manifest a graft versus host response (Rygaard, 1978; Reed and Manning, 1978). Nude mice also have significantly reduced or absent concentrations of IgA. Substantial numbers of T cell precursors exist as evidenced by partial restoration of helper and cytotoxic T cell activity following thymic transplants or administration of thymic factors (Kindred, 1978). Substantial reconstitution of T cell function is also achieved following in vitro incubation with or in vivo administration of interleukin 2 (IL-2). Therefore, the thymic defect in nude mice appears to result in failure to produce those T lymphocytes required for IL-2 synthesis and secretion (Baker and Smith, 1980; Smith et al., 1980).

In view of successful heterotransplantation of human neoplasms to nude mice (Sharkey et al., 1978), and the pur-ported role of T lymphocytes in surveillance of neoplastic cells, increased incidence of spontaneous neoplasia in nude mice may be expected. However, no significant increase in spontaneous neoplasia has been observed and, in general, nude mice develop neoplasms of the type and rate typical of the inbred strain into whose background the nude gene has been inserted (Stutman, 1978). Nude mice have been shown to express greater natural killer (NK) cell activity when compared to conventional mice. The increased NK cell activity is believed to be important in protecting nude mice from increased spontaneous neoplasia, and to retard the metastasis of heterotransplanted human neoplasms (Herberman, 1978).

Nude rats. Comparable immunological defects occur in nude rats. The athymic nude mutation was observed in 1953 in a colony of outbred hooded rats maintained at the Rowett Research Institute, Bucksburn, Aberdeen, U.K. The symbol rnu for Rowett nude was assigned to the recessive mutant gene. Festing et al. (1978) described the thymic abnormal-ities of these animals. At present, two athymic nude mutations are recognized in rats (Rowett and New Zealand). Nude rats have bent vibrissae and variable amounts of hair. The rats are nearly athymic, although a small highly dysplastic thymic rudiment is present in most animals (Vos et al., 1980a). Using monoclonal antisera to rat T lymphocyte antigens, investigators have shown that nude rats possess measurable numbers of lymphocytes carrying

T cell markers (Festing, 1981). Immunologic impairment is severe. Splenic lymphocytes do not respond to T cell mitogens or thymic dependent antigens. Lymph node cells, on the other hand, are able to respond at reduced levels to phytohemagglutinin and concanavalin A. Skin allografts are accepted, while xenografts may be accepted or rejected acutely or chronically by undefined mechanisms. Neoplastic xenografts have been grown in nude rats, but the comparability of nude rats to nude mice for growth and maintenance of human neoplasms remains to be defined. While nude rats are more susceptible to several experimental infections than conventional rats, they are apparently more hardy and survive longer than nude mice when raised in sub-optimal conditions. Because of their greater survivability and size, nude rats may be more suitable for several experiments which are technically difficult to perform in nude mice (Festing, 1981; Vos et al., 1980b).

Hairless immunodeficient guinea pigs. Reed and O'Donoghue (1979) observed hairlessness and immunodeficiency in a closed colony of Hartley guinea pigs. Affected animals were smaller than littermates and had wrinkled skin as well as stunted vibrissae. Hairlessness resulted from improper hair shaft development. Thymic development is abnormal, resulting in thymic hypoplasia or aplasia. Deficient immune responses are characterized by delayed graft rejection, hypogammaglobulinemia, and increased susceptibility to cytomegalovirus, systemic balantidiasis, and Pneumocystis carinii infections (O'Donoghue and Reed, 1981).

Lethal Trait A46 in Black Pied Danish Cattle
of Friesian Descent

In 1970, a lethal primary immunodeficiency disorder was described in Black Pied Danish Cattle of Friesian descent (Andresen et al., 1970). The disorder is inherited as an autosomal recessive trait (Andresen et al., 1970, 1974; Andresen, 1974). Affected calves appear normal at birth but develop skin lesions at 1 to 2 months of age, consisting of exanthema and alopecia, and parakeratosis around the eyes, mouth, and under the jaw. Without treatment, calves die within 4 months of age. Gross and microscopic examination of lymphoid tissues reveals marked hypoplasia of thymus, spleen, lymph nodes, and gut-associated lymphoid tissues with depletion of lymphocytes in the thymic dependent regions. Immunological studies indicate that cellular immunity is significantly decreased, while immunoglobulin concentrations and antibody titers following immunization are relatively normal (Flagstad et al., 1972; Brummerstedt et al., 1971). Affected calves form near-normal quantities of antibody to tetanus toxoid but respond weakly or negatively in delayed hypersensitivity skin tests using dinitrochlorobenzene (DNCB) and Mycobacterium tuberculosis. Susceptibility to infections is greater than for nonaffected calves.

Lethal trait A46 is one of very few immunodeficiencies of man or animals for which the metabolic basis of the disorder is understood. Oral treatment of affected calves with large quantities of zinc oxide or zinc sulfate results in full recovery, as evidenced by resolution of skin lesions, normal development of lymphoid tissues, recovery from infections, and ability to respond to DNCB and Fasciola hepatica larvae (Brummerstedt et al., 1971; Flagstadt et al., 1972). Cessation of supplementary zinc administration leads to relapse after one to three weeks. Available data indicate the basis of the disorder is an intestinal malabsorption defect for zinc which can be overcome by large oral doses of zinc ions (Brummerstedt et al., 1977). In this respect, lethal trait A46 of cattle closely resembles acrodermatitis enteropathica of man (Good et al., 1980).

This model should be highly useful for investigation of T lymphocyte deficiencies, zinc absorption, the role of zinc ions on cells and thymic factors involved in the immune system, and for comparative study of acrodermatitis enteropathica in man. Homozygous affected animals can be maintained to sexual maturity with appropriate zinc therapy and are fertile. Therefore it is possible to obtain a pure breeding herd of fertile individuals which are homozygous for the recessive trait (Brummerstedt et al., 1977).

B LYMPHOCYTE DEFICIENCIES OF ANIMALS

Table 4 lists the currently recognized immunodeficiencies of animals in which B lymphocytes are preferentially affected. Three of the disorders will be briefly discussed.

Table 4.   B Lymphocyte Deficiencies of Animals

Disorder	Reference
Agammaglobulinemia of horses	Banks et al., 1976; Perryman and McGuire, 1980
Dysgammaglobulinemia of chickens	Benedict et al., 1978; 1981
Immune defective CBA/N mice	Scher, 1981
Hereditary asplenia of mice	Welles and Battisto, 1981
Selective immunoglobulin deficiencies	
IgA deficiency in chickens	Luster et al., 1977
IgG_2 deficiency in cattle	Nansen, 1972
IgM deficiency in horses	Perryman and McGuire, 1980

Agammaglobulinemia of Horses

Sex-linked agammaglobulinemia was the first immuno-deficiency described in persons (Bruton, 1952). To date, the only animal model closely resembling this disorder is agammaglobulinemia in horses. Three cases have been described (Banks et al., 1976; McGuire et al., 1976; Deem et al., 1979; Perryman and McGuire, 1980) and all have been in males, suggesting the trait may be sex-linked in horses as well. Affected horses lack lymphocytes bearing surface immunoglobulin. In addition there is absence of IgM, IgA, and IgG(T). Small quantities of IgG are detectable but are of maternal origin. Other features include absence of specific antibody following immunization with a variety of antigens; absence of plasma cells, primary follicles, and germinal centers in lymph nodes following antigenic stimulation; absence of "natural" serum antibodies to rabbit erythrocytes which are easily detected in age-matched control horse serums; and increased susceptibility to infections. It is not known if agammaglobulinemic horses develop pre B cells as have been demonstrated in boys with agammaglobulinemia (Vogler et al., 1976; Fu et al., 1980).

Dysgammaglobulinemia of Chickens

Chickens can be manipulated by several procedures to achieve bursectomy, resulting in hypogammablogulinemia. Such chickens develop suppressor cells which, when adoptively transferred to normal birds, will result in hypogammaglobulinemia (reviewed in Lerman et al., 1978). These experimentally derived birds have been used to study mechanisms of B lymphocyte suppression.

An inherited, naturally occurring disorder of inbred UCD chickens has been characterized in which affected birds are dysgammaglobulinemic, have demonstrable suppressor T cell activity, and resemble the immunological features of common variable immunodeficiency of man (Benedict et al., 1977; 1978; 1981). The disorder in birds is clearly inheritable, but the precise mode of inheritance, number of genes involved, and their degrees of penetrance remain to be defined. Immunological abnormalities are late in onset. Immunoglobulin concentrations are normal for the first month after hatching. Shortly thereafter, IgG concentration decreases substantially, and IgM concentration is significantly increased. IgA may also be elevated. Although the general pattern is one of IgG deficiency with elevated IgM and IgA, several patterns of dysgammaglobulinemia may occur, including decreased IgM and IgG, decreased IgG with normal IgM, and dysgammaglobulinemia (Benedict et al., 1978). The decreased IgG concentrations suggest active suppression of immunoglobulin synthesis, and suppressor T cells have been demonstrated in affected birds (Benedict et al., 1981).

Immunological studies have shown effector T cells to be present in normal quantities. Delayed-type hypersensitivity to tuberculin is of the same intensity in sensitized dysgammaglobulinemic chickens as it is in normal chickens. Peripheral blood lymphocytes from affected birds proliferate normally when stimulated with phytohemagglutinin, pokeweed mitogen tuberculin, and rabbit anti-Fc antibody. Abnormalities are detected when B lymphocytes are evaluated. While normal numbers of B cells are present and immune responses are induced with a variety of immunogens, reduced quantities of specific antibody are produced. Only IgM antibody is synthesized in response to sheep red blood cells and dinitrophenyl-bovine gammaglobulin. In vitro immunoglobulin synthesis following pokeweed mitogen stimulation is also limited to IgM.

Co-cultivation of lymphocytes from normal chickens with those from abnormal chickens revealed the presence of cells in abnormal chickens which can suppress immunoglobulin synthesis. Suppression is selective for IgG synthesis. Through appropriate cell mixing experiments employing enriched B cell and enriched T cell populations from abnormal birds, it has been shown that the suppressor cell is of the T lymphocyte lineage. Selective treatment of cells with complement and antisera specific for T cells has confirmed the earlier experiments showing T cells to be responsible for suppression of immunoglobulin synthesis (Benedict et al., 1978; 1981).

Kinetic studies indicate that suppressor cells are detectable as early as 7 days post hatch, even though the immunoglobulin abnormalities are not apparent for another 3 to 5 weeks. In addition to dysgammaglobulinemia, autoimmune phenomena appear in birds at 6 months of age. They include immune complex disease, Coombs' positive hemolytic anemia, and serum rheumatoid factor. Terminally, birds have signs of anemia, congestive heart failure, and splenomegaly (Benedict et al., 1981).

Common variable immunodeficiency (CVID) occurs in people with high frequency. Because of the severity of resulting infections and the incidence of the disorder, it is probably the most significant immunodeficiency disease in people. CVID is a heterogeneous group of disorders, but in many of the patients studied, suppressor T cells have been incriminated as the basis for the disease (Walmann et al., 1974; 1980). Therefore, study of immunoregulatory disturbances in UCD dysgammaglobulinemic chickens may be of significant value in the management of patients with CVID.

Immune Defective CBA/N Mice

A vast literature exists concerning the immune defects in CBA/N mice (reviewed in Scher, 1981). These mice carry an X-linked gene, xid, that inhibits the normal development and maturation of B lymphocytes. Immune defective CBA/N mice display diminished antibody responses to thymic-dependent antigens, and fail to respond to certain thymic-independent antigens. These mice cannot generate B cell colonies in soft agar cultures, have reduced numbers of B cells in their spleens, produce subnormal antibody titers to a number of infectious agents, and possess markedly reduced levels of serum IgM and IgG_3 antibodies. Analysis of B lymphocytes for quantity and type of surface membrane immunoglobulin has revealed a basic abnormality in the immune defective CBA/N mice. The surface immunoglobulin pattern is that of a high ratio of IgM to IgD, a pattern typical of immature B lymphocytes (Finkelman et al., 1975). As normal B lymphocytes mature, a reversal of the ratio is expected so that IgD becomes the predominant surface immunoglobulin. Immune defective CBA/N mice lack the subpopulation of B cells with these characteristics.

CBA/N mice have been exceedingly useful for studying B lymphocyte maturation as well as B cell requirements for interaction with antigen, T lymphocytes and macrophages. CBA/N mice do not resemble known immune defects in man. However, they are mentioned in this review because of their use in crossbreeding with nude mice to produce offspring sharing some characteristics with children having severe combined immunodeficiency (Azar et al., 1980).

COMBINED T AND B LYMPHOCYTE DEFICIENCIES OF ANIMALS

Table 5 lists the currently recognized immunodeficiencies of animals in which both T and B lymphocytes are

Table 5.   Combined T and B Lymphocyte Deficiencies of Animals

Disorder	Reference
Combined immunodeficiency in horses	McGuire and Perryman, 1981
N:NIH(S)11-nu/nu mouse	Azar et al., 1980
Motheaten mouse	Kincade, 1981

significantly affected. Combined immunodeficiency of horses will be described in detail and the evidence for the metabolic basis of the condition presented.

Combined Immunodeficiency of Horses

Combined immunodeficiency (CID) in children is a heterogeneous group of diseases in terms of mode of inheritance, immunological expression, and underlying biochemical mechanisms. Investigations of affected children have contributed knowledge to the cellular basis and biochemical requirements for normal immune responsiveness. These studies have been impeded by the small number of affected children available for study. Availability of a relevant animal model would facilitate these studies and also allow evaluation of treatment modalities applicable to affected children. In 1973, an animal counterpart of severe combined immunodeficiency was reported in young horses (McGuire and Poppie, 1973). Additional studies indicated the disorder is inherited as an autosomal recessive trait, is limited to foals of Arabian breeding, and occurs with a frequency of about two percent of the Arabian foals produced in the United States and Australia (Poppie and McGuire, 1977; Perryman and Torbeck, 1980; Studdert, 1978). Because of the high frequency of the disorder, we have been able to assemble a large herd of Arabian horses heterozygous for the CID trait, from which affected foals are obtained for study.

The clinical and immunological features of CID in foals have been extensively reviewed (Studdert, 1978; Perryman, 1979; Perryman et al., 1979; Splitter et al., 1980; Perryman and McGuire, 1980; McGuire and Perryman, 1981). In brief, affected foals appear normal at birth but, under field conditions, invariably die before 5 months of age. Severe respiratory signs are associated with equine adenovirus and Pneumocystis carinii infections. Profound lymphopenia, absence of lymphocytes with surface markers characteristic of B lymphocytes, and failure to synthesize immunoglobulins in response to immunization are typical features of CID foals. In addition, functional T lymphocytes are markedly reduced or absent as evidenced by the absence of delayed hypersensitivity skin reactions, markedly reduced or absent lymphocyte response to phytolectin stimulation, and absence of lymphocyte response to allogeneic cells in mixed lymphocyte cultures. The total numbers, surface receptors, and phagocytic capacity of neutrophils and monocytes are usually within normal limits. No abnormalities of the complement system have been identified, and foals with CID synthesize secretory component.

Foals with CID have proven useful for evaluating immunotherapeutic procedures applicable to CID children lacking histocompatible bone marrow donors. Ontogeny of equine lymphocyte development has been characterized and the features of graft versus host reactions in CID foals determined (Ardans et al., 1977; Perryman et al., 1980; Perryman and Liu, 1980). Transplantation with fetal liver and thymus has been performed with varying degrees of success (Ardans et al., 1977; Perryman et al., 1979; Perryman, 1980).

Biochemical Aberrations in Combined Immunodeficiency

In addition to evaluation of therapeutic procedures, another use of the CID model in horses concerns the identification of metabolic defects that result in immuno-deficiency. We began a series of experiments focusing on abnormalities of purine metabolism prompted by the discoveries of altered purine metabolism in children with specific immunological deficiencies. The discovery of ADA deficiency in children with CID was important because it defined the first biochemical defect responsible for an immune disorder (Giblett et al., 1972). The resulting awareness that purine metabolism was important for lymphoid tissue development and function led to the identification of two other purine enzyme deficiencies in children with immunological disorders. These are PNP deficiency associated with T cell dysfunction (Giblett et al., 1975), and 5'-nucleotidase deficiency associated with primary immunoglobulin deficiency (Johnson et al., 1977; Edwards et al., 1978; Webster et al., 1978; Edwards et al., 1979a and 1979b). The actual relationship of 5'-nucleotidase deficiency to B lymphocyte dysfunction remains to be defined.

Approximately one-third of the children with severe combined immunodeficiency are ADA deficient. In these children who lack ADA activity, intracellular accumulation of adenosine, 2'-deoxyadenosine, and the corresponding nucleotides results. It is thought that these accumulated metabolites are responsible for inhibition of lymphocyte differentiation. Many mechanisms have been proposed to explain this inhibition (Fox, 1979; reviewed in Pollara et al., 1979) but only the two most popular will be discussed here.

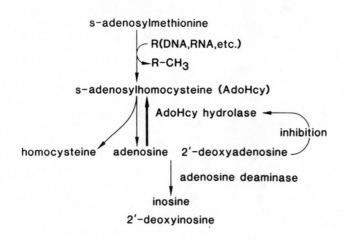

Figure 2.   Relationship of adenosine and 2'deoxyadenosine to s-adenosylmethionine-dependent methylation reactions.

ADA catalyzes the conversion of adenosine and 2'-deoxyadenosine to inosine and 2'-deoxyinosine, respectively (Figure 2). One theory proposes that when adenosine and 2'-deoxyadenosine accumulate in cells, transmethylation reactions are inhibited. Methylation usually involves transfer of a methyl group from S-adenosylmethionine (AdoMet) to a substrate (e.g., RNA, DNA, proteins and small molecules such as catechols, indoles, and phospholipids, Kredich et al., 1979). The products of this transfer are the methylated substrate and

S-adenosylhomocysteine (AdoHcy). The enzyme AdoHcy hydrolase (EC 3.3.1.1) converts AdoHcy to adenosine and L-homocysteine. Because of the reversibility of this reaction with a Keq that greatly favors synthesis of AdoHcy, net hydrolysis of AdoHcy can only occur upon efficient removal of the reaction products. Furthermore, AdoHcy hydrolase has a high affinity for adenosine so that in the presence of excess adenosine, AdoHcy may accumulate and inhibit methylation (Hershfield and Kredich, 1978). Unlike adenosine, 2'-deoxyadenosine is not a substrate for AdoHcy hydrolase. However, it appears to function as a "suicide" inactivator by binding to the enzyme and causing irreversible inactivation (Hershfield, 1979). One consequence of this inactivation may be AdoHcy accumulation with subsequent AdoHcy-mediated inhibition of methylation.

The second theory proposes that the deficiency of ADA leads to inhibition of ribonucleotide reductase, resulting in inadequate DNA synthesis. According to this theory, 2'-deoxyadenosine is the toxic metabolite (Cohen et al., 1978; Coleman et al., 1978). It is phosphorylated by deoxyadenosine kinase, and the resulting 2'-deoxyATP is a potent inhibitor of ribonucleotide reductase (Figure 3) (Moore and Hurlbert, 1966). Supporters of this theory propose that lymphoid tissues are selectively affected because they contain higher activities of deoxyadenosine kinase than other tissues and thus generate toxic quantities of 2'-deoxyATP, while other tissues remain generally unaffected.

PNP is closely related to ADA in the purine salvage pathway. It converts inosine, 2'-deoxyinosine, guanosine and 2'-deoxyguanosine to hypoxanthine and guanine (Figure 3). In children who lack PNP activity, 2'-deoxyGTP accumulates and is hypothesized to inhibit ribonucleotide reductase. Thus, the mechanism of immune dysfunction in PNP deficiency may resemble that in ADA deficiency, with a final common pathway via inhibition of ribonucleotide reductase (reviewed in Fox, 1979).

The first experiments performed in the biochemical evaluation of horses with CID demonstrated that both ADA and PNP activities were normal (McGuire et al., 1976; Castles et al., 1977). These results indicated that CID in horses was similar to the majority of CID children in whom ADA and PNP activities are also normal. This finding also

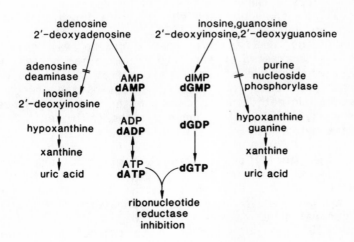

Figure 3.   Proposed pathways of dATP and dGTP formation in
            adenosine deaminase and purine nucleoside
            phosphorylase deficiency.

suggested that a defect in an enzyme other than ADA or PNP
might influence purine metabolism and cause CID.   The
subsequent studies on CID in horses were directed at
determining whether or not this hypothesis was correct.

One of the hallmarks of the immunodeficiency diseases
associated with either ADA or PNP deficiency is the
accumulation of certain purine metabolites in erythrocytes,
lymphocytes, plasma and urine of affected children
(reviewed in Hirschhorn and Martin, 1978; Polmar, 1980;
Mitchell and Kelley, 1980).   Abnormal concentrations of
metabolites have not been detected in any of these tissues
or fluids from horses with CID (Magnuson and Perryman,
1979; Magnuson et al., unpublished observations).   However,
altered purine metabolism has been observed in erythrocytes

from horses with CID following in vitro incubation with adenosine or 2'-deoxyadenosine in physiological concentrations of inorganic phosphate. This alteration was observed as a change in the relative amounts of the adenine nucleotides. These changes were assessed in several ways, including the energy charge relationship (Table 6) described by Shen et al., 1978; and Swedes et al., 1975. A significant decrease in energy charge was observed in nucleoside-treated erythrocytes from normal horses, whereas the energy charge of erythrocytes from CID horses remained unchanged. Other methods for assessing the change in the adenine nucleotide pools gave similar results (Magnuson and Perryman, 1979). These observations indicated a defect in purine metabolism existed in horses with CID.

The paucity of functional lymphocytes precludes many experiments involving the critical cell type. In two foals however, it was possible to study the effect of adenosine on mitogen responsiveness of lymphocytes. We found that peripheral blood lymphocytes (PBL) from these two foals with CID were more sensitive to adenosine than were PBL from normal horses (Table 7, Magnuson and Perryman, 1979). One proposed mechanism for growth inhibition resulting from adenosine treatment involves pyrimidine starvation (Green and Chan, 1973; Carson and Seegmiller, 1976; Ullman et al., 1976; Kredich and Martin, 1977; Gudas, et al., 1978). The adenosine-mediated inhibition of the mitogen response in normal horse PBL was prevented by addition of uridine (Table 8). In contrast, there was no concentration of uridine which was effective in preventing the adenosine-mediated inhibition in PBL from CID horses (Magnuson and Perryman, 1979). This suggests that while pyrimidine starvation occurred in normal horse lymphocytes, a different mechanism was operative in CID horse lymphocytes inhibited by adenosine.

Recent studies involving dermal fibroblasts from CID foals have revealed additional differences in purine metabolism. In examining the growth inhibitory effects of adenosine and 2'-deoxyadenosine on fibroblasts derived from CID horses, 2'-deoxyadenosine was found to be more inhibitory to CID fibroblasts than to fibroblasts from normal horses (Magnuson and Perryman, 1981). One of the postulated mechanisms for 2'-deoxyadenosine toxicity, as described earlier, involves phosphorylation of 2'-deoxyadenosine to 2'-deoxyATP, a potent inhibitor of

Table 6. Effect of Adenosine on Energy Charge of Erythrocytes*

Normal horses

Horse	Control	Adenosine
2	0.57	0.31
304	ND+	0.54
328	0.89	0.71
	0.80	0.66
	0.90	0.50
333	ND	0.39
333	ND	0.77
338	0.87	0.66
350	0.94	0.76
376	ND	0.46
Mean±SD	0.82±0.13	0.58±0.16

Foals with CID

Horse	Control	Adenosine
1082	0.90	0.88
1113	0.83	0.82
	0.89	0.82
	0.77	0.89
	0.94	0.85
	0.84	0.89
	0.91	0.45
	0.79	0.81
1146	0.91	0.86
	0.91	0.66
1150	0.88	0.82
	0.92	0.81
1161	ND	0.92
	0.94	0.79
Mean±SD	0.87±0.05	0.81±0.12

*Determined by the expression, energy charge = [ATP] + 1/2[ADP]/[ATP] + [ADP] + [AMP].
+ND, not done.
The extraction of the adenine nucleotides and chromatographic analysis are described elsewhere (Magnuson and Perryman, 1979).

Table 7. Effect of adenosine on ^{3}H-thymidine uptake by PHA-stimulated PBL

Adenosine concentration	% of normal PHA response			
	normal horse (n=10)	carrier (n=12)	CID (n=1)	human (n=4)
µM				
0.1	102.3 ± 18.7	97.9 ± 12.8	68.1	102.1 ± 30.9
1	96.7 ± 18.8	95.3 ± 18.1	74.3	93.7 ± 25.4
10	93.9 ± 16.6	92.2 ± 17.5	75.9	125.3 ± 40.6
100	44.0 ± 23.6	36.5 ± 15.1	3.8	133.1 ± 32.7
1000	1.2 ± 0.7	1.7 ± 1.3	2.3	66.8 ± 24.7

Cells were cultured as described (Magnuson and Perryman, 1979). Results are expressed as mean percentage of radioactivity incorporated by PHA- and adenosine-treated PBL divided by the radioactivity incorporated by PHA-treated PBL. The n indicates the number of separate experiments used to calculate the mean ± SD for each group of subjects.

Table 8. Uridine reversal of adenosine inhibition of ^{3}H-thymidine uptake in PHA-stimulated lymphocytes.

Uridine concentration	% of normal PHA response			
	normal horse (n=11)	carrier (n=10)	CID foal #1 (n=1)	CID foal #2 (n=3)
μM				
0.1	44.2 ± 13.2	35.5 ± 12.3	23.2	6.5 ± 1.3
1	56.9 ± 19.9	50.4 ± 16.5	21.5	7.4 ± 0.5
10	96.4 ± 33.1	85.7 ± 21.8	25.4	11.5 ± 6.1
100	58.9 ± 15.9	51.2 ± 15.8	22.0	7.0 ± 2.0
1000	30.5 ± 9.7	30.6 ± 10.3	19.5	5.6 ± 0.4

Cells were cultured as described (Magnuson and Perryman, 1979) with the indicated concentrations of uridine together with 100mM adenosine. Results are expressed as mean percentage of radio-activity incorporated by PHA and adenosine-treated PBL divided by the radioactivity incorporated by PHA-treated PBL. The n indicated the number of separate experiments for each group of subjects.

ribonucleotide reductase (Moore and Hulbert, 1966).
Consistent with this hypothesis, 2'-deoxyadenosine toxicity
in mitogen-stimulated human or mouse lymphocytes can be
reversed by addition of purine and/or pyrimidine deoxynucleosides (Bluestein and Seegmiller, 1978; Uberti et al.,
1979; Mitchell et al., 1979). In our experiments with
fibroblasts from CID horses, deoxycytidine in a wide range
of concentrations, or when in combination with deoxyguanosine and thymidine, did not prevent inhibition of
growth. In contrast to 2'-deoxyadenosine, adenosine
inhibited CID and normal fibroblast growth to the same
extent. Addition of uridine completely restored the
maximum growth rate of normal fibroblasts but restored only
60% of the maximum growth rate to CID fibroblasts. These
observations of altered responses to adenosine and
2'-deoxyadenosine by CID fibroblasts suggested that perhaps
AdoHcy hydrolase might be abnormal. Subsequent studies
showed, however, that values for activity and K_m were
normal (Magnuson and Perryman, unpublished observations).
Nevertheless, the possibility exists that the binding
activity for one of the many negative allosteric effectors
of this enzyme is altered and, thus, this aspect needs to
be examined (Ueland and Saebo, 1980).

In addition to the differences between CID and normal
horse metabolism previously discussed, variations in purine
metabolism exist between horses and other species. An
understanding of these differences may suggest site(s) at
which metabolic defects exist in CID horses and children
where ADA and PNP are normal. Some of the differences in
purine metabolism involve ADA. ADA activity in horse PBL
is approximately 10% of that found in human PBL (Magnuson
et al., 1981). This low activity correlates with the
observation that horse PBL are 10-fold more sensitive to
adenosine in mitogenic assays than are human PBL (Magnuson
and Perryman, 1979) and also require more time to degrade
inhibitory concentrations of adenosine before responding in
these assays (Magnuson et al., 1981; Uberti et al., 1977;
Hirschhorn and Sela, 1977). Furthermore, of the various
lymphoid tissues (spleen, lymph node, peripheral blood and
thymus), horse thymus appears to have the lowest ADA
activity. This is in contrast to rat and man where thymus
has the highest ADA activity (Barton et al., 1979; Adams
and Harkness, 1976; Hirschhorn et al., 1978; Carson et al.,
1977; Sullivan et al., 1977) For comparative purposes,
equine thymus has only 1% of the ADA activity reported for

human thymus (Adams and Harkness, 1976; Carson et al., 1977).

Other differences relate to the ability of lymphocytes from various tissues to phosphorylate 2'-deoxyadenosine. Human lymphocytes from spleen, thymus and peripheral blood carry out this phosphorylation reaction while, in horses, only lymphocytes from the thymus have this ability (Carson et al., 1977; Carson et al, 1980; Magnuson et al., 1981). Furthermore, horse PBL (which are primarily T cells, Magnuson et al., 1978; Banks and Greenlee, 1981) when treated with mitogen and 2'-deoxyadenosine will not respond to the mitogen even when purine and/or pyrimidine deoxynucleosides are added (Magnuson et al., 1981). Under identical conditions human PBL will respond (Bluestein and Seegmiller, 1978; Uberti et al., 1979; Mitchell et al., 1979). This indicates that in horse PBL, 2'-deoxATP inhibition of ribonucleotide reductase is not the mechanism by which 2'deoxyadenosine inhibits lymphocyte proliferation.

In summary, these results indicate that purine metabolism in horses is different from that of other species. In addition, tissues from CID foals metabolize adenosine and 2-deoxyadenosine differently from those of normal horses. These observations suggest CID in horses is associated with a defect in purine metabolism. However, the mechanism is not the same as those presently recognized in children.

SUMMARY

Significant contributions to understanding the role of lymphocyte subpopulations in the immune response and to the characterization of immunodeficiencies in children have been achieved through study of animal models of immunodeficiency. Additional contributions can be made in two important areas. One is through identification of relevant, naturally-occurring models of adenosine deaminase deficiency and purine nucleoside phosphorylase deficiency. The second, and potentially more important contribution, would be the identification of the metabolic basis for existing immune deficiencies. The necessary collaborative working arrangements should be established to achieve this objective. Demonstration of the metabolic basis for immune deficiencies in animals may enable the identification of similar defects in people, and eventually lead to enzyme or metabolite delivery schemes for treatment of affected children.

ACKNOWLEDGEMENT

Work performed by the authors was supported by National Institutes of Health Grant no. HD 08886 from the Institute for Child Health and Human Development, the Morris Animal Foundation, and the Arabian Horse Registry of America, Inc.

REFERENCES

Adams A, Harkness RA (1976). Adenosine deaminase activity in thymus and other human tissues. Clin Exp Immunol 26:647.

Andresen E, Flagstad T, Basse A, Brummerstedt E (1970). Evidence of a lethal trait, A46, in Black Pied Danish Cattle of Friesian descent. Nord Vet-Med 22:319.

Andresen E, Basse A, Brummerstedt E. Flagstad T (1974). Lethal trait A46 in cattle: Additional genetic investigations. Nord Vet Med 26:275.

Ardans AA, Trommershausen-Smith A, Osburn BI, Mayhew IG, Trees C, Park MI, Sawyer M, Stabenfeldt GH (1977). Immunotherapy in two foals with combined immunodeficiency, resulting in graft versus host reaction. J Am Vet Med Assoc 170:167.

Arroyave CM, Levy RM, Johnson JS (1977). Genetic deficiency of the fourth component of complement (C4) in Wistar rats. Immunology 33:453.

Asherson GL, Webster ADB (1980). "Diagnosis and Treatment of Immunodeficiency Diseases." Oxford: Blackwell Scientific Publications, p1.

Azar HA, Hansen CT, Costa J (1980). N:NIH(S)11-nu/nu mice with combined immunodeficiency: a new model for human tumor heterotransplantation. J Nat Cancer Inst 65:421.

Baker PE, Smith KA (1980). The potential therapeutic utility of T-cell growth factor. Fed Proc 39:803.

Banks KL, McGuire TC, Jerrells TR (1976). Absence of B lymphocytes in a horse with primary agammaglobulinemia. Clin Immunol Immunopathol 5:282.

Banks KL, Greenlee A (1981). Isolation and identification of equine lymphocytes and monocytes. Am J Vet Res 42:1651.

Barton R, Martiniuk F, Hirschhorn R, Goldschneider I (1979). The distribution of adenosine deaminase among lymphocyte populations in the rat. J Immunol 122:216.

Bennedict AA, Abplanalp HA, Pollard LW, Tam LQ (1977). Inherited immunodeficiency in chickens: a model for common variable hypogammaglobulinemia in man? In Benedict AA (ed): "Avian Immunology." New York: Plenum Press, p 197.

Benedict AA, Chanh TC, Tam LQ, Pollard LW, Kubo RT, Abplanalp HA (1978). Inherited immunodeficiency in chickens. In Gershwin ME, Cooper EL (eds): "Animal Models of Comparative and Developmental Aspects of Immunity and Disease." New York: Pergamon Press Inc, p 99.

Bennedict AA, Gershwin ME, Abplanalp H (1981). Inherited dysgammaglobulinemia of chickens. In Gershwin ME, Merchant B (eds): "Immune Defects of Laboratory Animals." New York: Plenum, vol 1, p 139.

Bitter-Suerman D, Hoffman T, Burger R, Hadding U (1981). Linkage of total deficiency of the second component (C2) of the complement system and of genetic C2-polymorphism to the major histocompatibility complex of the guinea pig. J Immunol 127:608.

Bluestein HG, Seegmiller JE (1978). Deoxynucleoside reversal of deoxyadenosine toxicity to PHA-stimulated adenosine deaminase-inhibited human lymphocytes. Fedn Proc 37:1465.

Brummerstedt E, Flagstad T, Basse A, Andresen E (1971). The effect of zinc on calves with hereditary thymus hypoplasia (lethal trait A 46). Acta Path Microbiol Scand Sect A 79:686.

Brummerstedt E, Basse A, Flagstad T, Andresen A (1977). Animal model of human disease: Acrodermatitis enteropathica, zinc malabsorption. Am J Path 87:725.

Bruton OC (1952). Agammaglobulinemia. Pediatrics 9:722.

Carson DA, Seegmiller JE (1976). Effect of adenosine deaminase inhibition upon human lymphocyte blastogenesis. J Clin Invest 57:274.

Carson DA, Kaye J, Seegmiller JE (1977). Lymphospecific toxicity in adenosine deaminase deficiency and purine nucleoside phosphorylase deficiency: Possible role of nucleoside kinase(s). Proc Natl Acad Sci USA 74:5677.

Carson DA, Kaye J, Wasson BB (1980). Differences in deoxyadenosine metabolism in human and mouse lymphocytes. J Immunol 124:8.

Castles JJ, Gershwin ME, Saito W, Ardans A, Osborn B. (1977). The activity of purine salvage pathway enzymes in murine and horse models of congenital and acquired dysimmunity. Dev Compar Immun 1:165.

Cohen A, Hirschhorn R, Horowitz SD, Rubinstein A, Polmar SH, Hong R, Martin DW Jr (1978). Deoxyadenosine triphosphate as a potentially toxic metabolite in adenosine deaminase deficiency. Proc Natl Acad Sci USA 75:472.

Coleman MS, Donofrio J, Hutton JJ, Hahn L (1978). Identification and quantitation of adenine deoxynucleotides in erythrocytes of patient with adenosine deaminase deficiency and severe combined immunodeficiency. J Biol Chem 253:1619.

Dale DC, Alling DW, Wolff SM (1972). Cyclic hematopoiesis: the mechanisms of cyclic neutropenia in grey Collie dogs. J Clin Invest 51:2197.

Deem DA, Traver DS, Thacker HL, Perryman LE (1979). Agammaglobulinemia in a horse. J Am Vet Med Assoc 175:469.

Duquesnoy RJ, Pedersen GM (1981). Immunologic and hematologic deficiencies of the hypopituitary dwarf mouse. In Gershwin ME, Merchant B (eds): "Immune Defects of Laboratory Animals." New York: Plenum vol 1, p 309.

Edwards NL, Magilavy DB, Cassidy JT, Fox IH (1978). Lymphocyte ecto-5'-nucleotidase deficiency in agammaglobulinemia. Science (Wash DC) 201:628.

Edwards NL, Gelfand EW, Burk L, Dosch H-M, Fox IH (1979). Distribution of 5'-nucleotidase in human lymphoid tissues. Proc Natl Acad Sci USA 76:3474.

Edwards NL, Cassidy JT, Fox IH (1979). Lymphocyte 5'-nucleotidase deficiency: Clinical characteristics of the associated hypogammaglobulinemia. Clin Res 27:324A.

Ellman L, Green I (1970). Genetically controlled total deficiency of the fourth component of complement in the guinea pig. Science 170:74.

Erickson KL, Gershwin ME (1981). Hereditarily athymic-asplenic (Lasat) mice. In Gershwin ME, Merchant B (eds): "Immune Defects of Laboratory Animals." New York: Plenum, vol 1, p 297.

Festing ME, Day D, Connors TA, Lovell D, Sparrow S (1978). An athymic nude mutation in the rat. Nature 274:365.

Festing MF (1981). Athymic nude rats. In Gershwin ME, Merchant B (eds): "Immune Defects of Laboratory Animals." New York: Plenum, vol 1, p 267.

Finkelman FD, Smith AH, Scher I, Paul WE (1975). Abnormal ratio of membrane immunoglobulin classes in mice with an X-linked B-lymphocyte defect. J Exp Med 142:1316.

Flagstad T, Andresen S, Nielsen K (1972). The course of experimental Fasciola hepatica infection in calves with a deficient cellular immunity. Res Vet Sci 13:468.

Flanagan SP (1966). "Nude": A new hairless gene with pleiotropic effects in the mouse. Genet Res 8:295.

Fogh J, Giovanella BC (1978). "The Nude Mouse in Experimental and Clinical Research." New York: Academic Press.

Fox IH (1979). Purine metabolism: Possible biochemical basis for immunodeficiency. In Pollara B, Pickering RJ, Meuwissen HJ, Porter IH (eds): "Inborn Errors of Specific Immunity," New York: Academic Press, p 93.

Fu SM, Hurley JN, McCune JM, Kunkel HG, Good RA (1980). Pre-B cells and other possible precursor lymphoid cell lines derived from patients with X-linked agammaglobulinemia. J Exp Med 152:1519.

Gershwin ME, Merchant B (eds) (1981). "Immune Defects of Laboratory Animals." New York: Plenum, vol 1 and 2.

Giblett ER, Anderson JE, Cohen I, Pollara B, Meuwissen HJ (1972). Adenosine-deaminase deficiency in two patients with severely impaired cellular immunity. Lancet 2:1067.

Giblett E, Ammann AJ, Wara D, Sandman R, Diamond LK (1975). Nucleoside-phosphorylase deficiency in a child with severely defective T-cell immunity and normal B-cell immunity. Lancet 1:1010.

Good RA (1972). Structure-function relations in the lymphoid system. Clin Immunobiol 1:1.

Good RA, West A, Fernandes G (1980). Nutritional modulation of immune responses. Fed Proc 39:3098.

Green H, Chan TS (1973). Pyrimidine starvation induced by adenosine in fibroblasts and lymphoid cells. Science 182:836.

Gudas LJ, Cohen A, Ullman B, Martin DW Jr (1978). Analysis of adenosine mediated pyrimidine starvation using culture wild type and mutant mouse T-lymphoma cells. Somat Cell Genet 4:201.

Hammer CH, Gaither T, Frank MM (1981). Complement deficiencies of laboratory animals. In Gershwin ME, Merchant B (eds): "Immune Defects of Laboratory Animals." New York: Plenum, vol 2, p 207.

Hansen CT (1978). The nude gene and its effects. In Fogh J, Giovanella BC (eds): "The Nude Mouse in Experimental and Clinical Research." New York: Academic Press, p 1.

Herberman RB (1978). Natural cell-mediated cytoxicity in nude mice. In Fogh J, Giovanella BC (eds). "The Nude Mouse in Experimental and Clinical Research." New York: Academic Press, p 136.

Hershfield MS, Kredich NM (1978). S-adenosyl homocysteine hydrolase is an adenosine binding protein: A target for adenosine toxicity. Science 202:757.

Hershfield MS (1979). Apparent suicide inactivation of human lymphoblast S-adenosyl homocysteine hydrolase by 2'-deoxyadenosine and adenine arabinoside: A basis for direct toxic effects of analogs of adenine. J Biol Chem 254:22.

Hirschhorn R, Sela E (1977). Adenosine deaminase and immunodeficiency: An in vitro model. Cell Immunol 32:350.

Hirschhorn R, Martin DW Jr (1978). Enzyme defects in immunodeficiency diseases. Springer Seminar Immunopath 1:299.

Hirshhorn R, Martinick F, Rosen FS (1978). Adenosine deaminase activity in normal tissues and tissues from a child with severe combined immunodeficiency and adenosine deaminase deficiency. Clin Immunol Immunopath 9:287.

Hobbs JR (1975). IgM deficiency. In Bergsma D (ed): "Immunodeficiency in Man and Animals." Sunderland, Mass: Sinauer Associates Inc, p 112.

Horowitz SD, Hong R (1977). The pathogenesis and treatment of immunodeficiency. Monographs in Allergy 10:1.

Johnson SM, Asheron GL, Watts RWE, North ME, Allsop J, Webster ADB (1977). Lymphocyte purine 5'-nucleotidase deficiency in primary hypogammaglobulinemia. Lancet 1:168.

Kincade PW (1981). Hemopoietic abnormalities in New Zealand Black and motheaten mice. In Gershwin ME, Merchant B (eds): "Immune Defects of Laboratory Animals." New York: Plenum, vol 2, p 125.

Kindred B (1978). The nude mouse in studying T cell differentiation. In Fogh J, Giovanella BC (eds). "The Nude Mouse in Experimental and Clinical Research." New York: Academic Press, p 111.

Kramer JW, Davis WC, Prieur DJ (1977). The Chediak-Higashi syndrome of cats. Lab Invest 36:554.

Kredich NM, Martin DW Jr (1977). Role of S-adenosyl-homocysteine in adenosine-mediated toxicity in cultured mouse T lymphoma cells. Cell 12:931.

Kredich NM, Hershfield MS, Johnston JM (1979). Role of methylation in adenosine toxicity in adenosine deaminase inhibited cells. In Pollara B, Pickering RJ, Meuwissen HJ, Porter IH (eds): "Inborn Errors in Specific Immunity," New York: Academic Press, p 261.

Lerman SP, Grebenau MD, Palladino MA, Galton J, Chi DS, Thorbecke GJ (1978). The agammaglobulinemic chicken as a model for T-cell mediated B-cell suppression. In Gershwin ME, Cooper EL (eds): "Animal Models of Comparative and Developmental Aspects of Immunity and Disease," New York: Pergamon Press Inc, p 110.

Luster MI, Bacon LD, Rose NR, Leslie GA (1977). Immunogenetic and ontogenetic studies of chickens with selective IgA-deficiency and autoimmune thyroiditis. Cell Immunol 32:417.

Lutzner MA, Lowrie CT, Jordan HW (1967). Giant granules in leukocytes of the beige mouse. J Hered 58:299.

Magnuson NS, McGuire TC, Banks KL, Perryman LE (1978). In vitro and in vivo effects of cortisosteroids on peripheral blood lymphocytes from ponies. Am J Vet Res 39:393.

Magnuson NS, Perryman LE (1979). In vitro effects of adenosine on lymphocytes and erythrocytes from horses with combined immunodeficiency. J Clin Invest 64:89.

Magnuson NS, Perryman LE (1981). Effects of adenosine and deoxyadenosine on growth of fibroblasts from CID horses. Fed Proc 40:763.

Magnuson NS, McConnell LA, Perryman LE (1981). Adenosine and deoxyadenosine metabolism in lymphocytes from horses, Equis cabalus. Comp Biochem Physiol (in press).

McGuire TC, Poppie MJ (1973). Hypogammaglobulinemia and thymic hypoplasia in horses: a primary combined immuno-deficiency disorder. Infect Immun 8:272.

McGuire TC, Pollara B, Moore JJ, Poppie MJ (1976). Evaluation of adenosine deaminase and other purine salvage pathway enzyme in horses with combined immunodeficiency. Infect Immun 13:995.

McGuire TC, Banks KL, Evans DR, Poppie MJ (1976). Agamma-globulinemia in a horse with evidence of functional T lymphocytes. Am J Vet Res 37:41.

McGuire TC, Perryman LE (1981). Combined immunodeficiency of Arabian foals. In Gershwin ME, Merchant B (eds): "Immune Defects of Laboratory Animals," New York: Plenum, vol 2, p 185.

Mitchell BS, Wilson JM, Mejias E, Kelley WN (1979). Differential effects of deoxyribonucleosides on human T and B lymphoblast cell lines. In Pollara B, Pickering RJ, Meuwissen HJ, Porter IH (eds): "Inborn Errors of Specific Immunity," New York: Academic Press, p 209.

Mitchell BS, Kelley WN (1980). Purogenic immunodeficiency diseases: clinical features and molecular mechanisms. Ann Intern Med 92:826.

Moore EC, Herlbert RB (1966). Regulation of mammalian deoxyribonucleotide biosynthesis by nucleotides as activators and inhibitors. J Biol Chem 241:4802.

Murphy S, Hayward A, Troup G, Devor EJ, Coons T (1980). Gene enrichment in an American Indian population: an excess of severe combined immunodeficiency disease. Lancet 2:502.

Nansen P (1972). Selective immunoglobulin deficiency in cattle and susceptibility to infection. Acta Path Microbiol Scand, Sect B 80:49.

O'Donoghue JL, Reed C (1981). The hairless immune-deficient guinea pig. In Gershwin ME, Merchant B (eds): "Immune Defects of Laboratory Animals," New York: Plenum, vol 1, p 285.

Ooi YM, Colten HR (1979). Genetic defect in secretion of complement C5 in mice. Nature 282:207.

Padgett GA, Leader RW, Gorham JR, O'Mary CC (1964). The familial occurrence of the Chediak-Higashi syndrome in mink and cattle. Genetics 49:505.

Pantelouris EM (1968). Absence of thymus in mouse mutant. Nature 217:370.

Perryman LE (1979). Primary and secondary immune deficiencies of domestic animals. Adv Vet Sci Comp Med 23:23.

Perryman LE, Magnuson NS, Torbeck RL (1979). Combined immunodeficiency in horses. In Pollara B, Pickering RJ, Meuwissen HJ, Porter IH (eds): "Inborn Errors of Specific Immunity," New York: Academic Press, p 391.

Perryman LE, Buening GN, McGuire TC, Torbeck RL, Poppie MJ, Sale GE (1979). Fetal tissue transplantation for immuno-therapy of combined immunodeficiency in horses. Clin Immunol Immunopathol 12:238.

Perryman LE (1980). Use of fetal tissues for immunoreconsti-tution in horses with severe combined immunodeficiency. In Lucarelli G, Fliedner TM, Gale RP (eds): "Fetal Liver Transplantation. Current Concepts and Future Directions," Amsterdam: Excerpta Medica, p 183.

Perryman LE, Liu IKM (1980). Graft versus host reactions in foals with combined immunodeficiency. Am J Vet Res 41:187.

Perryman LE, McGuire TC (1980). Evaluation for immune system failures in horses and ponies. J Am Vet Med Assoc 176:1374.

Perryman LE, Torbeck RL (1980). Combined immunodeficiency of Arabian horses: confirmation of an autosomal recessive mode of inheritance. J Am Vet Med Assoc 176:1250.

Perryman LE, McGuire TC, Torbeck RL (1980). Ontogeny of lymphocyte function in the equine fetus. Am J Vet Res 41:1197.

Pollara B, Pickering RJ, Meuwissen HJ, Porter IH (eds) (1979). "Inborn Errors of Specific Immunity." New York: Academic Press.

Polmar SH (1980). Metabolic aspects of immunodeficiency diseases. Seminars in Hematology 17:30.

Poppie MJ, McGuire TC (1977). Combined immunodeficiency in foals of Arabian breeding: evaluation of mode of inheritance and estimation of prevalence of affected foals and carrier mares and stallions. J Am Vet Med Assoc 170:31.

Reed C, O'Donoghue JL (1979). A new guinea pig mutant with abnormal hair production and immunodeficiency. Lab Anim Sci 29:744.

Reed ND, Manning DD (1978). Present status of xenotransplantation of nonmalignant tissue to the nude mouse. In Fogh J, Giovanella BC (eds): "The Nude Mouse in Experimental and Clinical Research," New York: Academic Press, p 167.

Renshaw HW, Davis WC, Renshaw SJ (1977). Canine granulocytopathy syndrome: defective bactericidal capacity of neutrophils from a dog with recurrent infections. Clin Immunol Immunopathol 8:385.

Roth JA Lomax LG, Altszuler N, Hampshire J, Kaeberle ML, Shelton M, Draper DD, Ledet AE (1980). Thymic abnormalities and growth hormone deficiency in dogs. Am J Vet Res 41:1256.

Rother K, Rother V, Muller-Eberhard HJ, Nilsson U (1966). Deficiency of the sixth component of complement in rabbits with an inherited complement defect. J Exp Med 124:773.

Rygaard J (1978). The nude mouse - background, some achievements, and implications. In Fogh J, Giovanella BC, (eds): "The Nude Mouse in Experimental and Clinical Research," New York: Academic Press, p 95.

Scher I (1981). B-lymphocyte development and heterogeneity: analysis with the immune-defective CBA/N mouse strain. In Gershwin ME, Merchant B (eds): "Immune Defects of Laboratory Animals," New York: Plenum, vol 1, p 163.

Seligmann M, Hitzig WH (1980). "Primary Immunodeficiences." Amsterdam: Elsevier North Holland, p 1.

Sharkey FE, Fogh JM, Hajdu SI, Fitzgerald PJ, Fogh J (1978). Experience in surgical pathology with human tumor growth in the nude mouse. In Fogh J, Giovanella BD (eds): "The Nude Mouse in Experimental and Clinical Research," New York: Academic Press, p 188.

Shen LC, Fall PL, Walton GM, Atkinson DE (1968). Interaction between energy charge and metabolite modulation in the regulation of enzymes of amphibolic sequences. Phosphofuctokinase and pyrvate dehydrogenase. Biochemistry 7:4041.

Smith KA, Baker PE, Gillis S, Ruscetti FW (1980). Functional and molecular characteristics of T-cell growth factor. Molec Immunol 17:579.

Splitter GA, Perryman LE, Magnuson NS, McGuire TC (1980). Combined immunodeficiency of horses: a review. Develop Comp Immunol 4:21.

Studdert MJ (1978). Primary, severe, combined immunodeficiency disease of Arabian foals. Aust Vet J 54:411.

Stutman O (1978). Spontaneous, viral, and chemically induced tumors in the nude mouse. In Fogh J, Giovanella BC (eds): "The Nude Mouse in Experimental and Clinical Research," New York: Academic Press, p 411.

Sullivan JL, Osborne WRA, Wedgwood RJ (1977). Adenosine deaminase activity in lymphocytes. Br J Hemat 37:157.

Swedes JS, Sedo RJ, Atkinson DE (1975). Relation of growth and protein synthesis to the adenylate energy charge in an adenine-requiring mutant of Escherichia coli. J Biol Chem 250:6930.

Taylor RF, Farrell RK (1973). Light and electron microscopy of peripheral blood neutrophils in a killer whale affected with Chediak-Higashi syndrome. Fed Proc 32:822.

Uberti J, Lightbody JJ, Johnson RM (1977). Determination of adenosine deaminase activity using high-pressure liquid chromatography. Analyt Biochem 80:1.

Uberti J, Lightbody JJ, Johnson RM (1979). The effect of nucleosides and deoxycoformycin on adenosine and deoxyadenosine inhibition of human lymphocyte activation. J Immunol 123:189.

Ueland PM, Saebo J (1979). S-adenosylhomocysteinase from mouse liver. Effect of adenine and adenine nucleotides on the enzyme catalysis. Biochemistry 18:4130.

Ullman B, Cohen A, Martin DW Jr (1976). Characterization of a cell culture model for the study of adenosine deaminase- and purine nucleoside phosphorylase deficiency immunologic disease. Cell 9:205.

Vogel SN, Weinblatt AC, Rosentreich DL (1981). Inherent macrophage defects in mice. In Gershwin ME, Merchant B (eds): "Immune Defects of Laboratory Animals," New York: Plenum, vol 1, p 327.

Vogler LB, Pearl ER, Gathings WE, Lawton AR, Cooper MD (1976). B lymphocyte precursors in bone marrow in immunoglobulin deficiency diseases. Lancet 2:376.

Vos JG, Berkvens JM, Kruijt BC (1980a). The athymic nude rat. I. Morphology of lymphoid and endocrine organs. Clin Immunol Immunopathol 15:213.

Vos JG, Kreeftenberg JG, Kruijt BC, Kruizinga W, Steerenberg P (1980b). The athymic nude rat. II. Immunologic characteristics. Clin Immunol Immunopathol 15:229.

Waldmann TA, Broder S, Blaese RM, Durm M, Blackman M, Strober W (1974). Role of suppressor T cells in pathogenesis of common variable hypogammaglobulinemia. Lancet 2:609.

Waldmann TA, Broder S, Goldman CK, Marshall S, Muul L (1980). Suppressor cells in common variable immunodeficiency. In Seligmann M, Hitzig WH (eds): "Primary Immunodeficiencies," Amsterdam: Elsevier North Holland, p 119.

Webster ADB, North M, Allsop J, Asherson GL, Watts REW (1978). Purine metabolism in lymphocytes from patients with primary hypogammaglobulinemia. Clin Exp Immunol 31:456.

Welles WL, Battisto JR (1981). The significance of hereditary asplenia for immune competence. In Gershwin ME, Merchant B (eds): "Immune Defects of Laboratory Animals," New York: Plenum, vol 1, p 191.

Winkelstein JA, Cork LC, Griffin DE, Griffin JW, Adams RJ, Price DL (1981). Genetically determined deficiency of the third component of complement in the dog. Science 212:1169.

DR. O'BRIEN: Have you excluded xanthine oxidase in these foals as being affected?

DR. PERRYMAN: That has been looked at, and the activity was normal.

DR. O'BRIEN: I have a second question which I will direct to you, but the other people possibly might know the answer, if you don't. There is a cat that does not have any hair, the sphinx cat. Is there anything known about the immunological status of that animal?

DR. PERRYMAN: I am not aware of any publications. Does anyone else know? I know anecdotally of two other defects that have been postulated. Some Burmese cats, according to the anecdote, are athymic. Another anecdotal T lymphocyte defect in animals occurs in male miniature dachshunds that have a high prevalence of Pneumocystis carinii infection.

DR. JEZYK: Since you mentioned my model, I thought I might take the opportunity to describe it a bit. It was first detected in a family of basset hounds. Affected animals were presented with a pyoderma early in life, about 2 weeks of age, and went on to very severe pyoderma, otitis externa and stomatitis. They eventually succumbed to distemper infection, which is a paramyxoviral infection. We managed to obtain the dogs and have bred them to reproduce the disease. The mode of inheritance is not yet clear. It is either an autosomal or an X-linked recessive. The disease is characterized by thymic and lymph node dysplasia, absence of T lymphocyte function, at least as we have crudely described it by response to lectins, and hypo-IgG, absent IgA and normal to increased IgM. So, it looks very much like there are abnormalities similar to those described in some of the variable combined immunodeficiencies in man. It also has similarities, except for the hairlessness, to either the nude mouse or the nude rat. We have some preliminary data which were done in conjunction with Dr. Michael Lennon indicating that, in fact, there may be a purine nucleoside phosphorylase deficiency in these animals. I think this is going to turn out to be a very interesting new model.

DR. DESNICK: In the human disorders you can show the accumulation of deoxyadenosine and other purine metabolites in ADA deficient urine by HPLC assay techniques. Have you looked at the urine of your affected foals? Perhaps you can identify the metabolites that are accumulated and then pursue the enzymatic defect.

DR. PERRYMAN: We have analyzed urine, red cell extracts, and fibroblast extracts, and found no evidence for accumulation of metabolites. We had an interesting peak on HPLC about which we became tremendously excited. However, we later found that it was an age-related phenomenon, that normal foals of the same age have it, and by twelve weeks of age it is undetectable. To answer your question directly, we have not found spontaneous accumulations of metabolites in the absence of manipulation of cells in vitro.

Animal Models of Inherited Metabolic Diseases, pages 309-313
© 1982 Alan R. Liss, Inc., 150 Fifth Avenue, New York, NY 10011

GENETIC REGULATION OF ERYTHROCYTE PURINE NUCLEOSIDE
PHOSPHORYLASE IN MICE

Floyd F. Snyder, Fred G. Biddle, Marcia J. Sparling
and Trevor Lukey
Depts. of Medical Biochemistry and Pediatrics,
University of Calgary, Faculty of Medicine,
Calgary, Alberta   T2N 1N4   Canada

Purine nucleoside metabolism acquired a new dimension
of significance with the discovery of adenosine deaminase
deficiency in two patients with severe combined immunodeficiency disease (Giblett et al 1972). Affected children
have a deficiency of both cellular and humoral immunity,
marked lymphopenia and are fatally susceptible to infection.
In 1975, a second disorder of purine metabolism associated
with immunodeficiency was discovered, that of purine nucleoside phosphorylase deficiency (Giblett et al 1975) which is
associated primarily with T cell dysfunction. Both adenosine deaminase and purine nucleoside phosphorylase are auto-
somally recessively inherited disorders, the loci for these
enzymes being on human chromosomes 20 (Creagan 1973) and 14
(Ricciuti, Ruddle 1973) respectively.

In attempts to establish an animal model for the enzyme
deficiencies associated with immunodeficiency, we have begun
screening for quantitative activity variants of adenosine
deaminase and purine nucleoside phosphorylase in Mus
musculus. Impetus for these studies comes from observations
of the mean frequency of null alleles for 25 enzyme loci in
Drosophila melanogaster being 0.002 (Voelker et al 1980).
In addition, evidence for a null allele or heterozygosity
was found in 1 of 214 families screened for adenosine
deaminase 3 years prior to the discovery of the complete
deficiency of this activity (Hopkinson et al 1969).

In screening for quantitative purine nucleoside phosphorylase activity in erythrocyte lysates of feral Mus musculus
we found greater than 3-fold range in activity. The

magnitude of this variability caused us to examine inbred
lines. Preliminary screening of inbred mouse strains revealed
two exclusive groups exemplified by C57BL/6J and DBA/2J, the
former having 2.5-fold greater activity than the latter
(Table 1). Offspring from matings between DBA/2J and C57BL/6J
had intermediate activity characteristic of the additive
contribution of both parents. The backcrosses of the Fl
with DBA/2J gave offspring with low and intermediate activity
and F2 offspring had either low, intermediate or high
activity. There is no evidence for varied reticulocyte
count or different red cell characteristics between the two
lines (Russell 1951) which could give rise to altered enzyme
activity. In addition, adenosine kinase which has been
assigned to chromosome 14 in the mouse (Leinwand et al 1977),
as has purine nucleoside phosphorylase (Womack et al 1977),
was not significantly different between C57BL/6J and DBA/2J
($p < 0.05$), being 0.72±0.21 and 0.66±0.08 nmol/min/mg protein,
respectively.

Table 1. Erythrocyte purine nucleoside phosphorylase activity.

Strain	Purine Nucleoside Phosphorylase nmol/ min/ mg protein	
DBA/2J	17.2 ± 1.4	(20)
C57BL/6J	43.2 ± 2.2	(20)
(DBA/2J X C57BL/6J) F_1	32.1 ± 2.7	(20)
(F_1 x DBA/2J) BC_1	15.8 ± 4.1	(7)
	35.2 ± 4.9	(13)
(F_1 X F_1) F_2	16.7 ± 1.8	(11)
	32.5 ± 3.1	(6)
	47.6 ± 3.4	(3)

Purine nucleoside phosphorylase was assayed in 100 mM
phosphate, pH 7.2, with 0.8 mM [8-^{14}C] inosine, essentially as previously described (Snyder et al 1976).

We examined a number of properties of the enzyme to
determine if differences between DBA/2J and C57BL/6J purine
nucleoside phosphorylase activity could be found. Mixtures
of DBA/2J and C57BL/6J lysates gave the expected additive
activity ruling out the possibility of endogenous inhibitors
or activators. The pH activity profiles for both strains were

identical with a broad peak of activity between pH 6.8 and
7.2. Differences were observed in the Michaelis constants
between DBA/2J and C57BL/6J; they were 99 and 136 μM for
inosine and 52 and 78 μM for deoxyguanosine, respectively.
The thermal inactivation profiles also had some unique
aspects. Purine nucleoside phosphorylase from both strains
was rapidly inactivated at 55^{0} C but was stable in the
presence of 100 mM phosphate even at 60^{0} C. Inactivation
at 50^{0} C in the absence of phosphate gave half lives of 15.5
and 18.0 min for DBA/2J and C57BL/6J, respectively, there
being evidence of a more stable component in C57BL/6J. Thus
there is evidence for differing kinetic and thermal stability
properties and our observations are consistent with there
being more purine nucleoside phosphorylase present in C57BL/6J
than DBA/2J erythrocytes.

DBA/2J and C57BL/6J have a common purine nucleoside
phosphorylase electrophoretic allele, Np-1^{a}, at the Np-1
locus, which shows linkage with esterase-10 on chromosome
14 (Womack et al 1977). In addition, C57BL/6J has a more
cathodally migrating band visible on starch gel electrophoresis, which is apparently not expressed in DBA/2J (Bremner
et al 1978).

We have now demonstrated that the quantitative activity
difference in purine nucleoside phosphorylase between DBA/2J
and C57BL/6J is associated with the absence and presence of
the more cathodally migrating Np-2 band by following criteria.
Offspring of the crosses between these strains, F1, all have
intermediate activity and exhibit the Np-2 electrophoretic
band. Backcrosses of the F1 with the low activity parent
(F$_1$ X DBA/2J)BC$_1$, had low and intermediate activity in the
expected 1:1 ratio. All of the backcrosses with intermediate
activity have the Np-2 band; none with low activity have the
Np-2 band. Thus the presence of the Np-2 allele may be
determined by either quantitative assay or starch gel electrophoresis, but heterozygosity at the Np-2 locus may only be
determined by quantitative assay. Although the quantitative
activity difference appears to be associated with the Np-2
band, staining of Np-2 relative to Np-1 is not sufficient
to account for the 2.5-fold difference in activity between
C57BL/6J and DBA/2J.

The foregoing quantitative and electrophoretic observations are consistent with there being two structural loci
for purine nucleoside phosphorylase in the mouse, Np-1 and

Np-2. The origin of this duplicity and the implications for protection from immunological dysfunction associated with a deficiency of purine nucleoside phosphorylase are of considerable interest. Further investigations now underway include characterization of the gene products of the Np-1 and Np-2 loci and mapping of the Np-2 locus.

Supported by the Medical Research Council of Canada and the Alberta Children's Research Foundation.

References

Bremner TA, Premkumer-Reddy E, Nayar K, Kouri RE (1978). Nucleoside phosphorylase 2 (Np-2) of mice. Biochem Genet 16:1143.

Creagan RP, Tischfield JA, Nichols EA, Ruddle FH (1973). Autosomal assignment of the gene for the form of adenosine deaminase which is deficient in patients with combined immunodeficiency syndrome. Lancet 2:1449.

Giblett ER, Ammann AJ, Sandman R, Wara DW, Diamond LK (1975). Nucleoside phosphorylase deficiency in a child with severely defective T-cell immunity and normal B-cell immunity. Lancet 2:1010.

Giblett ER, Anderson SE, Cohen F, Pollara B, Meuwissen HJ (1972). Adenosine deaminase deficiency in two patients with severely impaired cellular immunity. Lancet 2:1067.

Hopkinson DA, Cook PJL, Harris H (1969). Further data in the adenosine deaminase polymorphism and a report of a new phenotype. Am Hum Genet 32:361.

Leinwand L, Fournier REK, Nichols EA, Ruddle FH (1978). Assignment of the gene for adenosine kinase to chromosome 14 in Mus musculus by somatic cell hybridization. Cytogent Cell Genet 21:77.

Ricciuti F, Ruddle FH (1973). Assignment of nucleoside phosphorylase to D-14 and localization of X-linked loci in man by somatic cell genetics. Nature 241:180.

Russell ES, Neufeld EF, Higgins CT (1951). Comparison of normal blood picture of young adults from 18 inbred strains of mice. Proc Soc Exp Biol Med 78:761.

Snyder FF, Mendelsohn J, Seegmiller JE (1976) Adenosine metabolism in phytohemagglutinin stimulated human lymphocytes. J Clin Invest 58:654.

Voelker RA, Langley CH, Brown AJL, Ohnishi S, Dickson B, Mongtgomery E, Smith SC (1980). Enzyme null alleles in natural populations of Drosophila melanogaster: Frequencies in a North Carolina population. Proc Nat Acad Sci 77:1091.

Womack JE, Davisson MT, Eicher EM, Kendall DA (1977).
Mapping of nucleoside phosphorylase (Np-1) and esterase-10
(Es-10) on mouse chromosome 14. Biochem Genet 15:347.

Animal Models of Inherited Metabolic Diseases, pages 315–325
© **1982 Alan R. Liss, Inc., 150 Fifth Avenue, New York, NY 10011**

CHARACTERIZATION OF A MURINE MODEL (BEIGE) FOR A NATURAL
KILLER CELL IMMUNODEFICIENCY IN THE CHEDIAK-HIGASHI
SYNDROME OF MAN

John C. Roder, PhD
Asst. Prof.
Dept. of Microbiology and Immunology
Queen's University
Kingston, Ontario,
Canada   K7L 3N6

Natural killer cells are a recently described
(Kiessling et al, 1975) subpopulation of large granular
lymphocytes (Timonen et al, 1981) which are thought to play
an important role in immune surveillance against tumors
(Roder and Haliotis, 1980a) and some viral infections
(Shellam et al, 1981). Although poorly characterized in
mice, a new lineage specific marker (HNK-1), detected by
monoclonal antibodies, has recently been described on human
NK cells (Abo and Balch, 1981). The initial event in NK
mediated cytolysis of a tumor cell involves specific recognition of large molecular weight glycoproteins on the tumor
cell membrane (Roder et al, 1979a), followed by a firm and
dynamic cell-cell interaction as shown in figs 1 and 2.
This binding event triggers the NK cell, possibly through
the cyclic nucleotide system (Roder and Klein, 1979b), and
leads to the release of a hypothetical lytic moiety ("toxin")
from the NK cell. This lymphotoxin then binds to receptors
on the tumor cell and delivers the lethal hit which leads
to the destruction of the target cell by a process of
colloid-osmotic lysis, (Roder et al, 1981a), as shown in
fig 3. Due to the poorly understood nature of the events
occurring subsequent to target-effector contact, we began a
search for mutations which might block the cytolytic pathway.
Since indirect evidence suggested the lysosomal enzymes might
be involved in the lethal hit stage (Roder et al, 1980b) we
started our investigation with Chediak-Higashi patients.

The Chediak-Higashi syndrome in man is a rare,
genetically determined disease manifested clinically by

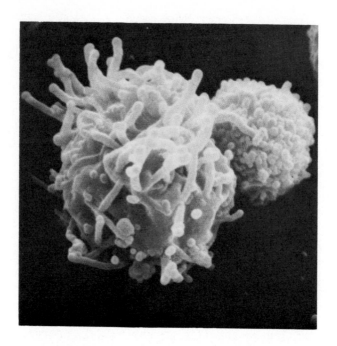

Fig. 1. Scanning electron micrograph showing an NK lymphocyte (upper right) bound to a murine thymoma cell, YAC (lower left) (X 8000).

abnormal leukocyte granulation, defective pigmentation and an increased susceptibility to infections. Humoral immunity and delayed type hypersensitivity are normal and children usually die of pyogenic infection, presumably resulting from a host defence abnormality related to defective granules in their polymorphonuclear (PMN) leukocytes. Survivors generally succumb to a lymphoproliferative disorder which may be malignant. The beige mutation in C57BI/6 mice occurred spontaneously in an autosomal recessive gene on chromosome 13 and is thought to provide an accurate model of the Chediak-Higashi syndrome in man. A detailed comparison of the beige mouse and CH syndrome has been made previously by Windhorst and Padgett (1973). Briefly the animal model is analogous to the human syndrome in terms of (i) increased susceptibility to infection, (ii) distribution, morphology and histochemistry of enlarged granules, (iii) pigment

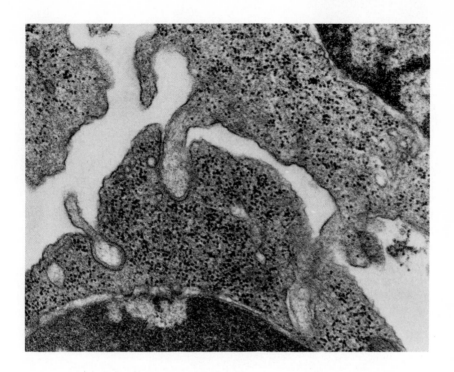

Fig. 2. Transmission electron micrograph of the contact area
between NK cells (lower) and YAC tumor cells (upper), formed
at 37° (X 54,000).

dilution, (iv) bleeding tendency, (v) immunological responses,
(vi) delayed chemotaxis, (vii) decreased serotonin levels,
but differs in some respects since the human but not the
mouse exhibits elevated muramidase levels and abnormal serum
lipid patterns. Humans exhibit a more pronounced accelerated
phase but a similar response could occur later in life in
beige mice, and has not yet been adequately investigated.
Chediak-Higashi disease has also been observed in mink,
cattle, cats and a killer whale.

Six patients carrying the autosomal recessive CH gene
were examined and found to have a profound defect in their
ability to spontaneously lyse various tumor cells by antibody dependent or independent mechanisms (Roder et al, 1980c).
As shown in fig 4 cytolysis of K562 cells by CH peripheral
blood lymphocytes was depressed 100-fold, in terms of lytic

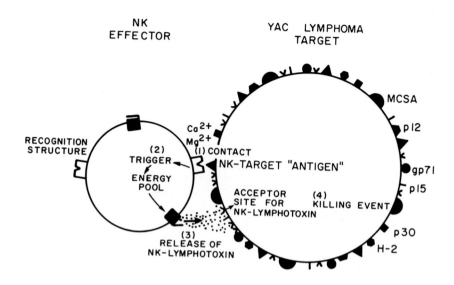

Fig. 3. A schematic model of NK cytolysis (working hypothesis).

units, compared to age and sex matched normals and an unaffected sibling control. In addition, lysis of tumor cells precoated with an optimum dose of rabbit antibody was also severely depressed which is understandable since this form of antibody-dependent cellular cytotoxicity (ADCC) is mediated by NK cells (Haliotis et al, 1980). The selectivity of the antibody-independent NK cell defect is summarized in Table 1. Lymphocytes were blocked in their ability to spontaneously lyse tumor cell targets whereas spontaneous cytolysis of tumor cells by monocytes was normal. Cytostasis by neutrophils from CH patients against K562 cells was also normal as was lectin generated killing by this cell type. The population of T killer cells, as measured by lectin dependent cytolysis was normal in 5 out of 6 patients tested (Klein et al, 1980). Others have previously observed normal mixed-lymphocyte culture (MLC) generated cytotoxic lymphocytes (CTL) in three CH patients and T cell mediated immunity in general, was previously shown to be normal in these and other CH patients as judged by skin testing and proliferative

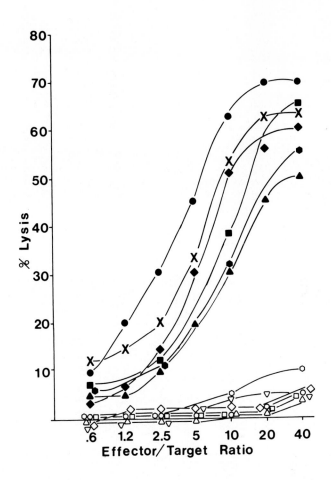

Fig. 4. Peripheral blood lymphocytes from six pre-lymphoma-
tous CH patients (open symbols) and six age and sex matched
normal donors (closed symbols) were incubated for 4 hr with
^{51}Cr labelled K562 cells, a human erythroleukemia cell line.
Values represent the mean percent lysis in triplicate wells.

responses to T dependent mitogens. Non-adherent lymphocytes
from CH patients were completely normal in their ability to
bind K562 and MOLT-4 tumor cells. In addition, the frequency
of cells bearing the NK specific marker, HNK-1, was normal in
CH patients as detected by analysis on the fluorescence

TABLE 1

IMMUNE FUNCTION IN BEIGE MICE AND CHEDIAK-HIGASHI HUMANS

Function	bg/bg Mice	CH Patients
NK cytolysis	low	low
Frequency of NK target-binding cells	normal	normal
ADCC vs tumor cells	low	low
ADCC vs erythrocytes	normal	normal
CTL - MLC	normal	normal
- in vivo alloimmune	normal	ND
- lectin induced	normal	normal*
Skin graft rejection	normal	normal
Delayed type hypersensitivity	normal	normal
T cell - mitogens	normal	normal
B cell - mitogens	normal	normal
- Ig production	normal	normal
Activated macrophage cytolysis	normal	normal
Promonocyte cytolysis - spontaneous	normal	normal
- ADCC	normal	ND
NK interferon boost	yes[†]	yes[†]
Interferon production	normal	ND
cGMP restoration of NK function	no	yes*
Lysosomal enzyme function	low	low

* In some but not all patients (Katz, P. and Haliotis, T.; unpublished observations).
[†] Does not approach level of untreated or IF boosted normal cells.

activated cell sorter (Abo et al, 1981). It was interesting to note that the HNK-1[+], NK cells from CH patients had a single giant granule instead of the 6-12 small granules found in HNK-1[+] cells from normal donors. These results suggest that NK cells are present in CH patients but do not function. Although the biochemical nature of the NK defect is unknown, recent success in restoring NK function to normal levels with cyclic GMP suggests that faulty cyclic nucleotide metabolism may be involved (Katz et al, 1981).

As shown in fig 5 (left panel), homozygous beige mutants (bg^J/bg^J) were markedly (but not completely) deficient in their ability to lyse YAC cells, a murine lymphoma, which is

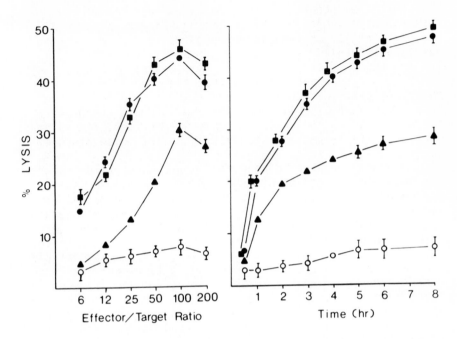

Fig. 5.   Spleen cells were incubated with ^{51}Cr labelled YAC
tumor cells at various effector-to-target ratios in a 4-hr
assay (left panel) or for various periods of time at a 100/1
effector/target ratio (right panel). ▲, A Sn; 0, C57Bl/6,
bg^J/bg^J; ●, +/bg^J littermates; ■ , age-matched +/+ controls.
Values represent the mean % specific lysis ± s.e. in quadru-
plicate wells.

one of the most sensitive NK targets in the mouse system.
The heterozygous littermate controls (+/bg^J) responded as
well as the wild type (+/+).   This impairment in NK function
could not be accounted for by a delayed kinetics of killing
or by an altered organ distribution, target selectivity or
ontogenesis (Roder et al, 1979c).   Interferon could improve
but not fully restore the response which suggests that the
defect does not result from a lack of endogenous interferon
stimulation in beige mice.   Recent findings show that bg/bg
mice produced normal amounts of interferon and virus upon
infection with LCMV (Welsh and Kiessling, 1980).   It is
important to note that the NK defect in beige mice, as in CH

patients, was selective. Other forms of cytolysis mediated by T cells, macrophages or promonocytes were normal as summarized in Table 1. The defect in NK cytolysis was predetermined at the level of progenitor cells in the bone marrow as revealed in radiation chimaeras (Roder et al, 1979d). The frequency of target binding cells was normal in all lymphoid organs which suggests that the defect is intrinsic to the NK cell and does not involve an altered population size or an inability to recognize and interact with the target. Rather, the defect may lie within the lytic pathway subsequent to target cell contact as in the human disease.

In summary, the beige mutant mouse provides an accurate analogue of the Chediak-Higashi syndrome in man in terms of the defect in granulation and the impairment in NK cell function. The two genes, bg and CH, may or may not be homologous (identical) but they provide the first defined genetic markers for sequencing the NK cytolytic pathway. Since the impairment in NK function is selective, these immunodeficiencies also provide the first opportunity to unequivocally assess the importance of NK cells in surveillance against tumor development. Preliminary results are encouraging and show that the beige mouse is more susceptible to the growth and dissemination of transplantable syngeneic tumors (Karre et al, 1980; Talmadge et al, 1980). It is also clear that most CH patients, with low NK activity, develop a lymphoproliferative disorder which may be malignant (Dent et al, 1966). Therefore, it is becoming increasingly certain that NK cells are important in host defense against tumors and a detailed study of NK cells in Chediak-Higashi patients or beige mice will help unravel the secrets of the cytolytic pathway. Human or animal diseases that lead to a block in NK differentiation would be equally helpful in clarifying the developmental lineage of NK cells and their relationship to other effectors in the lymphoid system.

Abo T, Balch CM (1981). A differentiation antigen of human NK and K cells identified by a monoclonal antibody (HNK-1). J Immunol 127:1024.
Dent PB, Fish LA, White JF, Good RA (1966). Chediak-Higashi syndrome. Observations on the nature of the associated malignancy. Lab Invest 15:1634.
Haliotis T, Roder JC, Klein M, Ortaldo J, Fauci AS, Herberman RB (1980). The Chediak-Higashi gene in humans. I. Impairment of NK function. J Exp Med 151:1039.

Karre K, Klein GO, Kiessling R, Klein G, Roder JC (1980).
Low natural in vivo resistance to syngeneic leukemias in
natural killer-deficient mice. Nature 284:624.

Katz P, Roder JC, Zaytoun A, Herberman RB, Fauci AS (1981).
Correction of a selective defect in natural killing. J
Immunol (submitted).

Kiessling R, Klein E, Wigzell H (1975). Natural killer cells
in the mouse. I. Cytotoxic cells with specificity for
mouse Maloney leukemia cells. Specificity and distribution according to genotype. Eur J Immunol 5:112.

Klein M, Roder JC, Haliotis T, Korec S, Jett J, Herberman RB,
Katz P, Fauci AS (1980). The Chediak-Higashi gene in
humans. II. The selectivity of the defect in NK and ADCC
function. J Exp Med 151:1049.

Roder JC, Rosen A, Fenyo EM, Troy FA (1979a). Target-effector
interaction in the natural killer cell system: the isolation of target structures. Proc Natl Acad Sci (USA) 76:
1405.

Roder JC, Klein M (1979b). Target-effector interaction in
the natural killer cell system. IV. Modulation by cyclic
nucleotides. J Immunol 123:2785.

Roder JC (1979c). The beige mutation in the mouse. I. A
stem cell predetermined impairment in natural killer cell
function. J Immunol 123:2168.

Roder JC, Lohmann-Matthes ML, Domzig W, Wigzell H (1979d).
The beige mutation in the mouse. II. Selectivity of the
natural killer cell defect. J Immunol 123:2174.

Roder JC, Haliotis T (1980a). Do NK cells play a role in
anti-tumor surveillance? Immunol Today 1:96.

Roder JC, Argov S, Klein M, Petersson C, Kiessling R,
Andersson K, Hansson M (1980b). Target-effector interaction
in the natural killer cell system. V. Energy requirements,
membrane integrity and the possible involvement of lysosomal enzymes. Immunol 40:107.

Roder JC, Haliotis T, Klein M, Korec S, Jett J, Ortaldo J,
Herberman RB, Katz P, Fauci AS (1980c). A new immunodeficiency disorder in humans involving NK cells. Nature
248:553.

Roder JC, Beaumont TJ, Kerbel RS, Haliotis T, Kazbor D (1981).
Selective natural killer resistance in a clone of YAC
lymphoma cells. Proc Natl Acad Sci (USA) 78:(10).

Shellam GR, Allan JE, Papadimitriou JM, Bancroft GJ (1981).
Increased susceptibility to cytomegalovirus infection in
beige mutant mice. Proc Natl Acad Sci (USA) 78:5104.

Talmadge JE, Meyers KM, Prieur DJ, Starkey JR (1980). Role
of natural killer cells in tumor growth and metastasis in
beige mice. Nature 284:622.

Timonen T, Ortaldo JR, Herberman RB (1981). Characteristics
   of human large granular lymphocytes and relationship to
   natural killer and K cells. J Exp Med 153:569.
Welsh R, Kiessling R (1980). Natural killer cell response
   to lymphocytic choriomeningitis virus in beige mice. Scand
   J Immunol 11:363.
Windhorst DB, Padgett G (1973). The Chediak-Higashi syndrome
   and the homologous trait in animals. J Invest Dermatol
   60:529.

DR. RATTAZZI: There are a number of mutants in the mouse that are similar to the beige mutant: pale, pink ears and so on that Dr. Paigen's group has studied. Have you any information as to whether the phenomenon that you just described is present in these other models?

DR. RODER: Some workers from Uppsala, Sweden, Anders Örn and Hans Wigzell, have looked at five pigment mutants in the mouse. Four of them had a concomitant depression in lysosomal enzyme function, and the fifth did not. The four with depressed lysosomal enzyme function had depressed natural killer cell activity, and the fifth had normal natural killer cell activity. This kind of co-relation strengthens the argument that secretion of lysosomal enzymes may be involved in NK mediated cytolysis.

Animal Models of Inherited Metabolic Diseases, pages 327–349
© **1982 Alan R. Liss, Inc., 150 Fifth Avenue, New York, NY 10011**

HISTOCOMPATIBILITY, DISEASE AND AGING

Edmond J. Yunis, M.D. and Ada L.M. Watson

Sidney Farber Cancer Institute and
Harvard Medical School (EJY)
44 Binney Street, Boston, MA 02115

The term'aging', normally applied only with reference
to long-lived members of a population, can be defined as a
slow, genetically-programmed decline in the functional effectiveness of the organism. It constitutes the collective set
of changes, occurring over the course of a life span, which
limit the duration of life.('Life span' is the duration of
life of one individual, but can be expressed, for a population, either as the duration of life of the longest survivors,
or as the median duration. This is an extremely complicated
process, involving numerous interactions which are extremely
sensitive to the environment.Much evidence indicates that both
genetic and environmental factors influence aging and life
span.(Yunis, J.J. et al.,1977)

Interactions between genotype and environment occur at
every level of the life of an individual. Consequently, explanations of aging must analyze the extremely complex interactions between purely hereditary factors and those environmental influences which affect such genetically determined
processes as differentiation, morphogenesis and metabolism.
These processes operate in the context of coordinated activity by the nervous and endocrine systems. It is possible,
also, that biologic control mechanisms may shift at any time
between fertilization and senescence. Thus, it is not surprising that no single theory of aging has provided an encompass-
ing explanation of that process. It is also not surprising
that responsibility for aging changes cannot be assigned to
any one system, organ or group of cells.

Generally, graying hair and wrinkling skin are considered

part of the aging process, while embryogenesis and subsequent stages in biologic maturation usually are not. In fact, however, death of individual cells, of the individuals themselves, may occur at any stage in development. Within a given genetic framework, organs develop and involute according to specific timetables. Schedules for organ development and involution in a given species, together with the limits imposed by a preordained proliferative capacity of cells, strongly suggest that life span must be under genetic control mediated via cell and organ 'clocks.'

Age-associated diseases, and physiological changes associated with the aging process, relate, at least in part, to changes in immune system function. With respect to etiology and pathogenesis of age-associated disease or dysfunction, two factors must be considered: (1) thymic involution, which may be accompanied by cell-mediated immune dysfunction, and (2) major histocompatibility complex (MHC)-associated genetic control of immune response and resistance to disease. Although deficiencies in immunologic function have not yet been proved to be fundamental in the etiology of such age-associated disease states as autoimmunity, vascular degeneration and insufficiency, or kidney or nervous system degeneration, most studies have been limited to correlation of diseases of aging with accumulating immunologic changes. Whether progressive changes in the immune system are responsible for the decline of functional effectiveness, or whether immune changes are a secondary effect, remains unknown.

Medical services, sanitation and nutrition have allowed mankind to manipulate the environment in ways which affect survival. In recent decades, survival curves have progressively approached rectangular form. The remaining population at about 80-85 years of age (5-8% of the original cohort) represents individuals of maximum genetically-determined life span, and is the most appropriate group in which to study the process of aging. (Walford, 1969) On the other hand, approximately 20% of the general population carry genetic defects which shorten life span; these individuals contribute substantially to mortality below 70 years of age. (Yunis, J.J. et al., 1977) Both of these observations emphasize difficulties in distinguishing between research on aging itself as opposed to research on diseases associated with aging. They also argue, in a general sense, in favor of the existence of genetically-determined physiologic and cellular clocks. In future, the number and nature of such clocks must be determined. Here, dis-

cussion will center on the so-called 'thymus clock'and its
relation to an immunologic theory of aging. The role of cellular immune functions and of the major histocompatibility
complex in the production of autoantibodies and in longevity
will also be reviewed.

In two diseases- 21 hydroxylase deficiency of man (Dupont, et al., 1977) and the neuraminidase deficiency of mice
(Womack, et al., 1981)- the MHC is the marker for enzyme deficiency. In many cases, major factors for susceptibility to human and animal diseases, immune disorders included, can be
identified. In addition, the MHC constitutes an important marker for longevity in mice, and should be significant in studies of aging in humans.

THE THYMUS CLOCK AND THE IMMUNOLOGIC THEORY OF AGING

Theories concerning the association of immunologic mal-
function with aging follow several directions. The immunologic interpretation of aging, first clearly stated by Walford
(1969) and extensively promulgated and developed by Burnet
(1971), holds that the immune system is essential for maintenance of health, its integrity determining survival. Walford
further suggested that aging results from somatic-cell changes
in the factors which determine self-recognition among cells,
progressive breakdown of that system then producing autoimmunity and autoimmune disease. In our studies, the decline of
vigorous immune function in aging man and mouse has been associated with the same diseases and immunologic abnormalities
found in individuals which lack normal T-cell systems. (Good
and Yunis, 1974) Observations of this type led Burnet
(1959)to suggest that clones of cells, ordinarily forbidden by
intact immune systems, appear by somatic mutation and persist
as immune functions become defective. Such events, he concluded
would explain the autoimmunity which is frequently observed
in both aging and immunodeficient individuals. (Burnet, 1970)
Alternatively, Good and Yunis (1974) have interpreted these
associations in terms of a"forbidden antigen" theory of autoimmunity, arguing that under immunodeficient circumstances,
antigens otherwise excluded from the body, or promptly eliminated, are permitted to enter and remain. Persisting, as a
consequence of inefficient or ineffective immune response,the
antibodies may either act as infectious agents or else generate cross-reacting antibodies.(Good and Yunis,1974;Yunis et
al., 1970; Yunis et al,1976)

One possible immunologic theory of aging based on thymic involution holds that the primary events of aging are embodied in a persistent, genetically-programmed process of declining function and control of the T-dependent lymphoid system. The genetically-programmed 'clock' operates at a rate consistent with the median life span of the species. For the longest-lived individuals or strains, the clock may adhere to limits imposed by the postulate of Hayflick. (1965)

Maturation of thymocytes by the thymus may cease as a consequence either of changes in CNS-endocrine control, or of intrinsic temporal limitations. Given that B-lymphocytes are regulated by T-cells, involution of the thymus would indirectly limit the vigor of B-lymphocyte differentiation, thus promoting further declines in humoral immunity. Involution of either or both controlling lymphoid systems, with consequent loss of their generating and supportive functions, would limit immunologic vigor during aging.

These considerations suggest that the primary age-related change in the immune system is a decrease in T-cell functional capacity. The resulting imbalanced systems, in which B-cells remain relatively normal while T-cells are deficient, may influence the appearance of autoantibody and of a number of diseases associated with aging. Observations of decreased life expectancy among old people with defective cell-mediated immunity (CMI) support the notion that T-cell deficiency is associated with the pathogenesis of age-related disease. (Roberts-Thomson, et al., 1974) Our own studies suggest that disturbance of T-cell subpopulation balance may further aggravate the situation. (Hallgren and Yunis, 1977) One type of T-cell deficiency may be a decrease in suppressor cell function which would allow autoimmune clones to form and to be expressed. Conversely, loss of self-tolerance and the development of autoimmunity could stimulate production of anti-T-cell antibodies, accelerating T-cell immunodeficiency as aging proceeds.

A progressive decrease in mass of both human and animal lymphoid systems generally begins at puberty and continues thereafter. Normally, there is a rather close correlation between lymphoid mass and immunologic function. Thymic involution precedes, and is probably the key determinant of, an age-dependent decline in the ability of the immune system to generate functional T-cells. Apparently, a T-cell differentiation pathway is affected. As the thymus ages, the relative

size of its cortex decreases while the absolute number of macrophages increases. Plasma cells and mast cells tend to in-
filtrate the thymic medulla, and secretory epithelial cells,
particularly those of the cortex, decrease in number with age.
Functional consequences include deficient lymphocyte population in T-cell-dependent areas of the lymph nodes, and also
declines in T-cell activity.

As shown by experiments with mice, the magnitude of immunologic activity in the aged is determined by the thymus, the
bone marrow, and the humoral environment of the lymphoid cells.
Among these, the thymus seems to be the limiting factor for
immunologic vigor since the immunologic capacity of aged animals can be restored by transplantation of young thymus together with young bone marrow. (Hirokawa,1977)

Decline of immune function reflects a decrease in both
the number and function of immunologically active cells, and
also alterations of the environment in which these cells function. As measured by antibody-forming capacity, approximately
10% of the age-dependent decline in immune function has been
attributed to environmental factors (i.e., to factors extrin-
sic to the cells), the remaining 90% apparently being a consequence of changes in the cells themselves.

THYMUS INVOLUTION IN SHORT-LIVED STRAINS OF MICE

Shrinkage of the thymus, and ensuing deficiency in cell-
mediated immune function, occur earlier in certain individuals
and inbred strains than others. For example, the immunodeficiency observed in strain A mice during the second year of
life is strikingly similar to that produced by neonatal thymectomy. (Good and Yunis,1974; Yunis, et al.,1970) Lymphoid neoplasms and lung tumors of mice occur at an early date when
life span is shortened by irradiation. (Alexander, 1964).Con-
versely, the CBA mouse strain, in which thymic involution is
relatively late, tends to be very long-lived and to maintain
immunologic function longer than many others.

AUTOIMMUNE STRAINS OF MICE

As found in 1963, Coombs positive hemolytic anemia regularly develops spontaneously in the New Zealand Black (NZB)
strain of mice. Neonatal thymectomy shortened the incubation

period for development of antinuclear antibodies and immune complex glomerular disease in both this strain and its (NZB xNZW)F_1 hybrids. The spontaneous development, by A/J mice, of antinuclear antibodies (Good and Yunis,1974; Fernandes,et al.,1977) likewise facilitated by neonatal thymectomy which also produces an extraordinary cell proliferation in the lymphoid tissues, similar to that observed in aging mice of autoimmune-susceptible strains. In contrast, CBA/H and C3H mice, which do not develop spontaneous autoimmunity during aging, exhibit lymphoid tissue atrophy, and show much less evidence of production of autoanibodies following neonatal thymectomy. The immunologic deficiencies, autoimmune hemolytic anemia, antinuclear and anti-DNA antibodies, and the hematologic, hepatic, splenic and renal lesion which appear early in life, following neonatal thymectomy in autoimmune-susceptible mice apparently represent an acceleration of the processes associated with cellular immunodeficiency during aging in these strains.

Attempts to correct immunodeficiency in thymectomized animals provide another line of evidence linking immunodeficiency to autoimmunity. In neonatally thymectomized mice, both immunodeficiency and autoimmunity can be prevented either by transplantation of syngeneic or allogeneic thymus from young mice, or by injection of thymus lymphocytes or spleen lymphocytes from syngeneic, semi-allogenic or allogeneic donors. (Good and Yunis, 1974; Fernandes, et al.,1977) To avoid Graft versus Host reaction (GVH), the injected thymus or peripheral lymphoid cells must be matched with the recipient at the major histocompatibility complex. (Yunis, et al.,1971) Even after wasting disease and autoimmune processes have appeared, effects in neonatally thymectomized mice can be reversed by treatment with multiple thymus grafts or by injections of large numbers of either thymus cells or peripheral lymphoid cells. (Fernandes, et al.,1977; Yunis, et al.,1971)

In young recipients, spleen cells from young A or NZB mice differentiate into antibody-producing cells, but spleen cells from an old donor in a young irradiated recipient, or from a young donor in an old irradiated recipient generated plague-forming cells inefficiently. These findings are consistent with the view that the immunodeficiency of aging, in short-lived or autoimmune-susceptible strains, involves not only the lymphoid cells themselves, but also the environment in which these cells function. (Makinodan, et al.,1975)

HUMAN IMMUNE RESPONSE

Disease of adult life, autoimmunity, infections and cancer in particular, have been linked to a decline in immune
function. However, it is not clearly demonstrable what general
aspects of immunity are impaired in old age, nor it is known how
pathologic conditions arise in any given 'immunodeficient' individual. This poses problems for clinicians who desire reliable assessment of immune function upon which to base prognoses.
Obviously, autoimmunity and infection result from inappropriate or inadequate immune responses; the role of the immune
system in tumor control is a subject of continuing debate.

In mice, humoral immunity is optimal during early life
but declines gradually with age (Makinodan,1978) with respect
to both primary and secondary responses to either thymus-dependent or thymus-independent antigens. Studies of congenic
mice, which have enabled investigators to examine the effects,
on longevity, of single changes in MHC, yield a few curious
results: Survival data indicate that median survival times
correlate with certain H2 haplotypes. (Smith and Walford,1977)

There may also be differences in immune response; thus,
in one study, the longest-lived strain was most responsive to
the mitogen phytohemagglutinin (PHA), and the shortest-lived
strain least responsive. It seems, therefore, that MHC might
influence longevity by means of immune competence.

In man, the percentage of lymphocytes with T-cell markers
does not seem to change with age, while the number of B-lymphocytes appears to remain constant or to increase. (Hallgren,
et al.,1974) Investigations of T-cell function have produced
conflicting results. In vitro studies often reveal that allo-
and mitogen-activation decline with age. (Hallgren, et al.,
1978) Because this does not result from decreased T-cell number, effects of age on T-cell function would appear to result
from changes in the relative properties of functional subpopulations. (Strelkauskas, et al.,1981) Humoral immunity does
decline with age, but in a process which appears to be exteme-
ly complicated. Although the influence of T-cell subsets on B-
cell function is of great importance, available methodology
has limited experimentation to assessments of subset function.
Age-dependent changes have been noted in serum levels of the
immunoglobulins, serum IgG and IgA increasing, and IgM and
IgE decreasing with age. The decline of IgE levels is greatest
in atopic individuals. (Table I) Natural antibodies for

anti-A isoagglutinins decrease with age, as primary antibody responses to a diversity of antigens. As measured by skin testing and radioallergosorobent test (RAST), levels of specific IgE antibody to the common aeroallergens tend to be lower in the older age groups.

TABLE I

ALTERATION OF IMMUNE PARAMETERS IN AGING MAN

	AGE GROUP	
	Young (20-39 years)	Old (80-99 years)
Cellular Immunity:		
Response to phytohemagglutinin	Normal	Decreased
Response to Concanavalin-A	Normal	Decreased
Response to allogeneic cells	Normal	Decreased
Suppressive action of Concanavalin-A stimulated lymphocytes	Normal	Decreased
Percentage of peripheral T-cells	Normal	Normal
T-cells identified by Juvenile Rheumatoid Arthritis autoantibody	Normal	Decreased
Humoral Immunity:		
Antibody response to heterologous antigens and iso-antigens	Normal	Decreased
Autoantibody production	Normal	Increased
Serum levels of IgG, IgA and IgE	Normal	Decreased
Percentage of peripheral B-cells	Normal	Normal

Although the regulation of immune response is predominantly under genetic control, the influence of non-lymphoid factors, such as nutrition, drugs and the condition of other organ systems, the neuroendocrine in particular, can affect the immune status of an experimental animal or patient. Since only non-genetic manipulation of the lymphoid system is possible, clinical experimentation on non-lymphoid factors is essential. Studies have shown that in autoimmune NZB mice, moderate calorie or protein restriction decreased levels of autoantibody formation, protected against glomerulonephritis, and prolonged life span. (Friend, et al.,1978)

THE MAJOR HISTOCOMPATIBILITY COMPLEX (MHC):

1. Genetics of MHC:

Humoral and cellular immune responses are based upon precisely integrated cooperative cellular interactions between macrophages, T-lymphocytes and B-lymphocytes.(Gershon,1975; Katz and Benacerraf,1976; Rosenthal,1978) Animal studies using molecules with single (or at most a few) antigenic determinants have revealed that these responses are under the control of genes within at least two separate linkage groups: Those controlling, at least, idiotypic specificities (and closely linked to immunoglobulin heavy chain genetic loci), and those of the MHC. (Levine. et al.,1963; McDevitt and Tyan, 1968; Benacerraf and McDevitt,1972; Grey, et al.,1965) MHC genes controlling the presence or absence, and magnitude, of the antibody response are called Ir genes. (Benacerraf and McDevitt,1972) In the animal with the best-characterized MHC, the mouse, Ir genes have been located, within the MHC, on the seventh chromosome between H-2K and the S (Ss-Slp) region. (The latter controls synthesis of the fourth component of murine complement, C4 or Ss, and also a closely similar molecule without C4 function, Slp. (Roos, et al.,1978;Ferreira, et al., 1978) The 'I' region, containing the Ir genetic loci, has been subdivided (proceeding from H-2K toward the S region and H-2D) into I-A, I-B, I-J and I-C. (Klein, et al.,1978) By immunizing inbred strains of mice with lymphocytes from other inbred strains which differ genetically on in the I-regions, antibodies have been obtained which react with surface determinants, the 'Ia antigens', produced by I-region genes. (David, et al.,1973; Hammerling, et al.,1974) It is now known that genes I-1, I-B and I-C code for structures on helper T-lymphocytes, whereas those in I-J control molecules on suppressor T-cells. (David, et al.,1976; Murphy, et al.,1976) Remarkably, antigen-specific helper and suppressor factors, secreted by respective subsets of T-lymphocytes, carry Ia antigenic determinants and idiotypic determinants without constant regions of heavy or light immunoglobulin chains. (Taussig, et al.,1974;Mozes and Haimovich,1979)

The MHC's of different mammalian species are strikingly similar. In the mouse, however, an inversion in the seventeenth chromosome has located the I-regions between, rather than outside, the two major serologically-defined histocompatibility loci (H-2K and H-2D). (Dorf, et al.,1975) In man, the MHC-linked genes for C4, Bf, and C2 possibly are located between HLA-B and HLA-D/DR.

2. HLA and Disease:

HLA antigens are associated with many diseases, a significant number of which are autoimmune in nature. To study a possible relationship, HLA tissue haplotypes of affected patients are compared with antigen frequencies in a large control group. For example, HLA-B27, found only in about 6% of the general Caucasian population, occurs in over 90% of patients with ankylosing spondylitis. (Dausset and Svejgaard, 1977) Other diseases with weaker but still significant HLA associations include rheumatoid arthritis, dermatitis herpetiformis, Addison's Disease, multiple sclerosis and myasthenia gravis.

Susceptibility in autoimmune or immune complex disease appears to be inherited, both in laboratory animals (Scher,et al.,1975; Young and Engleman,1980) and in man. Some of the responsible genes are MHC-linked, for studies of unrelated patients with these disorders show that specific MHC alleles occur with altered frequencies in comparison to matched populations. (Keck,1975; Bertrams, et al.,1976) (Table 2) In juvenile onset diabetes mellitus (IDDM), for example, there are increased frequencies of HLA-B8, B15 and B18, each with a relative risk (RR) of about 2.5, and also a decreased frequency of HLA-B7. (Ludvigsson, et al.,1977;Marsh, et al., 1978) Furthermore, there is an increased incidence of HLA-Dw3 and HLA-Dw4 (RR= 4.5) Gerrard, et al.,1978) a marked increase of the complement marker Bf F1 (RR+ 7.5). (Ott,1979) Similar findings, but different MHC associations, are obtained in patients with several autoimmune diseases thought to derive from unusual immune responses, possible to viruses. Keck,1975; Bertrams, et al.,1976) Certain autoimmune diseases of laboratory animals, such as experimental allergic encephalomyelitis in rats (Gasser, et al.,1973; Williams and Moore,

1973) and thyroiditis in mice (Vladutiu and Rose,1971) are clearly linked to MHC.

TABLE 2

ASSOCIATION BETWEEN HLA AND DISEASE

Disease	Antigen	Frequency of antigen (%)		Relative risk	Significance (P)
		Controls	Patients		
ALLERGY					
Ragweed hay fever	perhaps linked to HLA in family studies				
ARTHROPATHIES					
Ankylosing spondylitis	B27	9.4	90	87.4	$<10^{-10}$
Reiter's syndrome and	B27	9.4	79	37.0	$<10^{-10}$
reactive arthritis	B27 increased yersinia, salmonella, & shigella				
Psoriatic arthritis	B27	9.4	29	4.0	$<10^{-10}$
	B16	5.9	15	2.8	$<10^{-3}$
Juvenile arthritis	B27	9.4	32	4.5	$<10^{-10}$
Rheumatoid arthritis	Dw4	28.4	70	5.8	$<10^{-5}$
ENDOCRINE DISEASES					
Juvenile and/or insulin-	Dw2	25.8	0	0.0	$<10^{-6}$
dependent diabetes	Dw3	26.3	44	2.2	$<10^{5}$
	Dw4	19.4	49	4.0	$<10^{-10}$
Graves disease	Dw3	26.3	57	3.7	$<10^{-9}$
Idiopathic Addison's disease	Dw3	26.3	69	6.3	$<10^{-5}$
Congenital adrenal hyperplasia	Bw47				
	close linkage to HLA in family studies				
EYE DISEASES					
Acute anterior uveitis	B27	9.4	52	10.4	$<10^{-10}$
INFECTIONS					
Leprosy (Tuberculoid)	apparently linked to HLA in family studies				
Tuberculosis	B8	20.0	57	5.1	$<10^{-6}$
Subacute thyroiditis	B35	14.6	70	13.7	$<10^{-10}$
INTESTINAL DISEASES					
Coeliac disease	Dw3	26.3	79	10.8	$<10^{-8}$
LIVER DISEASES					
Chronic autoimmune hepatitis					
Childhood	B8	24.6	75	9.0	$<10^{-10}$
Adult	Dw3	19.0	78	13.9	$<10^{-6}$
	Dw4				
NEUROLOGICAL DISEASES					
Multiple sclerosis	Dw2	25.8	59	4.1	$<10^{-10}$
Cerebellar ataxia	perhaps linked to HLA in family studies				
SKIN DISEASES					
Psoriasis vulgaris	B13	4.4	18	4.8	$<10^{-10}$
	B17	8.0	29	4.8	$<10^{-10}$
	B37	2.6	11	4.4	$<10^{-6}$
	Cw6	33.1	87	13.3	$<10^{-10}$
Dermatitis herpetiformis	Dw3	26.3	85	15.4	$<10^{-10}$
	DRw3	25.0	97	56.4	$<10^{-10}$
Bechet's disease	B5	10.1	41	6.3	$<10^{-10}$
SYSTEMIC DISEASES					
Myasthenia gravis	B8	24.6	57	4.1	$<10^{-10}$
Sicca Syndrome	Dw3	26.3	78	9.7	$<10^{-9}$
Systemic lupus erythematosus	B8	24.6	41	2.1	$<10^{-10}$
Haemachromatosis	A3	28.2	76	8.2	$<10^{-10}$
	behaves as a recessive trait closely linked to HLA				

The H-2 complex also appears to be involved in susceptibility to oncogenic agents. The latter include Gross (Lilly,
et al.,1964; Lilly,1966), Tennant (Tennant,1968), Friend
(Chesebro, et al.,1974) Bittner (Muhlback and Dux,1974) radiation leukemia virus (Meruelo, et al.,1977; Lonai and Haran-
Ghera,1977) and Rous sarcoma virus. (Whitmore, et al.,1978)

One of the least understood relationships in genetically
associated disease is the nature of predisposition, by HLA,
to certain pathologic conditions. Despite extensive research,
the mechanisms of MHC-linked disease remain to be elucidated.
Models have been proposed to explain the observed phenomena.
Snell (1968) for example, has proposed that MHC gene products
could be the receptors for attachment of pathogens, or that
pathogens might be antigenically cross-reactive with a host,
thus escaping detection via tolerance. Nevertheless, no study
has yet shown an HLA gene product to be the basis for susceptibility to disease. However, MHC markers are closely linked
to genes controlling for susceptibility, possibly the Ir
genes and their products.

Many disease associations with HLA may, of course, result from linkage of HLA genes with genes responsible for the
disease. This is the case, for example, in hereditary ataxia.
(Nino et al.,1980) Family studies of such diseases demonstrate
that the conditions travel with parental haplotypes, as opposed to any given HLA antigen.

The fact that many HLA-associated diseases are autoimmune in nature may suggest that some HLA genes are active in
the etiology of a give disease. If the MHC regulates immune
response, perhaps specific MHC products can be implicated in
cases for which autoimmunity is an improper response. Also,
since the frequency of autoantibodies increase in old age, it
may be that some MHC genes affect longevity via the suppression of enhanced autoimmune reactions.

One hope of gerontological researchers is that etiology
of the so called 'progeroid' or 'accelerated aging syndromes'
could be attributed to heritable   alterations in immune competence and function, thus implying a role of the immune system in aging. Martin's (1978) exhaustive treatise of age-related genetic syndromes discusses certain diseases which may
have immunologic components. Once again, these are diseases
thought to be autoimmune in nature. Included in Martin's list
are alopecia areata, Hashimoto's struma, pernicious anemia,

autoimmune thyroiditis, hypoadrenocorticism, diabetes mellitus with Addison's disease and myxedema, and Turner's and
Down's syndromes. Some other conditions, such as amyeloido-
sis and Parkinsonism, may also be classified as diseases of
aging, but are less well characterized with respect to mechanism. Other genetic syndromes without overt evidence of autoimmunity which could be classified as 'progeroid' include
Alzheimer's disease, the DNA repair diseases, and the immunodeficiencies, such as ataxia-telangiectasia. All are generally thought to represent prematurely senescent phenotypes.
Nevertheless, the vast majority of progeroid syndromes are
thought to arise from abnormalities at non-immune related
loci.

Evidence presented at the recent Eighth International
Histocompatibility Workshop Conference demonstrated an association of HLA-B7 with Alzheimer's disease, (Walford and
Hodge, 1980) a condition which is characterized by specific
pathologies including widespread neurofibrillar degeneration
and senile plaques in the brain. Reports were also made on
the absence of an HLA link to aged humans (Hodge and Walford,
1980) and an inconclusive study was presented on HLA influences on the four DNA repair diseases, Bloom's syndrome. Fanconi's anemia, Werner's syndrome, and xeroderma pigmentosum.
(Hodge, et al.,1980) Xeroderma ia a particularly interesting
ailment in that immunologic studies remain inclusive even
while many syndromes and the basic defect itself have been
identified.

The problem of HLA associations is further complicated by
an as yet unexplained genetic phenomena, linkage disequilibrium, which is extremely prevalent in the HLA system. Two
alleles of different loci normally recombine over generations
so that the assortment of haplotypes in a given population is
relatively random; that is, no two alleles are disproportiona-
tely expressed, unless their combination affords some sort of
selective advantage during the reproductive period of the
species' lifetime. For example, HLA-A1 and B8 are in linkage
disequilibrium with each other and with HLA-Dw3, accounting
he fact that many of the HLA-B8 pathologies are also associa
ted with Dw3.

The clinical implications of HLA disease associations are
many. In cases of very strong associations, such as those of
the B27 pathologies, physicians can be aided in the diagnosis
of rather infrequent disorders. Also, a patient's family his-

tory and HLA types may provide the clinician with a'blueprint' for the pathological conditions likely to develop during the course of a lifetime. Finally, knowledge of the genetic etiology of a disease provides a basis for rational management.

GENETIC ASPECTS OF AGING:INFLUENCE OF THE MAJOR HISTOCOMPATIBILITY COMPLEX

Observations of progeroid syndromes, and of the increasing occurrence, with age, of autoantibody or autoimmunity favor the immunologic theory of aging. A distinction should be made, however, between autoimmunity as a primary or secondary event. Clearly, as vast number of hormonal changes occur during aging, as evidenced,in particular, by neuroendocrine influences on thymic involution. The latter may, in fact, represent an aging of the immune system which manifests itself in autoimmunity. The corollary, that autoantibodies produce the pathologic manifestations of aging, is definitely not the only possibility, and in fact, cannot be demonstrated in all aged individuals. Further information is still needed to clarify the relationships of immunologic factors and aging.

Immune deficiency states (both acquired and congenital) observed in man and animals, at whatever age, are associated with autoimmunity and malignant tumors. Although diseases of these types are more prevalent in the aged, it is still uncertain whether they result from aging per se or reflect more basic genetic defects. One example of immune deficiency in adult life is that of thymic deficiency and congenital viral infection in the NZB mouse. NZB hybrids with concomitant correction of the thymic defect by the breeding manipulation live longer than the parent strain. Although this finding does not prove that thymic involution shortens life span, it serves to emphasize the fact that both longevity and thymic involution are under genetic influence.

Since the MHC represents the main genetic control or regulator of the immune system, it should influence life span. (Greenberg and Yunis,1975)

Evidence that this is the case comes from recent studies of congenic mice with three different strain backgrounds: C57BL, C3H and A. Despite definite background-dependent differences in longevity when the H-2 allele was the same, the distinct differences appear among different H-2 congenics

with the same background genome. (Smith and Walford,1977;1978)
It is of interest also, that on the C57B1/10 background, the
longest-lived strain, B10.R111, displayed the highest response
to phytohemagglutinin throughout most of life, whereas, the
shortest-lived strain, B10.AKM, was least responsive. (Meredith
and Walford,1977)   Recent work by Popp shows that B10.F mice
($H-2^n$) are particularly short-lived (90% are dead by 17 months).
Curiously, less than 50% of the $H-2^{n/n}$ homozygous backcross
animals were dead at this time, even though there was some
indication that inheritance of the $H-2^n$ allele in the backcross to B10 results in earlier demise. (Popp,1978) These observations emphasize the requirement for cautious interpretation of data based solely on strain distribution of life span
in congenics, since possible maternal influences and failure
of expected simple H-2 segregation of longevity can occur in
genetic crosses. We anticipate that the genetic component
provided by the H-2 markers only suggests the multifactorial
genetic basis of longevity, and that life span is determined,
subsequently by interactions between genome and environment.
Furthermore, the hereditary component, may be polygenic, reflecting the activity of many genes in addition to the MHC.

To further study the role of the MHC in longevity, Williams, et al. (in press) sought to ask whether a single copy
of a particular H-2 haplotype might confer a survival advantage in hybrid animals under normal mouse colony circumstances.
All experimental animals were F_1 hybrids with a DBA/2J mother
and a B10-background H-2 congenic father. Because hybrids differed only with respect to various portions of the paternally-
derived H-2 haplotype, these experiments were designed to
detect possible effects of H-2 subregions (and linked Qa-Tla
genes). Paternal strains were B10.BR ($H-2^k$), B10 ($H-2^b$),2R
($H-2^{h2}$), B10.D2 ($H-2^d$), B10.A ($H-2^a$) and 5R ($H-2^{i5}$).   The
$H-2^k$ haplotype of the B.10BR paternal strain produced a mean
survival time of 964 days for (D2xB10.BR)F_1 mice, as compared
to 786 days for the next longest lived hybrid (D2xB10), which
has the $H-2^b$ paternal haplotype. The $H-2^b$ paternal chromosome
was superior to $H-2^{h2}$, $H-2^d$, $H-2^a$ and $H-2^{i5}$ as a paternal haplotype with no significant differences in mean survival times
among hybrids with these latter paternal haplotypes.

This experiment was designed to test the influence of a
single H-2 haplotype when present on an otherwise long-lived
background nearly equivalent to that of the hearty B6D2F_1
mouse. In numerous studies B6D2F_1 has been consistently long-
lived mouse (Myers,1978); thus, any dominant genetic control

oversurvival by H-2, should be due to H-2^b or H-2^d. Since H-2^b appears to be a particularly long-lived haplotype (Smith and Walford,1978), hybrids were constructed with one H-2^d parent (DBA/2J) and one H-2 congenic parent in which H-2 was some combination of H-2^k, H-2^b and/or H-2^d. Since these experiments were begun, it has become evident that commonly used H-2 congenics may differ by genes outside the boundaries of H-2K and H-2D, but still closely linked to the MHC.

To continue the investigation of the role of MHC in longevity, we undertook experiments in which B6D2F$_1$ (H-2$^{b/d}$) was backcrossed to the DBA/2J (H-2^d) parental strain. Backcross offspring (208 males and females) were examined for H-2 markers of chromosome 17, brown fur color of chromosome 4 and dilute fur color of chromosome 9. There were two possible H-2 types: heterozygous H-2$^{b/d}$ and homozygous H-2^d, and four possible coat color haplotypes: b/b,+/d (brown); +/b,+/d (black); +/b,d/d (dilute black); and b/b,d/d (dilute brown). Preliminary results at 650 days, showed a significant (p<.02) difference between the percent survival of H-2$^{b/d}$ heterozygous mice (86%) and H-2^d homozygous mice (72%). Sex of mice had no significant effect on survival. The coat color alleles of the brown locus of chromosome 4, as a genetic marker, did not significantly affect survival, but the dilute fur color marker of chromosome 9 did. The +/d mice show an 87% survival compared to 72% for the d/d mice (p<.01).

These preliminary results also indicate a significant survival advantage when the H-2 and dilute locus genetic markers are considered together. The survival of the H-2$^{b/d}$,+/d mice was 93% compared to 65% survival of the H-2^d,d/d mice. The H-2$^{b/d}$,d/d mice also showed a significantly higher survival than H-2^d, d/d; but were not significantly higher than mice genotyped H-2^d,+/d.

These results from backcross breeding between a long-lived F$_1$ hybrid and an intermediate-lived strain, corroborate the importance of the MHC in survival. We were also able to investigate the role of two additional genetic markers that are important in fur color. The calculations of survival advantage between H-2^b and +/d versus H-2^d and d is higher than that of of the H-2^b alone or +/d alone, suggesting that these two markers amy act synergistically in favor of survival.Additional crosses and investigation will be necessary to establish the importance of the MHC and dilute locus and the synergy of these two loci in survival of mice.

The knowledge and understanding of the genetic mechanisms involved in the diseases of aging and other diseases that shorten life span is increasing. This knowledge offers a potential improvement in the quality and length of life span.

ACKNOWLEGMENT: This research was supported by NIH grants # CA 20531, AG 02329 and CA 06516.

REFERENCES

1. Alexander P (1967). The role of DNA lesions in processes leading to aging in mice. Symposium of the Soc of Exp Biol 21:29-50.
2. Awdeh ZL, Alper CA (1980). Inherited polymorphism óf human C4 as revealed by desialyzation. Immunobiology 158: 35-41.
3. Benacerraf B, McDevitt HO (1972).Histocompatibility-linked immune response genes. Science 175:273-279.
4. Bertrams J, Jansen FK, Grunneklee D, Reis HE, Drost H,Beyer J, Gries FA, Kuwert E (1976). HLA antigens and Immunoresponsiveness to insulin in insulin-dependent diabetes mellitus. Tissue Antigens 8:13-19.
5. Burnet FM (1959). "The Clonal Selection Theory of Acquired Immunity",Nashville, Tennessee:Vanderbilt and Cambridge University Presses.
6. Burnet FM (1970). "Immunological Surveillance", New York Pergamon Press.
7. Burnet FM (1971). An immunological approach to aging. Lancet 2:358-360.
8. Chesebro B, Weherly K, Stimpfling J (1974). Host genetic control of recovery from Friend leukemia virus-included splenomegaly. Mapping of a gene within the major histocompatibility complex. J.Exp Med 140:1457-1467.
9. Dausset J, Svejgaard A (eds): (1977)."HLA and Disease", Copenhagen: Munksgaard, p 316.
10. David CS, Meo T, McCormick J, Shreffler DC (1976). Expression of individual Ia specificities on T and B cells. J Exp Med 143:218-224.
11. David CS,Shreffler DC,Frelinger JA (1973). New Lymphocyte antigen system (Lna) controlled by the Ir region of the mouse H-2 complex. Proc Nat'l Acad Sci USA 70:2509-2514.
12. Dorf ME, Balner H, Benacerraf B (1975). Mapping of the immune response genes in the major histocompatibility complex of the Rhesus monkey. J Exp Med 142:673-693.

13. Dupont B, Oberfield SE, Smithwick EM, Lee TD, Levine LS (1977). Close genetic linkage between HLA and congenital adrenal hyperplasia (21-hydroxylase deficiency). Lancet 2:1309-1311.

14. Fernandes G, Good RA, Yunis EJ (1977). Attempts to correct age-related immunodeficiency and autoimmunity by cellular and dietary manipulation in inbred mice. In Makinodan T and Yunis EJ (eds): "Immunology and Aging", New York: Plenum, pp 111-133.

15. Ferreira A, Nussenzweig V, Gigli IL (1978). Structural and functional differences between the H-2 controlled Ss and Slp proteins. J Exp Med 148:1186-1197.

16. Friend PS, Fernandes G, Good RA, Michael AF, Yunis EJ (1978). Dietary restrictions early and late: Effects on the nephropathy of NZBxNZW mouse. Lab Invest 38(6):629-632.

17. Gasser DI, Newlin CM, Palm J, Gonatas NK (1973). Genetic control of susceptibility to experimental allergic encephalomyelitis in rats. Science 181:872-873.

18. Gerrard JW, Rao DC, Morton NE (1978). A genetic study of immunoglobulin E. Am J Hum Genet 30:46-58.

19. Gershon RK (1975). A disquisition on suppressor T-cells. Transpl Rev 26:170-185.

20. Good RA, Yunis EJ (1974). Association of autoimmunity, immunodeficiency and aging in man, rabbits and mice. Fed Proc 33:2040-2050.

21. Greenberg LJ, Yunis EJ, (1975). Immunopathology of aging. Human Pathol 5:122-124.

22. Grey H, Mannick M, Kunkel HG (1965). Individual antigenic specificity of myeloma proteins. Characteristics and localization to subunits. J Exp Med 121:561-575.

23. Hallgren HM, Kersey JH, Dubey DP, Yunis EJ (1978). Lymphocyte subsets and integrated immune function in aging humans. Clin Immunol Immunopathol 10:65-68.

24. Hallgren HM, Kersey JH, Gajl-Peczalska K, Greenberg LJ, Yunis EJ (1974). T and B cells in aging humans. Fed Proc 33:646.

25. Hallgren HM, Yunis EJ (1977). Suppressor lymphocytes in young and aged humans. J Immunol 118:2004-2008.

26. Hammerling GJ, Deak BD, Mauve G, Hammerling U, McDevitt HO (1974). B lymphocyte alloantigens controlled by the I region of the major histocompatibility complex in mice. Immunogenetics 1:68-81.

27. Hayflick L (1965). The limited in vitro lifetime of human diploid cell strains. Exp Cell Res 37:614-636.

28. Hirokawa K (1977). The thymus and aging. In Makinodan T, Yunis EJ (eds): "Immunology and Aging", New York: Ple-

num, pp 51-72.

29. Hodge SE, Degos L, Walford RL (1980). Four chromosomal instability syndromes: Bloom's syndrome, Fanconi's anemia, Werner's syndrome, and xeroderma pigmentosum. In Terasaki PI (ed): "Histocompatibility Testing 1980", UCLA Tissue Typing Laboratory, Los Angeles, CA, pp 730-733.

30. Hodge SE, Walford RL (1980). HLA distribution in aged normals. In Terasaki PI (ed): "Histocompatibility Testing 1980", UCLA Tissue Typing Laboratory, Los Angeles, CA, pp 722-726.

31. Katz DH, Benacerraf B (eds): (1976). "The Role of Products of the Histocompatibility Gene Complex in the Immune Response". New York: Academic Press.

32. Keck K (1975). Ir-gene control of immunogenicity of insulin and A-chain loop as carrier determinant. Nature 254:78-79.

33. Klein J, Flaherty L, Van de Berg JL, Shreffler DC (1978). H-2 haplotypes, genes, regions and antigens: First Listing. Immunogenetics 6:489-512.

34. Levine BB, Ojeda A, Benacerraf B (1963). Studies on artificial antigens. III. The genetic control of the immune response to hapten-poly-L-lysine conjugates in guinea pig. J Exp Med 118:953-957.

35. Lilly F (1966). The inheritance of susceptibility to the Gross leukemia virus in mice. Genetics 53:529-539.

36. Lilly F, Boyce EA, Old LJ (1964). Genetic basis of susceptibility to viral leukemogenesis. Lancet 2: 1207-1209.

37. Lonai P, Haran-Ghera N (1977). Resistance genes to murine leukemia in the I immune response region of the H-2 complex. J Exp Med 146:1164-1168.

38. Ludvigsson J, Safwenberg J, Heding LG (1977). HLA-types, C-peptide, and insulin antibodies in juvenile diabetes. Diabetologia 13:13-17.

39. Makinodan T (1978). Mechanism, prevention and restoration of immunologic aging. In "Genetic Effects of Aging", National Foundation-March of Dimes, Birth Defects:Original Article Series, New York:Liss XIV, pp 197-212.

40. Makinodan T, Heidrick ML, Nordin AA (1975). Immunodeficiency and autoimmunity in aging. In Bergsma D, Good R, Finstad J (eds):"Birth Defects 11 (1)", Sunderland, MA: Sinauer Association, pp 193-198.

41. Marsh DG, Bias WB, Ishizaka K (1978). Genetic control of basal serum immunoglobulin E level and its effect on specific reaginic sensitivity. Proc Nat'l Acad Sci, USA, 71:3588-3592.

42. Martin GM (1978).Genetic Syndromes in man with potential relevance to the pathobiology of aging.In "Genetic Effects on Aging", National Foundation, March of Dimes, Birth Defects: Original Article Series, New York:Liss, Vol. XIV, pp 5-39.

43. McDevitt HO, Tyan ML (1968). Genetic control of the antibody response in inbred mice: Transfer of response by spleen cells and linkage to the major histocompatibility (H-2) locus. J Exp Med 128:1-11.

44. Meredith PJ, Walford RL (1977). Effect of age on response to T- and B-cell mitogens in mice congenic at the H-2 locus. Immunogenetics 5:109-128.

45. Meruelo D, Lieberman M, Ginzton N, et al., (1977).Genetic control of radiation leukemia virus-induced tumorigenesis. I. Role of the major histocompatibility complex, H-2. J Exp Med 146:1079-1087.

46. Mozes E, Haimovich J (1979). Antigen specific T-cell helper factor cross reacts idiotypically with antibodies of the same specificity.Nature 278:56-57.

47. Muhlbock O, Dux A (1974). Histocompatibility genes (the H-2 complex) and susceptibility to mammary tumor virus in mice. J Nat'l Cancer Inst 53:993-996.

48. Murphy DB, Herzenberg LA, Okumura K, Herzenberg LA, McDevitt HO (1976). A new subregion (I-J) marked by a locus (Ia-4) controlling surface determinants on suppressor T lymphocytes. J Exp Med 144:699-712.

49. Myers DD (1978). Review of disease patterns and life span in aging mice: Genetic and environmental interactions. In Bergsma D, Harrison DE (eds): "Genetic Effects on Aging", New York: Alan Liss, Inc.pp 41-53.

50. Nino HE, Noreen HJ, Dubey DP, Resch JA, Namboodiri K, Elseon RC, Yunis EJ (1980). A family with hereditary ataxia: HLA typing. Neurology 30:12-20.

51. Olaisen B, Teisberg P, Janassen R, Gedde-Dahl T, Jr,Moen T, Thorsby E. Human Immunology (in press).

52. Ott J (1979). Maximum likelihood estimation by counting methods under polygenic and mixed models in human pedigrees. Am J Hum Genet 31:161-175.

53. Popp DM (1978) Use of congenic mice to study the genetic basis of degenerative disease.In "Genetic Effects of Aging",National Foundation, March of Dimes, Birth Defects: Original Series, Vol. XIV, No.1:261-279.

54. Raum DD, Awdeh ZL, Glass E, Yunis EJ, Alper CA (1981). The location of C2, C4 and BF relative to HLA-B and HLA-D. Immunogenetics 12:473-483.

55. Roberts-Thomson I, Whittingham S, Youngchaiyud U, MacKay IR (1974). Aging, immune response and mortality. Lancet 2:368-370.

56. Roos MH, Atkinson JP, Shreffler DC (1978). Molecular characterization of the Ss and Slp (c4) proteins of the mouse H-2 complex: Subunit composition, chain size polymorphism, and an intracellular (Pro-Ss) precurson. J Immunol 121:1106-1115.

57. Rosenthal AS (1978). Determinant selection and macrophage function in genetic control of the immune response. Immunol Rev 40:136-152.

58. Scher I, Berning AK, Strong DM, Green I.(1975). The immune response to a synthetic amino acid terpolymer in man: Relationship to HLA-A type. J Immunol 115:36-40.

59. Smith GW, Walford RL (1977). Influence of the main histocompatibility complex on aging in mice. Nature 270: 727-729.

60. Smith G, Walford RL (1978). Influence of the H-2 and H-1 histocompatibility systems upon life span and spontaneous cancer incidences in congenic mice.In "Genetic Effects of Aging", National Foundation, March of Dimes, Birth Defects: Original Article Series, New York: Liss Vol. XIV, No. 1:281-312.

61. Snell GD (1968). The H-2 locus of the mouse: Observation speculations concerning its comparative genetics and polymorphism. Folia Biol 14: 335.

62. Strelkauskas AJ, Andrew JA, Yunis EJ (1981). Autoantibodies to a regulatory T cell subset in human aging. Clin Exp Immunol 45 (2): 308-315.

63. Taussig MJ, Munro AJ, Campbell R, David CS and Staines NA (1974). Antigen-specific T-cell factor in cell cooperation. J Exp Med 142:694-700.

64. Tennant JR, Snell GD (1968). The H-2 locus and viral leukemogenesis as studied in congenic strains of mice. J Nat'l Cancer Inst. 41:597-604.

65. Vladutiu AO, Rose NR (1971). Autoimmune murine thyroiditis relation to histocompatibility (H-2) type. Science 174:1137-1138.

66. Walford RL (1969). "The Immunologic Theory of Aging" , Copenhagen: Munksgaard.

67. Walford RL, Hodge SE (1980). HLA distribution in Alzheimer's disease. In Terasaki PI (ed): "Histocompatibility Testing 1980", UCLA Tissue Typing Laboratory, Los Angeles, CA pp 727-729.

68. Whitmore AC, Babcock GF, Haughton G (1978). Genetic control of susceptibility of mice to Rous sarcoma virus

tumorigenesis. II. Segregation analysis of strain A.
S.W.-associated resistance to primary tumor induction.
J Immunol 121:213-220.
69. Williams RM, Kraus LJ, Lavin PT, Steele LL, Yunis EJ
Genetics of survival in mice: Localization of dominant effects to subregions of the major histocompatibility complex. In Segre D (ed): "Immunological Aspects of Aging", (in press).
70. Williams RM , Moore MJ (1973). Linkage of susceptibility
to experimental allergic encephalomyelitis to the major histocompatibility locus in the rat. J Exp Med
138:775-783.
71. Womack JE, Yan DLS, Potier M (Oct 19 &20, 1981). Liver
neuraminidase deficiency inherited as a single gene on
mouse chromosome 17. Poster, presented at: International Symposium: Animal Models of Inherited Metabolic
Disease.
72. Young E, Engleman EG (1980). Human peripheral blood lymphocyte responses to sythetic antigens (T,G) -A-L and
GAT. Clin Histocompat Testing 4:174-177.
73. Yunis EJ, Fernandes G, Greenberg LJ (1976). Tumor immunology, autoimmunity and aging J Am Geriatric Soc 6:
258-263.
74. Yunis EJ, Fernandes G, Stutman O (1971). Susceptibility
to involution of the thymus-dependent lymphoid system
and autoimmunity. Am J Clin Pathol 56:280-292.
75. Yunis EJ, Fernandes G, Teague PO, et al., (1970). The
thymus, autoimmunity and the involution of the lymphoid system. In Siegel M, Good RA (eds): "Tolerance,
Autoimmunity and Aging", Springfield, Ill.: Thomas,
pp 62-120.
76. Yunis JJ, Greenberg LJ, Yunis EJ (1977). Genetic, developmental and evolutionary aspecsts of life span. In
Makinodan T, Yunis EJ (eds): "Immunology and Aging",
New York: Plenum pp 91-98.

DR. BALAZS: It now is recognized that several chemically induced immunotoxicological effects are linked to the major histocompatibility complex: for example, hydralazine and procainamide-induced lupus-like autoimmune reaction, nitrofurantoin-induced hepatitis, and organic gold-induced renal lesions in humans. The best experimental example is mercuric chloride-induced glomerulonephritis in the rat, which has been shown to be linked to the histocompatibility complex.

We tried to reproduce the procainamide-induced autoimmune response in dogs of about 1 year of age and failed. Then we repeated the study with dogs that were 4 to 5 years old and in one month began to detect the presence of the antinuclear antibody in their sera.

DR. YUNIS: In relation to that, it has been shown that schizophrenic patients treated with chlorpromazine develop autoantibodies and high immunoglobulin levels. We have found that the antigen BW44 is a good marker for patients with the autoimmune syndrome. It appears that in addition to exposure to a drug, one also must have susceptibility to produce autoimmunity.

DR. GUÉNET: In your talk you indicated that you performed back-cross matings to test for the possible role of the H-2 haplotype in the control of life span. Why did you not take advantage of the recombinant inbred lines which have been developed by Ben Taylor, Don Bailey and others?

DR. YUNIS: I am sorry, perhaps you missed it, because time constraints did not permit me to discuss it in more detail but some of the experiments showed that we used recombinant lines.

DR. GUÉNET: You speak of recombinant lines inside of the H2 locus, do you not?

DR. YUNIS: Yes.

DR. GUÉNET: I am thinking of those particular inbred strains that are called recombinant inbred strains which have two inbred lines as original parents, and are inbred from the F_1 generation onwards.

DR. YUNIS: Yes, you are correct. We have not used such animals. The reason we tried to approach it differently is because we wanted to have an experimental model in which we could study other genetic systems in addition to H2.

SECTION VI.
INBORN ERRORS OF HORMONE ACTION

Animal Models of Inherited Metabolic Diseases, pages 353–368
© 1982 Alan R. Liss, Inc., 150 Fifth Avenue, New York, NY 10011

INHERITED DISORDERS OF HORMONE RESISTANCE

G. D. Aurbach, M.D.

National Institute of Arthritis, Diabetes, and
Digestive and Kidney Diseases, NIH
Bethesda, Maryland 20205

In 1942 Albright and his colleagues reported on pseudohypoparathyroidism, the first documented clinical syndrome
of resistance to hormone action. These patients displayed
certain constitutional features and chemical hypoparathyroidism resistant to the effects of exogenous parathyroid
hormone. They also termed this disorder the "Seabright
Bantam syndrome," after the Sebright /* Bantam cock, which
displays the tail-feathering pattern of a hen instead of
that of the normal male rooster. They assumed that the
disorder in the rooster was due to resistance to the effects
of androgen. We review here several classes of hormone-
resistant states that produce clinical disease with particular emphasis on disorders of vitamin D and parathyroid hormone function. The reader is referred to an article by
Verhoeven and Wilson (1979) for a general review of hormone
resistant states.

There are two general classes of hormones in terms of
mechanism of action. Certain amine and peptide hormones
interact at the cell surface with a highly specific receptor
linked to the membrane-bound enzyme adenylate cyclase which
in turn catalyzes the formation of cyclic 3',5'-AMP from
ATP. The overall response of the cell to the hormone is
secondary to generation of cyclic AMP which in turn activates other enzyme and transport systems leading to the
ultimate physiological response to the hormone. Another
class of hormones must first penetrate the cell membrane to

/* The standard spelling is Sebright; Albright used
    "Seabright."

interact with intracellular cytoplasmic receptors for the hormone. The cytoplasmic receptor-hormone complex is then transported to the nucleus where new protein synthesis is activated. In this instance the overall response of the hormone is dependent upon synthesis of new proteins or enzymes that bring about the cell response to the hormone. These concepts are illustrated in Figure 1.

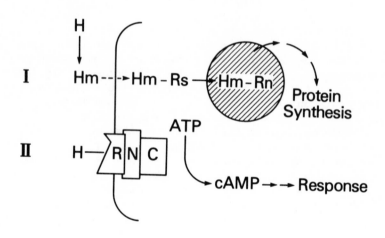

Figure 1. General mechanisms of hormone action. Type I mechanism: The hormone or its metabolite enters the cell, there to interact with a cytoplasmic receptor for the hormone. The hormone-cytoplasmic-receptor complex (H_m-R_s) is then transported to the nucleus where the complex activates protein synthesis. Hormones that act through type II mechanism interact with a receptor that is an integral component of the cell membrane facing the exterior. Interaction of the hormone with receptor (R) is coupled to C, the catalytic unit of adenylate cyclase, through a coupling factor known as N or G. The overall effect of hormone-receptor interaction thus is activation of adenylate cyclase (C) with con-

sequent generation of cyclic AMP from ATP, the enzyme substrate.

Hormone resistant states conceivably can develop
through an abnormality in any number of steps, from defective biosynthesis of hormone, to abnormalities in receptor
interaction, to problems at the post-receptor level. A
list of such possible defects is given in Table 1.

Table 1

Mechanisms in Apparent Hormone Resistant States

    Defective biosynthesis of hormone*
       (competitive inhibitor)

    Defective conversion to active form

    (Abnormal carrier protein)*

    Defective receptor
       plasma membrane, cytosolic, nuclear

    Abnormal coupling protein

    Antibodies
       a) to hormone   b) to receptor

    Post-receptor defect

* Mechanisms in parentheses have not been proven to exist.

In Table 2 are listed well-described syndromes involving
hormone-resistant states that are representative of several
of the types of abnormalities classified in Table 1.

Table 2

Hormone Resistant States

Hormone	Syndrome	Comment
Parathyroid hormone	Pseudohypoparathyroidism (Albright et al, 1942)	
Vasopressin	Nephrogenic diabetes insipidus (Williams and Henry, 1947)	
Growth hormone	Laron dwarfism (Laron et al, 1966)	Lack somatomedin
	African pigmy (Rimoin et al, 1967)	? Lack somatomedin receptor
Insulin	Diabetes with extreme insulin resistance (Flier et al, 1977)	Antibody to receptor
	Leprechaunism (Kobayashi et al, 1978)	Post-receptor defect
ACTH	Childhood adrenal crisis and death (Migeon et al, 1968)	Heterogenous pathophysiology
Androgens	Testicular feminization (Verhoeven and Wilson, 1979)	5-α-reductase deficiency
		deficient receptor
		post-receptor defect
Vitamin D	Vitamin D resistant rickets (Glorieux et al, 1972)	Phosphate transport defect

Table 2 (continued)

Hormone	Syndrome	Comment
	Vitamin D dependent rickets (Fraser et al, 1973)	D metabolism defect - reduced formation of $1,25(OH)_2D$
	$1,25(OH)_2$ resistant osteomalacia (Eil et al, 1981)	Receptor defect (another form may represent post-receptor defect)
Cortisol	Hypercortisolism without Cushing's syndrome (Chrousos et al, 1982)	Deficient cytosolic receptor
T_3, gonadotropins, aldosterone, progesterone	Diverse hormone resistant states (Verhoeven and Wilson, 1979)	

TESTICULAR FEMINIZATION

This is a group of clinical disorders that illustrates well classes of resistance to steroid hormone action (see Table 2). Testosterone production in all of these syndromes is normal. In one form of the syndrome, 5-α-reductase deficiency, the enzyme required for intracellular conversion of testosterone to dihydrotestosterone, the active form, is abnormal or deficient in quantity. In another form of the syndrome, complete testicular feminization, there is a deficiency of dihydrotestosterone receptor content in the cell cytosol. Still another form of androgen resistance causing male pseudohermaphroditism shows normal binding of dihydrotestosterone to the cytosolic receptor and normal translocation of the complex to the nucleus. It is suspected that the defect in these cases must lie at some point distal to interaction with the receptor.

GENETIC DEFECTS IN THE ACTION OF VITAMIN D

Dietary and environmental deficiency of vitamin D produces rickets in children and osteomalacia in adults, disorders that usually can be corrected by giving physiological
amounts of vitamin D. With the advent of general availability of active vitamin D preparations, most of nutritional
rickets and osteomalacia has been eliminated at least in
the Western world. Treatment of obvious nutritional vitamin
D deficiency with physiological replacement amounts of the
vitamin, however, has allowed recognition of vitamin D-resistant forms of osteomalacia and rickets. The first form
to be recognized of vitamin D resistance has been termed
vitamin D resistant rickets and was orginally recognized
by Albright and his associates (Albright and Reifenstein,
1948). The predominant form of this disorder is a sex-linked disorder of phosphate wasting due to an abnormality of
phosphate transport, particularly evident in the kidney
with renal loss of phosphate. This disorder represents,
thus, an abnormality of phosphate transport (Glorieux et al,
1972) and not strictly target tissue resistance to effects
of vitamin D.

Another disorder, a form of true resistance to the
actions of vitamin D, has been termed "vitamin D dependent
rickets" (Fraser et al, 1973). This is an autosomal recessive disorder attributable to defective conversion of 25-
hydroxycholecalciferol to 1,25-dihydroxycholecalciferol in
the kidney. The ultimate expression of vitamin D action is
dependent upon formation of the latter metabolite, 1,25-
dihydroxy-D. Ingested or endogenous vitamin D is converted
to 25-hydroxy-D in the liver and a second hydroxylation at
the 1-alpha position is carried out in the kidney. The
activity of this enzyme (1-α-hydroxylase) is also controlled
by parathyroid hormone. In vitamin D-dependent rickets, it
is this renal 1-α-hydroxylase step that is defective. Treatment of these subjects with 1,25-dihydroxy-D corrects the
disorder (Fraser et al, 1973).

A third form of abnormality in vitamin D response has
been discovered by Marx et al (1978) and Brooks et al (1978).
This appears to be an autosomal recessive disorder and is
characterized by classical rickets and osteomalacia with
high plasma levels of 1,25-dihydroxyvitamin D. Some of
these patients also show total alopecia. The work of Eil
et al (1981) has proven that this disorder can be attributed

to a defect at the receptor level. The latter investigators have cultured skin fibroblasts from these subjects and shown that there is defective nuclear uptake of labeled 1,25-dihydroxyvitamin D in vitro. There is also a suggestion that this disorder can be attributed to three different classes of receptor response abnormality. The first category includes those with a defective cytosolic receptor for 1,25-dihydroxy-D. The second class shows an abnormality in transfer of the receptor-hormone complex to the nucleus, and the third class putatively reflects a defect at the post-receptor level.

Note that the above abnormalities in vitamin D responsiveness parallel strikingly the abnormalities discussed earlier in characterizing testicular feminization syndromes. Each syndrome reflects defects at one of several classical steps required for steroid hormone action: 1) conversion of a precursor steroid to the active form; 2) receptor binding of the active steroid metabolite; 3) transfer of the steroid cytosolic receptor complex to the nucleus; and 4) post-receptor events. The reader will note one obvious difference between activation of a vitamin D precursor and that of testosterone. Testosterone is converted to dihydrotestosterone in the receptor tissue itself, whereas the active metabolite of vitamin D is formed in a distant tissue before entering the target tissue cell. There are other examples of abnormalities in sterol hormone metabolism and action (Table 2). Thyroid hormone action also parallels that of the sterol class in that conversion to an active form (T_4 to T_3) and nuclear binding are required for action. Thyroid hormone resistant states have been identified clinically, but distinct abnormalities in metabolism and receptor binding have yet to be clearly and uncontroversially identified.

RESISTANCE TO PEPTIDE HORMONE RESPONSIVENESS - PSEUDOHYPOPARATHYROIDISM

Several examples of clinical states with resistance to the action of peptide hormones are listed in Table 2. Certain types of resistance to growth hormone and insulin appear attributable to defects at the receptor level. In the Introduction, it was noted that the earliest form of hormone resistance identified clinically was that of pseudohypoparathyroidism (Albright et al, 1942). They defined

this syndrome in subjects with the chemical characteristics
of hypoparathyroidism (hypocalcemia and hyperphosphatemia)
who also showed certain constitutional features, short
stature, round faces, skeletal abnormalities, and mental
retardation, with resistance to effects of exogenous parathyroid extract. They proposed that this disorder was
attributable to target organ resistance to the effects of
parathyroid hormone. Bony abnormalities in the disorder
include shortening of the metacarpals, metatarsals and
phalanges, as well as in some cases exostoses, actual sub-
cutaneous bone formation and bowing of the long bones. This
complex of bony abnormalities has been termed Albright's
hereditary osteodystrophy (AHO).

In 1969 Chase et al found that subjects with pseudohypoparathyroidism are resistant to exogenous parathyroid
hormone in terms of urinary excretion of cyclic 3',5'-AMP.
Since the mechanism of action of parathyroid hormone is
mediated through activation of adenylate cyclase and generation of cyclic AMP in target tissues, this observation suggested that the metabolic abnormality in pseudohypoparathyroidism was attributable to a defect in the receptor-ade-
nylate cyclase complex in parathyroid hormone receptor
tissues. Subsequently in two different laboratories (Marcus
et al, 1971 and Drezner and Burch, 1978), samples of renal
tissue were obtained from subjects with pseudohypoparathyroidism. In each instance a distinct in vitro response of
renal adenylate cyclase to parathyroid hormone in vitro
was observed. In the study of Drezner and Burch the effect
on adenylate cyclase depended upon addition of guanosine
triphosphate (GTP) at low ATP concentrations. These authors
suggested that there might be an abnormal affinity of the
guanine nucleotide regulatory unit (N unit in Figure 1) for
GTP. In 1979 Farfel et al identified the guanine nucleotide
regulatory protein (N) in human erythrocyte membranes (human
erythrocyte membranes do not contain receptors or adenylate
cyclase catalytic units). This finding made it possible to
assay a readily obtainable human tissue for N unit content
as well as test affinity of the unit for guanine nucleotides.
Assays were performed by extracting human erythrocyte membranes with Lubrol PX, a nonionic detergent. The extract
contains N units which can be assayed by addition to preparations containing free catalytic units. Two preparations
useful for this purpose are turkey erythrocyte adenylate
cyclase catalytic (C) units or the catalytic units in the

S-49 cell mutant called AC⁻. This mutant lymphoma cell
contains catalytic units but no N units. Results of assays
on normal subjects and those with classical pseudohypoparathyroidism with AHO are illustrated in Figure 2. Farfel
et al (1980) have reported virtually identical results
using the AC⁻ assay system.

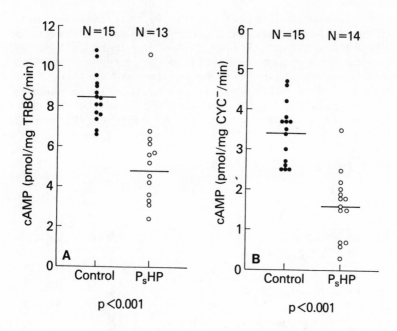

Figure 2. Guanine nucleotide regulatory component in red
cells from control and pseudohypoparathyroid subjects. The
component in extracts of human red cell membranes were incubated with GTP-S and mixed with the adenylate cyclase
catalytic unit from turkey erythrocyte membranes (A) or
AC⁻ membranes (B). Results are expressed as cAMP produced
per mg of protein in membrane extract. Human red cells
contain the regulatory unit but negligible amounts of the
adenylate cyclase catalytic component. Red cells from
subjects with pseudohypoparathyroidism show significantly
(p < .001) reduced content of the regulatory component.
Modified from Levine et al (1980).

Our studies show that there is no change in affinity
of the N unit for guanine nucleotides, a finding contrary
to the suggestion made by Drezner and Burch (1978). The
latter investigators, however, had available to them only
limited amounts of renal tissue from their patient and thus
were able to test guanine nucleotide (GTP) at only one
concentration and one time point.

The guanine nucleotide regulatory unit is ubiquitous
and, common to all receptor systems, linked to activation
of adenylate cyclase. It was thus of interest to test subjects with pseudohypoparathyroidism for responsiveness to
several hormones in addition to parathyroid hormone. Hypothyroidism indeed has been observed frequently in pseudohypoparathyroidism. Tests for responsiveness to TRH reveal
a hypothyroid response in a number of subjects (Figure 3).

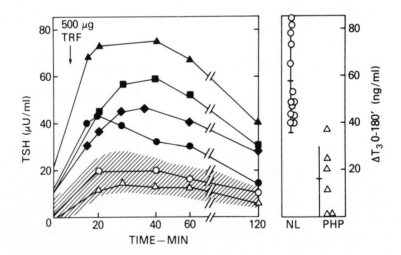

Figure 3. Response of normal subjects and those with
pseudohypoparathyroidism to intravenous injection of 500 μg

of thyrotropin-releasing hormone (labeled TRF in figure).
Normal response is shown by the shaded area and open
circles. The response of four subjects with pseudohypoparathyroidism is represented by results indicated by closed
symbols. Hyperresponsiveness to TRH is characteristic of
hypothyroidism with resistance to the action of thyrotropin.
Subjects with pseudohypoparathyroidism similarly show
diminished T_3 response to TRH (shown in figure at right).
Modified from Levine et al (1981).

There is evidence for resistance to still other hormones in pseudohypoparathyroidism. Glucagon testing in
classical pseudohypoparathyroidism shows diminished plasma
cyclic AMP responses to glucagon. Still another series of
tests had been carried out by culturing skin fibroblasts
from these subjects. Fibroblasts cultured from patients
with pseudohypoparathyroidism show a diminished cyclic AMP
response in vitro to prostaglandin E_2 as compared to fibroblasts cultured from normal subjects. It has also been
shown that the cultured fibroblasts in pseudohypoparathyroidism contain a diminished complement of the N unit.
Gonadal dysfunction, in particular oligomenorrhea, has been
described in pseudohypoparathyroidism and one case reported
showed elevated gonadotropin in plasma associated with
oligomenorrhea. Thus it is possible that the ovary may
show resistance to gonadotropins analogous to the hormone
resistance of other tissues described above. These several
findings with abnormalities of responsiveness in diverse
tissues indicate that pseudohypoparathyroidism is a more
generalized hormone-resistant state than was appreciated
in the original description of the disease. This more generalized abnormality is what would be expected with a disorder
attributable to a reduced complement of N units, since such
a reduction would be expected to affect generally all
hormonally responsive tissues in the body. Studies are in
progress to determine the extent of N unit deficiency
throughout various receptor tissues.

Another form of pseudohypoparathyroidism has been postulated by Drezner et al (1973). In rare cases of pseudohypoparathyroidism the urinary cAMP response is normal. Drezner
et al proposed that in these subjects there is an abnormal
cAMP-dependent kinase system.

We have reviewed here a number of abnormalities of

hormonal responsiveness with particular attention to those causing disorders in regulation of calcium metabolism. Much of the interest in studies on hormone-resistant syndromes was prompted by the initial report of Albright and his co-workers on "Sebright Bantam syndrome." In this concluding section, it is of particular interest to cite new work on this abnormality of the Sebright chicken. It has recently been discovered that the original concepts of this abnormality were incorrect. In chickens, the female feathering pattern is mediated by estrogens; castration of either male or female chickens leads to production of the male feathering pattern. The defect in the Sebright Bantam cock is not at all attributable to resistance to androgens. Rather it has been shown that there is an enzymatic abnormality in the skin of the Sebright bird, such that there is increased conversion of androgens to estrogens in the skin. The abnormal increased rate of production of estrogens from androgen in the skin produces the female feathering pattern in the Sebright rooster (George and Wilson, 1980).

REFERENCES

Albright F, Burnett CH, Smith PH, Parson W (1942). Pseudo-hypoparathyroidism - An example of "Seabright-Bantam syndrome. Endocrinology 30:922.
Albright F, Reifenstein EC Jr (1948). "The Parathyroid Glands and Metabolic Bone Disease." Baltimore: Williams and Wilkins.
Brooks MH, Bell NH, Love L, Stern PH, Orfei E, Queener SF, Hamstra AJ, DeLuca HF (1978). Vitamin D-dependent rickets type II: resistance of target organs to 1,25-dihydroxy-vitamin D. N Engl J Med 298:966.
Chase LR, Melson GL, Aurbach GD 1969). Pseudohypoparathy-roidism: defective excretion of 3',5'-AMP in response to parathyroid hormone. J Clin Invest 48:1832.
Chrousos GP, Vingerholds A, Brandon D, Eil C, Pugeat M, Loriaux DL, Lipsett MB (1982). Primary cortisol resistance in man: a glucocorticoid receptor mediated disease. J Clin Invest (In Press).
Drezner MK, Burch WM Jr (1978). Altered activity of the nucleotide regulatory site in the parathyroid hormone-sensitive adenylate cyclase from the renal cortex of a patient with pseudohypoparathyroidism. J Clin Invest 62: 1222.

Drezner M, Neelon FA, Lebovitz HF (1973). Pseudohypoparathyroidism type II: a possible defect in the reception of the
cyclic AMP signal. N Engl J Med 289:1059.

Eil C, Liberman UA, Rosen JF, Marx SJ (1981). A cellular
defect in hereditary vitamin D–dependent rickets type II:
defective nuclear uptake of 1,25-dihydroxyvitamin D in
cultured skin fibroblasts. N Engl J Med 304:1558.

Farfel Z, Brickman AS, Kaslow HR, Brothers VM, Bourne HR
(1980). Defect of receptor–cyclase coupling protein in
pseudohypoparathyroidism. N Engl J Med 303:237.

Farfel Z, Kaslow HR, Bourne HR (1979). A regulatory component of adenylate cyclase is located on the inner surface of human erythrocyte membranes. Biochem Biophys Res
Commun 90:1237.

Flier JS, Kahn CR, Roth J, Bar RS (1975). Antibodies that
impair insulin receptor binding in an unusual diabetic
syndrome with severe insulin resistance. Science 190:63.

Fraser D, Kooh SW, Kind HP, Holick MF, Tanaka Y, DeLuca HF
(1973). Pathogenesis of hereditary vitamin D dependent
rickets. An inborn error of vitamin D metabolism involving
defective conversion of 25-hydroxyvitamin D to 1 ,25-
dihydroxyvitamin D. N Engl J Med 289:817.

George FW, Wilson JD (1980). Pathogenesis of the henny
feathering trait in the Sebright Bantom chicken. J Clin
Invest 66:57.

Glorieux F, Scriver CR (1972). Loss of a parathyroid hormone
sensitive component of phosphate transport in X-linked
hypophosphatemia. Science 175:997.

Koyayashi M, Olefsky JM, Elders J, Mako M, Given BD,
Schedwie HK, Fiser RH, Hintz RL, Horner JA,
Rubenstein AH (1978). Insulin resistance due to a
defect distal to the insulin receptor: demonstration
in a patient with leprechaunism. Proc Natl Acad Sci USA
75:3469.

Laron Z, Pertzelan A, Mannheimer S (1966). Genetic pituitary dwarfism with high serum concentration of growth
hormone: a new inborn error of metabolism? Isr J Med Sci
2:152.

Levine MA, Downs RW Jr, Singer M, Marx SJ, Aurbach GD,
Spiegel AM (1980). Deficient activity of guanine nucleotide regulatory protein in erythrocytes from patients
with pseudohypoparathyroidism. Biochem Biophys Res Commun
94:1319.

Levine MA, Downs RW Jr, Marx SJ, Lasker RD, Aurbach GD, Spiegel AM (1981). Clinical and biochemical features of pseudohypoparathyroidism. In Cohn DV, Talmage RV, Matthews JL (eds): "Hormonal Control of Calcium Metabolism," Amsterdam: Excerpta Medica, p. 95.

Marcus R, Wilber JF, Aurbach GD (1971). Parathyroid hormone sensitive adenyl cyclase from the renal cortex of a patient with pseudohypoparathyroidism. J Clin Endocrinol Metab 33:537.

Marx SJ, Spiegel AM, Brown EM, Gardner DG, Downs RW Jr, Attie M, Hamstra AJ, DeLuca HF (1978). A familial syndrome of decrease in sensitivity to 1,25-dihydroxyvitamin D. J Clin Endocrinol Metab 47:1303.

Migeon CJ, Kenny FM, Kowarski A, Snipes CA, Spaulding JS, Finkelstein JW, Blizzard RM (1968). The syndrome of congenital adrenocortical unresponsiveness to ACTH. Report of six cases. Pediatr Res 2:501.

Rimoin DL, Merimee TJ, Rabinowitz D, McKusick VA, Cavalli-Sforza LL (1967). Growth hormone in African pygmies. Lancet 2:523.

Verhoeven GFM, Wilson JD (1979). The syndromes of primary hormone resistance. Metabolism 28:253.

Williams RH, Henry C (1947). Nephrogenic diabetes insipidus transmitted by females and appearing during infancy in males. Ann Intern Med 27:84.

DR. CARRIG: Is there any understanding of the mechanism whereby the fourth and fifth metacarpal bones specifically are shortened in pseudohypoparathyroidism?

DR. AURBACH: No, unfortunately there is no information at all about the cause of these developmental abnormalities or their causative relationship, if any, to abnormalities in quanine nucleotide regulatory protein. The only thing that one can say is there is a very high correlation between the bony abnormalities and the reduced content of the regulatory protein.

DR. SEGAL: Dr. Aurbach, how does this stack up with what Albright called pseudo-pseudohypoparathyroidism?

DR. AURBACH: In my brief presentation I left much undefined or unsaid. After his original report, Albright described something called "pseudo-pseudohypoparathyroidism." This is a disorder in which one finds the exact same types of constitutional abnormalities, but they do not have hypocalcemia. They do not have total resistance or even marked resistance to exogenous parathyroid hormone. We have seen one or two of these people, who are in the same families as progeny with the fullblown syndrome. In one case, at least, the mother with pseudo-pseudohypoparathyroidism showed a reduced complement of the quanine nucleotide regulatory unit but not as great a reduction as her daughter with pseudohypoparathyroidism. We do not have a good explanation, other than to say that the deficiency in the mother is less severe than that in the daughter and does not totally compromise the regulation of calcium metabolism. To go along with that, the mother has showed a modestly elevated basal urinary cyclic AMP concentration and high plasma levels of parathyroid hormone, suggesting that the abnormality is less severe, and that compensation can be achieved by secreting more parathyroid hormone. Thus pseudo-pseudohypoparathyroidism may simply represent a less severe form of pseudohypoparathyroidism.

DR. K. SMITH: How many patients with insulin-resistant diabetes are also deficient in responsiveness to TSH, or show similar membrane receptor protein defects?

DR. AURBACH: As far as I know they have not shown abnormalities in responsiveness to other hormones, but it has been primarily limited to insulin. They have shown certain other abnormalities like acanthosis nigricans and a variety of autoimmune phenomena.

DR. HIGAKI: Are membrane defects and receptor defects considered the same?

DR. AURBACH: Of course, I mentioned that there are two

classes of hormone receptor interactions. One is the steroid class which interacts with cytosolic receptors. Parathyroid hormone, TSH, glucagon, and β-adrenergic agonists, all of which act through the adenylate cyclase-cAMP system, interact with cell membrane receptors. Those receptors are linked through two other components of the complex, the G unit and the catalytic unit which also are components of the membrane. The defects we discussed seem to be defects (mutations?) of specific proteins that are components (integral proteins) of membranes.

Animal Models of Inherited Metabolic Diseases, pages 369–379
© 1982 Alan R. Liss, Inc., 150 Fifth Avenue, New York, NY 10011

MODELS OF ANDROGEN INSENSITIVITY IN THE STUDY OF ANDROGEN ACTION

Leslie P. Bullock, D.V.M.
Associate Professor, Comparative Medicine
Senior Research Associate, Medicine
The Milton S. Hershey Medical Center
Hershey, PA 17033

In the human, androgen resistance has been associated with several different defects which result in complete to partial insensitivity to male hormones (Verhoeven and Wilson, 1979). These disorders include 5α-reductase deficiency, complete and incomplete forms of testicular feminization (Tfm), Reifenstein's syndrome and a post receptor defect. Patients with these syndromes have a normal male XY karyotype but varying degrees of deficiency of male sex characteristics. Well characterized animal models of androgen resistance are available only for testicular feminization. These models have contributed a great deal toward our understanding of the mechanism of action of androgens as well as other steroids.

The major steps in the activation of eukaryotic cells by androgens are similar to those followed by other classes of steroids (Higgins and Gehring, 1978). After entry into the cell, the active steroid is bound by a specific cytoplasmic receptor. For androgens, the active steroid may be testosterone or a metabolite, 5α-dihydrotestosterone, depending on the tissue. The steroid-receptor complex is translocated into the nucleus where it is bound to chromatin at specific acceptor sites. Chromatin template and polymerase activities are increased leading to RNA and DNA synthesis which is, in turn, manifested by specific end organ responses.

One of the best ways to understand the relative importance of each of these steps in mediating steroid action is through the use of appropriate mutants. Although this approach has been used successfully for the study of bacterial metabolism, regulatory mutants are rare in eukaryotes.

One such example, the Tfm mutation, results in inherited, body wide end organ insensitivity to androgens. It has been identified in the rat (Tfm) (Stanley, et al., 1973), mouse (Tfm/Y) (Lyon and Hawkes, 1970), cow (Nes, 1966) and dog (Schultz, 1962), as well as man. This defect is associated with a deficiency in effective androgen receptors. This review will summarize the studies of the physiological and biological characteristics of the Tfm mutation in rodents and present examples of how these studies have added to our understanding of the mechanism of androgen action in both differentiating and mature tissues.

THE TFM RAT AND TFM/Y MOUSE

The androgen insensitive Tfm rat originated from a mutation occurring in a colony of King-Holtzman rats and was described by Stanley and Gumbreck in 1954 (Stanley et al., 1973). The Tfm/Y mouse arose in an outbred strain of mice and was described by Lyon and Hawkes in 1970. To our knowledge, all the androgen insensitive rodents in use today are descendents of these two original mutations. The physical abnormalities are similar in affected rats and mice. The Tfm mutation is on the X-chromosome and is transmitted by carrier females. Androgen insensitive rats and mice are male pseudohermaphrodites with similar gross abnormalities of sexual differentiation. Despite an XY karyotype and a chromatin negative nuclear sex, affected animals have a female phenotype which includes a well developed nipple line and a short, blind vagina. There is no evidence of a reproductive tract other than bilateral, inguinal, or abdominal testes. The absence of mullerian derivatives suggests the normal production of "mullerian-inhibiting substance" by the testes. Although microscopic epididymides have been reported in the Tfm/Y mouse (Blecher, 1978), they, and the rest of the wolffian duct, do not develop due to the androgen insensitivity of fetal anlagen. Although mutant animals do not have male secondary sex tissue, much information on the physical and biochemical parameters of androgen action has been obtained through the use of tissues, such as preputial gland, kidney, submaxillary gland, and brain. These tissues do not require androgens for differentiation but are, nevertheless, responsive to these hormones in normal animals.

IN VIVO STUDIES OF ANDROGEN ACTION

The androgen insensitivity in the Tfm rat (Reviewed in Bullock and Bardin, 1977) is similar to some forms of testicular feminization in that it is only partial. There is little evidence of response to endogenous androgens in the Tfm rat. This is shown not only by the anatomical defects but also by biochemical parameters. The activities of several sexually dimorphic enzymes in skin, liver, preputial glands and adrenal glands from Tfm rats are similar to those of female rather than male rats. There is, however, some evidence that endogenous androgens may have slight effects on some tissues. The body and organ weights of Tfm rats are intermediate between males and females. The late opening and need for estrogen to maintain patency of the vagina in some pseudohermaphrodites, as well as the complete absence of the vagina in others, suggests that this tissue may have been masculinized during differentiation. The defeminization of the hypothalamic-pituitary axis in the Tfm rat has been used as additional evidence of androgenic effects. However, recent data suggest that this is probably due to conversion of androgens to estrogens (McEwen, 1981, Shapiro et al., 1980) (Discussed below). The unresponsiveness of Tfm rats to exogenous androgens has been shown for multiple end points including body and organ weights, nitrogen metabolism, and the activities of a number of enzymes. Nevertheless, administration of large doses of androgens can stimulate some target organs including the preputial gland and the hypo-thalamic-pituitary axis. The responses induced, however, are never as great as in the normal animal.

The Tfm/Y mouse represents a complete form of androgen insensitivity. It has been studied in even greater detail than the Tfm rat through the use of several different tissues and multiple end points (Reviewed by Bullock and Bardin, 1977). In the submaxillary gland, morphology, nerve growth factor, epidermal growth factor, and total esteroproteolytic activity were studied. Gonadotropin values were used to evaluate the hypothalamic-pituitary axis. In the kidney, weight as well as the activities of several enzymes including -glucuronidase, ornithine decarboxylase (L. Bullock - un-published results), and RNA polymerase I and II, have been analyzed. Despite the use of large doses of androgen, no response was detected in any study. The insensitivity of the RNA polymerases, which is normally one of the earliest responses of target organs to androgens, supported other evidence that a pretranscription regulatory defect was involved.

IDENTIFICATION OF THE DEFECT IN TFM ANIMALS

The primary defect in Tfm animals is a lack of effective androgen receptors. This has been confirmed by numerous investigators. Although no receptors were detected in early studies, which used rather crude techniques (Reviewed in Bullock and Bardin, 1977), the development of more sensitive assays has allowed the detection of small concentrations of androgen receptors in both Tfm rats and mice. The androgen receptor in Tfm rats is thought to be normal (Naess et al., 1976), while the receptor in Tfm/Y mice has slightly altered biochemical characteristics (Attardi and Ohno, 1974; Gehring and Tomkins, 1974; Attardi and Ohno, 1978; Wieland and Fox, 1979).

The absence of effective androgen receptors in target organs results in an inability of Tfm animals to concentrate androgens at the active site in the cell, the nucleus. As a result, androgenic responses are not initiated. The deficient nuclear androgen accumulation in Tfm rats was first demonstrated by Bullock and Bardin (1970). The retention of ^{3}H-dihydrotestosterone by preputial gland nuclei from Tfm rats was deficient as compared to that in castrate males. These results have been confirmed and expanded by other investigators who have shown deficient nuclear androgen accumulation in kidney (Ritzen et al., 1972), preputial gland (Bullock and Bardin, 1973), and testis (Smith et al., 1975). Androgen uptake is also defective in kidney (Bullock et al., 1971), and submaxillary gland (Goldstein and Wilson, 1972) nuclei of Tfm/Y mice.

Cultured fibroblasts have been used to determine the defect in androgen action in humans with testicular feminization. In most studies defective androgen receptors have been found. There are some instances, however, where the androgen receptor is apparently normal but the retention of the androgen-receptor complex within the nucleus is defective (Amrhein et al., 1976; Collier et al., 1978). This suggests a defect in the acceptor site in chromatin. An animal model for this type of defect has not been identified.

USE OF ANDROGEN INSENSITIVE ANIMALS AS PROBES FOR UNDER-
STANDING BIOLOGICAL PROBLEMS

Tfm rats and mice provide unique opportunities to study
biological responses in the absence of androgenic effects.
They are also useful in identifying those responses that are
mediated via the androgen receptor. A few of the ways these
animals have been used are reviewed here. Others have been
reviewed in Bullock and Bardin, 1977.

Abnormality of the Tfm Nucleus

Since the primary defect in Tfm animals is in the
androgen receptor, it has been difficult to evaluate the
responsiveness of their target organ nuclei to normal androgen-receptor complexes. In vitro studies combining cytoplasm
containing normal receptors with nuclei from Tfm animals are
subject to many artifacts. Recently Drews and colleagues
used the autosomal sex reversed factor (Sxr) to convert
females, heterozygous for Tfm, into "males" (Thiedemann and
Drews, 1980; Thiedemann et al., 1981). X-inactivation
resulted in a mosaic animal with androgen sensitive wild type
and androgen insensitive Tfm cells. The androgen dependent,
striated urethral muscle, in which Tfm and wild type cells
fuse to form multinucleate muscle fibers, was then analyzed.
The Tfm nuclei in these fibers were exposed to androgens and
normal testosterone receptors coded for by the wild type
nuclei. Two classes of muscle nuclei could be identified by
morphological analysis or evaluation of RNA synthesis. These
classes corresponded to nuclei from insensitive Tfm or
androgen stimulated male controls. These results suggest
that Tfm nuclei are not stimulated by intact testosterone-
receptor complexes. It is not known if this represents a
second primary defect in Tfm animals or if it is secondary to
the receptor defect.

Epithelio-mesenchymal Interactions

Several laboratories have used the Tfm/Y mouse in
studies of the role of mesenchyme and epithelium in regulating the differentiation of androgen responsive embryonic
tissues. Cunha and colleagues (Cunha et al., 1980) used
combinations of epithelium and stroma from embryonic and
neonatal urogenital rudiments from normal and Tfm/Y mice.
The tissues were grown as grafts in intact male mice. When
wild type mesenchyme was combined with Tfm/Y epithelium, the

formation of prostatic buds by the Tfm/Y epithelium was induced. However, when Tfm/Y mesenchyme was paired with normal epithelium, vaginal-like histogenesis occurred. These results were confirmed by Lasnitzki and Mizuno (1980). Other investigators have used a similar approach to demonstrate the role of mesenchyme in mediating the testosterone dependent regression of the mouse mammary gland (Kratochwil and Schwartz, 1976; Drews and Drews, 1977).

Sexual Differentiation of the Brain

The Tfm rat has been an important tool in studies designed to elucidate the factors regulating sexual differentiation of the brain in male rats (Reviewed in McEwen, 1981). In rats, a combination of androgen pathways and aromatization of androgen to estrogen is involved in masculinization of the brain. In the normal rat both defeminization and masculinization of the brain occur during the neonatal period. Testosterone is thought to defeminize the rat brain via aromatization and the estrogen receptor. One piece of evidence for this is that in Tfm rats, with no androgen receptor but normal aromatization and estrogen receptor function, the brain is defeminized. The process of masculinization, on the other hand, involves the combination of aromatization and androgen receptor pathways. As a result, there is only partial masculinization of the Tfm rat brain. Regulation of male behavior by the CNS extends beyond the brain. There is evidence of masculinization of the spinal cord and penile reflexes by androgens. Furthermore, androgen concentrating cells in the spinal cord that project to muscles of the penis show marked sexual dimorphism and are absent in Tfm rats. Although the Tfm rat has provided a great deal of information concerning the differential roles of estrogens and androgens in the sexual differentiation of the brain in the rat, it should be remembered that much of this may be species specific. Masculinization of hamsters involves primarily the aromatization pathway while behavior of guinea pigs and rhesus monkeys is masculinized primarily through the direct action of androgens.

H-Y Antigen

The H-Y antigen has recently received a great deal of attention for its role in regulating testicular differentiation. Although the correlation between the presence of testes and the Y chromosome was noted in the early studies, it was not clear as to whether this male characteristic was related to androgens or the Y chromosome itself. The fact that the H-Y antigen and testes are present in Tfm/Y mice (Bennett et al., 1975) suggests that the expression of H-Y is related to the Y chromosome and is not androgen dependent.

Determining the Role of the Androgen Receptor

The Tfm/Y mouse has been used in several studies designed to determine the role of the androgen receptor in mediating the biological effects of various steroids. Two such examples will be given here.

Many progestins induce androgenic-type responses. We wanted to determine if these effects were mediated via the androgen receptor or the progesterone receptor (Bullock et al., 1977). The fact that Tfm/Y mice were unresponsive to the androgenic effects of progestins suggested that these steroids were **acting** via the androgen receptor. Subsequent studies demonstrated that in kidney and submandibular gland of normal mice the androgenic progestin, ^{3}H-medroxyprogesterone acetate, was bound to a cytoplasmic macromolecule that had the characteristics of the androgen receptor and was concentrated in nuclei. In contrast, there was no cytoplasmic binding or nuclear retention of this ^{3}H-steroid in Tfm/Y mice. These observations support the concept that the androgenic effects of progestins are mediated via the androgen receptor.

Androgens as well as nonandrogenic 5β-androstanes and 5-pregnanes are known to stimulate erythropoiesis. We used the Tfm/Y mouse as one of several probes to determine if the androgen receptor was involved in mediating the erythropoietic effects of any of these classes of steroid (Besa and Bullock, 1981). The response of the Tfm/Y mouse was similar to that of normal when the ability of 5α- and 5β-dihydrotestosterone to stimulate overall erythropoiesis in vivo and the pluripotential bone marrow stem cell in vitro was determined. These data suggest that the androgen receptor might not be essential for the effects of androgens or 5β-steroids on erythropoiesis.

As of this writing, the Tfm rat must be obtained from the International Foundation for the Study of Rat Genetics and Rodent Pest Control in Oklahoma City. In contrast, there are numerous colonies of Tfm/Y mice under the care of individual

investigators throughout this country and abroad. In most
instances, investigators are willing to provide a few animals
for study or breeding pairs.

REFERENCES

Amrhein JA, Meyer III WJ, Jones Jr HW, Migeon CJ (1976).
Androgen insensitivity in man:Evidence of genetic heterogeneity. Proc Nat Acad Sci USA 73:891.
Attardi B, Ohno, S (1974). Cytosol androgen receptor
from kidney of normal and testicular feminized (Tfm)
mice. Cell 2:205.
Attardi B, Ohno S (1978). Physical properties of androgen
receptors in brain cytosol from normal and testicular
feminized (Tfm/Y) mice. Endocrinology 103:760.
Bennett D, Boyse EA, Lyon MF, Mathieson BJ, Scheid M,
Yanagisawa K (1975). Expression of H-Y (male) antigen in
phenotypically female Tfm/Y mice. Nature 257:236.
Besa EC, Bullock LP (1981). The role of the androgen receptor in erythropoiesis. Endocrinology (In press).
Blecher SR (1978). Microscopic epididymides in testicular
feminisation. Nature 275:748.
Bullock L, Bardin CW (1970). Decreased dihydrotestosterone
retention by preputial gland nuclei from the androgen
insensitive pseudohermaphrodite rat. J Clin Endocrinol
Metab 31:113.
Bullock LP, Bardin CW (1973). In vivo and in vitro testosterone metabolism by the androgen insensitive rat. J
Steroid Biochem 4:139.
Bullock LP, Bardin CW (1977). Androgen-insensitive animals
as a tool for understanding the mode of androgen action.
In Martini L and Motta M (eds): "Androgens and Antiandro-
gens," New York: Raven Press, p 91.
Bullock LP, Bardin CW, Ohno S (1971). The androgen insensitive mouse:absence of intranuclear androgen retention in
the kidney. Biochem Biophys Res Commun 44:1537.
Bullock LP, Lin YC, Jacob S, Bardin CW (1977). Progestin
simulation and alteration of androgen action in rodent
tissues. In Garattini S and Berendes HW (eds): "Pharmacol-
ogy of Steroid Contraceptive Drugs," New York: Raven Press,
p 353.
Collier ME, Griffin JE, Wilson JD (1978). Intranuclear
binding of (^{3}H) dihydrotestosterone by cultured human
fibroblasts. Endocrinology 103:1499.
Cunha GR, Chung LWK, Shannon JM, Reese BA (1980). Stromal-
epithelial interactions in sex differentiation. Biol of

Repro 22:19.

Drews U, Drews U (1977). Regression of mouse mammary gland anlagen in recombinants of Tfm and wild-type tissues: Testosterone acts via the mesenchyme. Cell 10:401.

Gehring U, Tomkins GM (1974). Characterization of a hormone receptor defect in the androgen-insensitivity mutant. Cell 3:59.

Goldstein JL, Wilson JD (1972). Studies on the pathogenesis of the pseudohermaphroditism in the mouse with testicular feminization. J Clin Invest 51:1647.

Griffin JE, Punyashthiti K, Wilson JD (1976). Dihydrotestosterone binding of cultured human fibroblasts. Comparison of cells from control subjects and from patients with hereditary male pseudohemaphroditism due to androgen resistance. J Clin Invest 57:1342.

Higgins SJ, Gehring U (1978). Molecular mechanisms of steroid hormone action. Adv in Cancer Res 28:313.

Kratochwil K, Schwartz P (1976). Tissue interaction in androgen response to embryonic mammary rudiment of mouse: Identification of target tissue for testosterone. Proc Natl Acad Sci USA 73:4041.

Lasnitzki I, Mizuno T (1980). Prostatic induction:Interaction of epithelium and mesenchyme from normal wild-type mice and androgen-insensitive mice with testicular feminization. J Endocr 85:423.

Lyon MF, Hawkes SG (1970). X-linked gene for testicular feminization in the mouse. Nature 227:1217.

McEwen BS (1982). Sexual differentiation of the brain: Gonadal hormone action and current concepts of neuronal differentiation. In Brown I (ed): "Molecular Approaches to Neurobiology," New York: Academic Press, p 195.

O, Haug E, Attramadal A, Aakvaag A, Hansson V, French F (1976). Androgen receptors in the anterior pituitary and central nervous system of the androgen "insensitive" (Tfm) rat:Correlation between receptor binding and effects of androgens on gonadotropin secretion. Endocrinology 99:1295.

Nes N (1966). Testikulaer feminisering hos Storfe. Nord Vet Med 18:19.

Ritzen EM, Nayfeh SN, French FS, Aronin PA (1972). Deficient nuclear uptake of testosterone in the androgen-insensitive (Stanley-Gumbreck) pseudohermaphrodite male rat. Endocrinology 91:116.

Schultz MG (1962). Male pseudohermaphroditism diagnosed with aid of sex chromatin technique. J Am Vet Med Assoc 140:241.

Shapiro BH, Levine DC, Adler NT (1980). The testicular
  feminized rat:A naturally occurring model of androgen
  independent brain masculinization. Science 209:418.
Smith AA, McLean WS, Nayfeh SN, French FS (1975). Androgen
  receptor in rat testis. In French FS, Hausson U, Ritzen
  EM, Nayfeh SN (eds): "Hormonal regulation of spermatogenesis," New York: Plenum Press, p 257.
Stanely AJ, Gumbreck LG, Allison JE, Easley RB (1973).
  Male pseudohermaphroditism in the laboratory Norway rat.
  Recent Progress in Hormone Research 29:43.
Thiedemann K-U, Drews U (1980). Nuclei in testicular feminization (Tfm) are not activated by intact testosterone
  receptor complexes:A morphometric study in striated
  urethral muscle of mosaic mice. Cell Tissue Res 212:127.
Thiedemann K-U, Schleicher G, Drews U (1981). Intact
  testosterone receptor complex does not induce RNA synthesis of Tfm-nuclei in multinucleated urethral muscle
  fibres of mosaic mice. Histochemistry 70:123.
Verhoeven GFM, Wilson JD (1979). The syndromes of primary
  hormone resistance. Metabolism 28:253.
Wieland SJ, Fox TO (1979). Putative androgen receptors
  distinguished in wild-type and testicular-feminized
  (Tfm) mice. Cell 17:781.

DR. AURBACH: Is there a postulate concerning how androgens work in promoting erythropoietin synthesis that is not via the androgen receptor?

DR. BULLOCK: Right now I would not want to say whether the androgen receptor is needed for androgen stimulation of erythropoietin production or not.   I do not believe that the site of origin of erythropoietin has been completely resolved.   It could come directly from the kidney or originate following the cleavage of a plasma precursor by a renal enzyme.   In either case the kidney is involved and androgen receptors are present in the mouse kidney.   This makes it possible that the androgen receptor is involved.   On the other hand, the results of our in vivo studies suggest something different.   The assay we used, ^{59}Fe incorporation into RBC's in posthypoxic mice, integrates the effects of androgens on erythropoietin production and on the stem cell.   The fact that the in vivo erythropoietic response of the Tfm/Y mouse to stimulation by 5 α-dihydrotestosterone was as good as that of a normal mouse suggested that the androgen receptor may not be involved.

To answer this question specifically we need to evaluate erythropoietin production directly.   Right now there is no specific assay for mouse erythropoietin.   I have serum saved from androgen treated normal and Tfm/Y mice in the hope that an antibody with high specificity and cross reactivity with mouse erythropoietin eventually will be found.

A number of investigators, both hematologists and endocrinologists, have studied the effects of androgen on the stem cell and have tried to identify a mechanism.   So far, however, they have not been successful.

DR. AURBACH: Have they have looked specifically for receptors in this stem cell?

DR. BULLOCK: Yes.   In no case has a binder with the characteristics of the classical androgen receptor been identified.   Evidence of nuclear androgen accumulation in bone marrow has been reported but a soluble cytoplasmic binder with the characteristics of the androgen receptor has not been found.   Evidence of binders with intermediate to high affinity for 5 β-steroids has been reported for chick blastoderm and embryonic liver but there are no data that androgens are acting on mammalian pluripotential stem cells via similar mechanisms.   The mechanism of androgen action on the stem cell is apparently a difficult problem that still awaits solution.

Animal Models of Inherited Metabolic Diseases, pages 381–418
© **1982 Alan R. Liss, Inc., 150 Fifth Avenue, New York, NY 10011**

H-Y ANTIGEN AND SEX DETERMINATION IN ANIMALS

Jules R. Selden, V.M.D.

Memorial Sloan-Kettering Cancer Center

New York, New York 10021

A.   SEX DETERMINATION IN MAMMALS

The attainment of normal sexual development in
mammals involves a series of three highly integrated
events (Jost, 1970). At fertilization, the genetic
constitution of the developing organism is established (genetic sex), dictating whether testes or
ovaries develop (gonadal sex). Gonadal hormones
mediate both male genital tract development and the
secondary sex characteristics of both males and
females (body sex).

Genetic Sex and Gonadal Sex

In mammals, the genetic sex of the conceptus is determined by the fertilizing sperm (McClung, 1902). Mature
spermatozoa contain either an X or Y sex chromosome whereas
ova contain only an X (Boveri, 1909). Thus union of an
ovum with a Y-bearing sperm generally results in a male
zygote, while union of an ovum with an X-bearing sperm generally results in a female zygote.

In humans, the first signs of sexual development are
observed during the fifth week of gestation (van Wagenen
and Simpson, 1965). An indifferent gonad comprising elements
of coelomic epithelium and mesenchymal cells arises along
the medial aspect of the mesonephric kidney. The epithelial
cells give rise to primary sex cords, which become the seminiferous tubules in males and the primary ovarian follicles

in females. The mesenchymal cells differentiate into either
Leydig cells in the testis or theca and stromal cells in the
ovary (Arey, 1965). Primordial germ cells originate in the
yolk sac endoderm. These cells migrate to the embryonic
gonad, proliferating during their journey (Witschi, 1948).

The events associated with differentiation of the gonad
coincide with arrival of the germ cells, yet the factor(s)
responsible for gonadal development are present within the
genital ridge (indifferent gonad). Neither elimination of
migrating germ cells by busulphan (Merchant, 1975) nor severe
depletion by the mutant W gene in mice (Coulombre and Russell,
1954) thwart testicular or ovarian organogenesis.

Development of the testis generally precedes development
of the ovary. In humans, for example, distinct testicular
architecture is observed around the seventh week of gestation, but ovarian differentiation is not observed until the
tenth to twelfth week (see for example, Jost, 1953).

Body Sex

Like the gonads, the external genitalia of both sexes
arise from common anlagen, first noted at the eighth week of
gestation in man (Grumbach and Ducharme, 1960). However,
distinct female (Mullerian) and male (Wolffian) duct systems,
which become the internal genital tracts, co-exist at the
eighth week of fetal life in man (Jirásek, 1971). The
Wolffian duct elements give rise to the epididymides, vas
deferens and accessory sex glands, whereas the Mullerian duct
elements give rise to the fallopian tubes, uterus and cranial
vagina.

Male and female rabbit and mouse fetuses gonadectomized
during the sexually indifferent stage develop internal genital tracts and external genitalia of females (Jost, 1947 and
1953; Raynaud and Frilley, 1947). Thus, there exists a
passive inclination towards the female phenotype in all
mammalian embryos independent of their karyotype. Maleness
is superimposed upon this passive inclination by testicular
secretions. Testicular secretions serve a dual function in
this regard: (1) they induce Wolffian duct differentiation
and male development of the external genitalia, and (2) they
suppress the Mullerian duct system. Testosterone (a Leydig
cell product) and dihydrotestosterone stimulate male

differentiation of the internal genital tract and external genitalia, respectively (Wilson and Lasnitzki, 1971; Siiteri and Wilson, 1974); whereas anti-Mullerian hormone, a Sertoli cell product, prevents differentiation of the Mullerian duct system (Tran et al, 1977). Androgen biosynthesis by Leydig cells is detectable at the eighth week of fetal life in male human fetuses (Pelliniemi and Niemi, 1969). Secretion of anti-Mullerian hormone coincides with development of seminiferous tubules in male fetal pigs (Tran et al, 1977).

B. HISTOCOMPATIBILITY-Y (H-Y) ANTIGEN

"Some triggering mechanism seems to divert the male gonad from this slow ovarian evolution and to impose a more rapid and early testicular differentiation."

A. Jost (1970)

Discovery of H-Y Antigen in the Laboratory Mouse

It is a dictum of transplantation biology that tissue grafts exchanged between genetically identical individuals such as monozygotic twins, should be accepted. Genetic differences between two individuals are responsible for the rejection of a donor's tissue by the recipient.

Today there are more than 250 inbred strains of laboratory mice. These strains were developed by brother-sister matings for twenty generations or more. Theoretically each member of a particular strain is more than 98% likely to be homozygous for every autosomal locus in its genome, barring mutation.

Within certain inbred strains of laboratory mice (e.g., C57BL) male skin grafts are rejected by females, but female-to-female, female-to-male and male-to-male grafts are routinely accepted (Eichwald and Silmser, 1955). Two explanations for this phenomenon were immediately apparent (Hauschka, 1955): (1) chronic male skin graft survival is androgen-dependent and (2) the skin of these males contains an antigen determined by genes on the Y chromosome. Female recipients of male skin grafts accordingly respond to this foreign substance by rejecting the graft. This rejection of male-to-female skin grafts is prolonged (about 25-30 days) in comparison to rejection of skin grafts in donor-host combinations involving differences at the major histocompatibility complex (7-12 days). For that reason it was speculated that the immunological response mounted by these female mice is generated against a 'weak' or minor histocompatibility antigen (Snell, 1956).

The hormonal hypothesis of male-to-female graft rejection was tested by ovariectomizing female mice and inoculating them with testosterone proprionate before and during their exposure to male skin isografts. The duration of transplant survival appeared unchanged overall, but instances of extended acceptance were noted (Eichwald et al, 1958). Vojtíškova and Poláčková (1972) attempted to simulate a male hormonal environment in C57BL females by injecting them weekly with testosterone, starting at birth and continuing for nine weeks. After completion of the hormonal regimen, skin from C57BL males was grafted on these females. The grafts survived an average of 54 days; seven of the 18 grafts persisted for more than 200 days.

One explanation for the extended survival of these male grafts is that non-specific immunological suppression occurred with the administration of androgens. Hirota et al (1976) found that humoral antibody production (specifically IgG) is suppressed in chickens treated with testosterone proprionate. Additional evidence that these female mice were immunologically compromised was provided by a study in which skin from B10.LP-a female mice was grafted onto testosterone-treated C57BL females. These two laboratory mouse strains differ at the H-3 and H-9 loci, thus these grafts should be rapidly rejected. The grafts survived on the hormonally-treated females for a significantly longer period (21 days) than was observed on non-treated C57BL females (16 days), (Vojtíškova and Poláčková, 1972). In addition, skin from these testosterone-treated females showed no evidence of intrastrain histoincompatibility when grafted onto non-treated female mice (Vojtíškova and Poláčková, 1972).

Castration of adult C57BL male mice two or three weeks before receiving male skin homografts did not result in the rejection of any of the grafts (Eichwald et al, 1958; Bernstein et al, 1958). In another study, neonatal C57BL male mice were castrated and their spleens still expressed the male-specific antigen three months later (Celada and Wlshons, 1963).

The hormonal hypothesis was likewise tested on <u>donors</u>. Vojtíšková and Poláčková (1966) grafted skin from adult castrated C57BL males (neutered before they were two days old) onto female C57BL recipients. The mean survival time of these grafts was prolonged--50 days, and 14% of the grafts (3/21) were not rejected after a period of 200 days. Skin from male donors castrated within 12 hours after birth had a mean survival time of 45 days, and 50% (11/22) of these grafts were not rejected after 200 days (Poláčková and Vojtíšková, 1968). The authors claimed that these male skin grafts nonetheless contained the male-specific antigen. Their evidence was based on the observation that female C57BL mice which chronically harbored grafts from these castrated males rejected skin grafts from intrastrain intact males in an accelerated (second-set) manner. It is perhaps noteworthy though, that the original transplants were undisturbed even after the second panel of grafts had been rejected. Conflicting results were reported by Weissman (1973).

Conflicting data have also been reported on the fate of newborn C57BL skin transplanted to adult C57BL males for periods up to 100 days and subsequently retransplanted to adult C57BL females presensitized to H-Y antigen. In one study (Engelstein, 1967), the mean survival time of these grafts was 16.5 days, but Silvers <u>et al</u> (1968) and Poláčková (1969) proposed that graft rejection observed by Engelstein (1967) was directed against contaminating male passenger cells. Using H-2 incompatible donor-host combinations Poláčková (1969) reported acute rejection in 14/16 cases in which neonatal C57BL female skin grafts were briefly harbored on (C57BLxA) F_1 females before being transferred to adult C57BL females.

The hypothesis that male-to-female graft rejection was the result of a Y-linked antigen was tested using two approaches. Secondary exposure to a particular antigen by a primed immune system generates an immune response of greater magnitude than that observed after primary exposure (Medawar, 1944). This indication of an immune 'memory' is called an anamnestic response (or 'second set' reaction as compared to the initial or 'first set' reaction). When C57BL females received a second male skin isograft shortly after rejecting the first, the period of second graft survival was much shorter (averaging 12-15 days), indicating that a second set reaction had taken place (Eichwald et al, 1957).

In contrast to the above, C57BL newborn females inoculated with male C57BL spleen cells accepted male skin isografts as adults, indicating that they had become tolerant to the male transplants (Billingham and Silvers, 1958). Since both second set reactions and tolerance were observed with male-to-female isografts, the existence of a Y-associated histocompatibility antigen was confirmed. The antigen was called Histocompatibility-Y (H-Y) antigen by Billingham and Silvers in 1960.

In a study of acquired tolerance, Billingham and Silvers (1960) found no strain specificity for H-Y antigen in mice. Neonatal C57BL females were inoculated with bone marrow cells from males of strains A, C3H, CBA and AU. Neonatal C57BL females which were injected with bone marrow cells from females of strains A and AU served as controls. As adults, all mice were challenged with skin grafts from C57BL males. If the H-Y of any of the four strains tested were identical to the H-Y of C57BL males, then these female mice should exhibit tolerance to the C57BL skin graft. In fact, all females that had received male bone marrow inoculations as neonates were tolerant to the male isografts as adults; the females that served as controls unanimously rejected the male skin isografts. The authors surmised that H-Y antigen is perhaps the same in all male mice.

H-Y Antigen as a Male-Specific Transplantation Antigen in Laboratory Rats

In 1959 Billingham and Silvers demonstrated that female BN rats reject skin grafts from males of the same strain. To date, male-to-female skin graft rejection has been reported in 9 strains of the laboratory rat (Wachtel, personal communication). H-Y antigen has not been found in the kidneys of male Lewis and Fischer rats (Mullen and Hildemann, 1972) and HS rats (Heslop, 1973), yet additional experiments for determining the H-Y antigen phenotypes of the tissues of these rats (i.e., development of tolerance/second set reactions) need to be performed.

H-Y antigen may exist in more than one form in the rat

according to a study involving Lewis (Le) and Fischer (Fi) rats (Mullen and Hildemann, 1972). Skin transplants from Lewis males were placed on males produced from mating Fischer males with Lewis females. Thus donor ($X^{Le}Y^{Le}$) and recipient ($X^{Le}Y^{Fi}$) differ with respect to their Y chromosomes. Rejection was observed in 2 of 14 skin grafts. These findings are not supported by similar studies performed on male Lewis and BN rats (Billingham et al, 1962), and BS and HS males, BS and AS males, BS and $\overline{AS2}$ males and HS and Lewis males (Heslop, 1973). Moreover, HS females inoculated as newborns with AS2 male cells were tolerant of HS male skin grafts as adults (Heslop, 1968).

Heslop (1973) and Silvers et al (1977) observed that H-Y antigen expression in rats is independent of the presence of androgens. Heslop (1973) transplanted adult HS female skin on adult HS males and 6 months later transferred the grafts to adult HS females not presensitized to H-Y antigen. 100% of the grafts survived a 350-day observation period. Silvers et al (1977) compared H-Y antigen expression in adult Lewis and BN males castrated before they were 1 and 2 hours old, respectively, with H-Y in intact male littermates. Skin from members of each group was grafted on intrastrain adult females. The Lewis females were additionally presensitized to H-Y antigen. Neonatal castration did not significantly increase either graft survival time or the proportion of grafts that were accepted.

Homology of H-Y Antigen in Rats and Mice Revealed in Transplantation Studies

C57BL adult female mice rejected male skin homografts in an accelerated fashion when presensitized with injections of male rat lymph node cell suspensions in four of the nine rat strains tested (Lewis, Fischer, BH and August). Inoculations with lymph node cell suspensions from female rats in all nine strains failed to sensitize C57BL females against male C57BL skin transplants. Thus an identical or cross-reactive H-Y antigen molecule is shared by rats and mice (Silvers and Yang, 1973).

Investigating a Sex-Specific Transplantation Antigen in
Other Laboratory Animals

Intrastrain skin transplantation studies performed on
two lines of laboratory rabbits demonstrated the presence
of a male-specific antigen (Chai, 1968 and 1973). No sex-
specific skin transplantation antigen was detected in
Syrian hamsters (Adams, 1958; Billingham and Hildemann,
1958), nor was this observed in two lines of laboratory
guinea pigs (Bauer, 1960).

Summary of Transplantation Studies on H-Y Antigen

Presence of a male-specific transplantation
antigen (H-Y antigen) was detected in the laboratory
mouse, rat and rabbit. As a general rule, males
from any strain can serve as a source of H-Y
antigen (although H-Y alleles have been reported
in certain strains of the laboratory rat). Homology of rat and mouse H-Y antigen has been
demonstrated. Evidence is lacking for a sex-
associated transplantation antigen in inbred hamsters and guinea pigs.

The section which follows details the significant findings to date of serological assays
using antisera containing 'H-Y antibody'. Although it is not known if the cell surface antigen
recognized serologically is the same as the antigen
recognized in the aforementioned transplantation
studies, it is clear that both are identifying a
sex-specific antigen. Thus the term 'H-Y antigen'
will be used to describe the sex-specific antigen
identified serologically.

Phylogenetic Conservation of H-Y Antigen and its Presumptive
Role in Primary Sex Determination

With the development of serological assays, the search
for H-Y antigen in a variety of species of animal was initiated. Mouse H-Y antiserum was absorbed with male and
female cells of rats, guinea pigs, rabbits, humans (Wachtel
et al, 1974).   To date, male and female cells from 16
species of mammals and 19 species of fish, amphibians, birds
and reptiles have had H-Y antigen phenotypes assigned

(Wachtel, personal communication).

In every mammalian species studied only male cells absorbed H-Y antibody. H-Y antigen has been detected on virtually all cells of the male mouse. Exceptions are mature erythrocytes (Sachs and Heller, 1958; but see Furasawa et al, 1963 and Shalev et al, 1978) and prepachytene spermatocytes (Koo et al, 1979). H-Y antigen has been detected on the cell surfaces of 8-cell mouse embryos (Krco and Goldberg, 1976; Epstein et al, 1980). Twenty three strains of the laboratory mouse have been evaluated for the presence of H-Y antigen (Wachtel, personal communication). Like the mouse, H-Y antigen appears to be distributed throughout the tissues of the male rat, but premeiotic male rat germ cells apparently do not express H-Y antigen (Zenzes et al, 1978).

In non-mammalian vertebrates, H-Y antigen is always present on the cell surfaces of the heterogametic sex (XY or ZW). Thus, the heterogametic male (XY) leopard frog, Rana pipiens, and the heterogametic female (ZW) South African clawed frog, Xenopus laevis, have H-Y+ phenotypes (Wachtel et al, 1975a).

The presence of H-Y antigen on the cell surface of all male mammals led to the proposal that H-Y antigen is responsible for development of testes in mammals whereas the corresponding antigen (often referred to as H-W antigen) in heterogametic females is responsible for development of ovaries (Wachtel et al, 1975b).

C. THE XX MALE SYNDROME AND XX TRUE HERMAPHRODITISM

Environmental or genetic factors may affect sexual development. Sexually ambiguous individuals are called 'intersexes' or 'hermaphrodites.' Intersexes are classified as either true hermaphrodites, male pseudohermaphrodites or female pseudohermaphrodites according to gonadal sex. Intersexes possessing bilateral testes are called male pseudohermaphrodites. Intersexes possessing bilateral ovaries are called female pseudohermaphrodites. True hermaphrodites have both ovarian and testicular tissues which may reside either as distinct organs (an ovary on one side

and a testis contralaterally) or co-exist in a
gonad (called an ovotestis).

Although female pseudohermaphrodites generally
have XX karyotypes, a variety of sex chromosome
complements may be observed in male pseudohermaphrodites and true hermaphrodites. The latter,
for example in man, exhibit a spectrum of karyotypes: 46,XX; 46,XY; 46,XX/46XY; 46,XX/47XXY
(van Niekerk, 1974); 45X/46,XY (van Niekerk,
1974); 46,XX/48,XXYY (Blank et al, 1964); 46,XX/
47,XYY (Buyse, 1975). The phenotypes observed
within each intersex class likewise are diverse,
ranging from slightly virilized females to nearly
normal males.

The XX Male Syndrome and XX True Hermaphroditism in Man

Testicular development in the absence of a Y chromosome
is observed in XX true hermaphroditism and in the XX male
syndrome. Human 46,XX males were first identified in 1964
(Court Brown et al, 1964; de la Chapelle et al, 1964;
Therkelsen, 1964). These individuals possess unambiguous
male genitalia, but they may be characterized by gynecomastia,
decreased facial hair and a female-type distribution of body
and pubic hair. The incidence of XX males has been estimated
at about 1 in 20,000 male babies (Jacobs et al, 1974; Evans
et al, 1979; de la Chapelle, 1981).

Adult XX males exhibit a male psychosexual orientation
(de la Chapelle, 1972). Their testes are hypoplastic and
are frequently cryptorchid. Microscopic examination of the
gonads reveals absence of spermatogenic activity, small
hyalinized seminiferous tubules, peritubular fibrosis and
Leydig cell hyperplasia (Simpson, 1976).

XX true hermaphrodite humans were first described in
1959 (Hungerford et al, 1959; Harnden and Armstrong, 1959;
Ferguson-Smith et al, 1960). Some 302 cases of human true
hermaphroditism have been documented since the turn of the
century by van Niekerk (1974). Of the 91 subjects whose
chromosomes were studied, 55 (60%) had a 46,XX karyotype.
The external genitalia of human XX true hermaphrodites are
either predominantly male or markedly ambiguous. Breast
development and menarche occur typically at puberty.

Microscopic examination of the gonads reveals no spermatogenic activity in the testicular regions although follicular
development is often normal in the ovarian regions. Pregnancy and childbirth have been reported in two XX true
hermaphrodites (Narita et al, 1975; Mayou et al, 1978).
Reconstructive vaginal surgery and removal of testicular
tissue were necessary in both cases to facilitate impreg-
nation, and the babies were delivered by Caesarean section.

Familial Incidence of XX Male and XX True Hermaphrodite
Humans

Although nearly all intersex humans are isolated cases,
a number of studies have documented families with more than
one affected member:

1) two families with two XX true hermaphrodite sibs
(Mori and Mitzutani, 1968; Fraccaro et al, 1979), and two
families with three XX true hermaphrodite sibs (Rosenberg
et al, 1963; Armendares et al, 1975).

2) a family with monozygotic XX male twins (Nicolis
et al, 1972) and another family with two XX male children
(Minowada et al, 1979). A third family contained three XX
males. In this last study, two of the affected members were
first cousins who were related to the third affected person
through an ancestor born in 1668 (de la Chapelle et al, 1978).

3) a family with two intersex children (an XX male
and an XX true hermaphrodite) and two normal offspring (a
girl and a boy). A paternal uncle was purported to be an
XX male (Kasdan et al, 1973).

4) a high incidence of 'isolated' cases of XX true
hermaphroditism has been reported in the Bantu tribe of
South Africa (van Niekerk, 1974).

The mode of inheritance of intersexuality in these
families is unknown. In the last part of this section,
possible explanations for the origin and inheritance of these
conditions are presented.

Autosomal Recessive Sex Reversal in Polled Goats

Intersex goats range in appearance from nearly normal males to slightly abnormal females. Regional estimates of the incidence of intersexuality among newborn goats vary from 2% (Davies, 1913) to 10% (Buechi, 1963). In the United States, the incidence of intersexuality among certain herds of Toggenburg and Saanen goats is as high as 6 and 11%, respectively (Eaton and Simmons, 1939). Evidence that intersexuality in these animals is genetically determined was provided by the observation that all intersex goats are hornless (polled) (Asdell, 1944). Since all intersex goats are hornless but not similarly masculinized, it would appear that either the polled gene has a pleiotropic effect upon sexual development, or that other genes closely linked to the polled gene produce intersexuality in polled goats.

The polled condition (P) is inherited as an autosomal dominant gene. Heterozygotes at the polled locus (P/+) are hornless but otherwise phenotypically normal, whereas homozygotes (P/P) are hornless and exhibit aberrant sexual development. Only homozygous P/P XX goats are intersexes (Nes et al, 1963; Basrur and Coubrough, 1964). Approximately 10-30% of the P/P XY goats are infertile males. The lesion in these infertile males is an occlusion of the caput epididymis (Widmaier, 1957).

The P/P XX goats usually have bilateral testes which are often atrophic, but true hermaphrodites have also been described (Asdell, 1936; Eaton, 1945; Kondo, 1952; Hamerton et al, 1969). Histologically, the testes contain reduced numbers of hypoplastic hyalinized seminiferous tubules, devoid of spermatogenic activity. Production of mature sperm by intersex polled goats has been reported (Basrur and Coubrough, 1964, Basrur and Kanagawa, 1969) and has been attributed to the presence of XO spermatocytes (Lyon, 1974).

A heterozygote advantage may be conferred by the polled gene since larger litters are produced when either parent is a carrier (Soller and Angel, 1964; Soller and Kempenich, 1964; Ricordeau and Lauvergne, 1967). When homozygous males are mated with heterozygous females, an excess of males has been observed at the expense of normal and intersex females (Ricordeau and Lauvergne, 1967). It has also been noted that multiparous deliveries produce a greater frequency of intersex goats than do single births; this implies that intrauterine events also influence the sexual development of the fetal goat (Laor et al, 1962).

Autosomal Recessive Inheritance of XX True Hermaphroditism and the XX Male Syndrome in the Pig

Intersexuality has been reported to affect between 0.2 and 0.5% of swine populations (Andersson, 1956; Freudenberg, 1957; Breeuwsma, 1969) with incidences approaching 20% in some herds (Baker, 1928; Gerneke, 1967). Intersex pigs are generally genetic females (38,XX), but occasionally are mosaic (38,XX/38,XY) (McFee et al, 1966; Bruere et al, 1968; Vogt, 1968; Somlev, et al, 1970; Breeuwsma, 1970). These intersex pigs routinely appear as females with an enlarged clitoris, a 'fishhook' vulva or vestigial prepuce and rudimentary scrotum, sometimes containing gonads. Their internal reproductive tract normally contains a cranial vagina, uterine horns, bilateral vas deferens and epididymides. Their gonads usually are testes. However, ovotestes have been observed (Hammond, 1912; Corner, 1920; Crew, 1923). The birth of an XX male and an XX true hermaphrodite in the same litter has been described (Gerneke, 1967). Testes or ovotestes of affected pigs usually contain azoospermic seminiferous tubules, but normal oogenesis with formation of corpora lutea is routinely described. There are several reports of pregnancy and farrowing by true hermaphrodite pigs (Petersen, 1952; Hulland, 1964; Cox, 1968).

Intersexuality in pigs is inherited as an autosomal recessive defect. There is evidence favoring a simple recessive mode of inheritance (Johnston et al, 1958; Basrur and Kanagawa, 1969; Bishop, 1972), although a segregation analysis suggested recessive genes at two autosomal loci may be involved (Sittman, 1973). In the single locus hypothesis, females homozygous for the recessive gene are abnormal, whereas heterozygous females are phenotypically normal carriers. Males, whether heterozygous or homozygous for the mutation, would be sexually normal carriers. According to the latter explanation (two autosomal loci), only females homozygous for recessive mutations at both loci would be sex-reversed. All other genotypes would result in phenotypically normal male and female pigs.

Autosomal Dominant Sex Reversal in Mice

An autosomal dominant mutation, Sxr (sex-reversed) causes genetic female mice (40,XX) to develop as phenotypic males with testes of approximately one-fifth normal size (Cattanach et al, 1971). Histologic studies reveal Leydig cell hyperplasia and small seminiferous tubules devoid of spermatogenic activity. One Sxr embryo was a true hermaphrodite, possessing bilateral ovotestes (Mittwoch and Buehr, 1973).

The appearance of the 40,XX Sxr/- fetal testis however, is not grossly abnormal. Testicular development is similar in 40,XX Sxr/- embryos and 40,XY -/- littermates (Spoljar and Drews, 1978). Testicular induction, indicated by the appearance of testis cords, occurs in both groups on the thirteenth day of gestation. In addition, overall testicular growth is similar in both groups between days 13 and 17 in utero.

The testes of 16 day old 40,XX Sxr/- fetuses contain as many primordial germ cells as are found in comparably developed genetic males. In contrast with normal female germ cells, none of the germ cells of these sex-reversed fetuses enter meiotic prophase. Cattanach and colleagues (1971) speculated that these gonocytes may also have been functionally sex-reversed by the Sxr mutation. They reported marked germ cell degeneration perinatally and found no spermatogonia in mice 10 days of age and older. McLaren (1980) observed oocytes in 6 of 21 40,XX Sxr/- mice, examined between 8 and 18 days of age. The oldest mouse with testes containing oocytes was 15 days of age. The oocytes were found within the seminiferous tubules and were surrounded by an incomplete layer of cells which resembled granulosa cells. The follicular growth evident in three day old mouse ovaries was never observed, although the oocytes found in these testes were as large as the oocytes present in the ovaries of mice of comparable age. Testes from 12 adult (6 to 9 weeks) 40,XX Sxr/- mice were also studied and none possessed germ cells.

The 40,XY Sxr/- males are phenotypically normal but have smaller testes than 40,XY -/- littermates. Males with the smallest testes produce fewest sperm, most of which are morphologically abnormal (Cattanach, 1975).

Sxr sex-reverses XO mice. Usually XO mice are phenotypic females having brief reproductive lifespans (Lyon and Hawkes, 1970) but 39,XO Sxr/- mice are phenotypic males with larger testes than their 40,XX Sxr/- counterparts (Cattanach, 1975).

Inherited Intersexuality in the Dog

Hare (1976) reviewed 48 spontaneous cases of intersexuality in the dog. There were 13 true hermaphrodites,
25 male pseudohermaphrodites and 2 female pseudohermaphrodites; eight purported intersex dogs could not be classified by the author.

Sixteen dog breeds were represented among the 48 cases
(Table 1). Most striking was the preponderance of cocker
spaniels (16/48). The frequencies of affected Chinese pugs
(5/48) and beagles (5/48) may also be noteworthy. More
recent papers have documented four isolated cases of intersexuality in miniature schnauzers (Brown et al, 1976;
Salkin, 1978) and the familial occurrence of intersexuality
in kerry blue terriers (Williamson, 1979).

TABLE 1

Breeds of Dogs Represented in Survey
of Canine Intersexuality[a]

Breed	Number of Cases Reported
Beagle	5
Bull Terrier	1
Chinese Pug	5
Cocker Spaniel	16
Collie	1
German Shepherd Dog	2
Golden Retriever	1
Irish Setter	1
Kerry Blue Terrier	1
Miniature Schnauzer	2
Norwegian Elkhound	1
Poodle	2
Schipperke	1
Springer Spaniel	1
Toy Terrier	1
Yorkshire Terrier	1
Mixbreed	6
	Total - 48

[a] From Hare, 1976

Two of the sixteen cocker spaniels were true hermaphrodites. Both dogs were described as phenotypic females posessing a hypertrophied clitoris containing a bony structure normally found in the dog penis (os penis); neither dog was karyotyped. The internal genital tract was Mullerian-derived and the gonads were situated in the usual ovarian position. Four of the five beagles were true hermaphrodites. The appearance of these beagles was similar to that of true hermaphrodite cocker spaniels. One beagle true hermaphrodite was reported to be an XX/XY mosaic, but may in fact have been only XX since a putative Y chromosome was found in only one of the 50 cells studied. Another beagle true hermaphrodite was reported to be sex chromatin positive. One Chinese pug was a true hermaphrodite. This intersex pug was a phenotypic female with a hypertrophied clitoris; the internal genital tract was composed of both Mullerian and Wolffian duct derivatives.

Nine of the sixteen cocker spaniels possessed bilateral testes. Five were karyotyped and all were chromosomal females. All dogs were cryptorchid, most possessing bilateral abdominal testes. Included among the nine testicular intersexes were three XX male siblings (Hare et al, 1974). One beagle intersex had bilateral abdominal testes. This beagle was a phenotypic female with a hypertrophied clitoris containing an os; the internal genital tract was composed of both Mullerian and Wolffian duct derivatives. Two Chinese pugs had bilateral abdominal testes. These pugs were phenotypic females who possessed an enlarged clitoris (one which contained an os). The reproductive tract of one Chinese pug was composed almost exclusively of Mullerian duct derivatives, save for the presence of a left epididymis; the other Chinese pug possessed only Wolffian duct derivatives.

All intersex miniature schnauzers and kerry blue terriers had bilateral testes. One kerry blue terrier was karyotyped and was 78,XX; none of the miniature schnauzers were karyotyped. All miniature schnauzers were phenotypic males who possessed a uterus and Sertoli cell tumors. The phenotypes of the kerry blue terriers varied from dog to dog.

SUMMARY. Sex-reversed males occur in man, mouse, goats, pigs and dogs. XX true hermaphrodites have also been reported in these species. Since both XX males and XX true hermaphrodites have been reported in the same family, the two conditions may share a

common genetic origin. The mode of inheritance
varies between species (e.g., simple autosomal
recessive in polled goats vs. simple autosomal
dominant in Sxr mice). Thus different genetic
mechanisms may be generating grossly similar
defects in mammals. Fertility is recognized
among XX true hermaphrodite swine and humans
(and dogs, see Section D).

Causes of XX Sex Reversal and XX True Hermaphroditism in
Mammals

Four hypotheses have been advanced to explain the development of testes, either exclusively or in association
with ovaries, in the absence of a conspicuous Y chromosome.
All four conserve the Y chromosomal function(s) considered
necessary for testicular organogenesis.
1. Cryptic mosaicism or Y chromosomal elimination.
According to this hypothesis, male development can be im-
printed upon rudimentary XX gonads by subpopulations of
cells possessing a Y chromosome. These Y-bearing cells may
be so few in the adult organism as to escape detection in
routine cytogenetic studies. Alternatively, such a Y-
containing subpopulation may have had a transient but critical influence in the developing organism prior to its elimination or early loss of the Y chromosome.

Cytogenetic investigations have revealed minor XXY
cell populations in human XX males (Court Brown et al, 1964;
Lindsten et al, 1966; Hecht et al, 1966; de la Chapelle,
1972; Dosik et al, 1976; Miró et al, 1978) and XY cell populations in human XX true hermaphrodites (Waxman et al,
1962; Brøgger and Aagenaes, 1965).

Loss of the Y chromosome with persistence of XX cells
is possible in XY zygotes. Mitotic nondisjunction, incor-
porating Y elimination could conceivably produce XX and YY
daughter cells. The latter would not be expected to survive.
Ultimate loss of the original XY cell line would create an
exclusive XX cell presence. XX cell lines could also be
produced from the fertilization of an XX ovum (meiotic nondisjunction) by a Y-containing sperm. Elimination of the Y
which lags at anaphase or by mitotic nondisjunction of the
Y chromosome in the original XXY cells could result in an
eventual population of XX cells. In the former instance
(anaphase lag), elimination of the parental cells (XXY)

would be necessary and in the latter (mitotic nondisjunction), elimination of both parental and XXYY cell populations would be necessary (de la Chapelle, 1972).

The theory of Y elimination has support from studies involving the human Xg blood group, the locus for which is on the X chromosome. Anomalous inheritance of Xg in XX males can be explained by nondisjunction. For example, the birth of an Xg(a-) XX son of an Xg(a+) father and an Xg(a-) mother could be explained if both X chromosomes of the child were maternally derived by either mitotic or meiotic nondisjunction (de la Chapelle, 1972).

Rare situations involving unexpected inheritance of two X-linked genes, Xg and Xm, could also be the result of abnormal chromosomal inheritance. The gene for the serum group, Xm is located on the X chromosome but is not closely linked to the Xg locus (Berg and Bearn, 1968; Berg, 1969). The anomalous inheritance of both loci simultaneously should involve a substantial portion of the X chromosome, large enough to be detected cytologically. In the instance of the birth of an Xg(a-), Xm(a-) XX male by an Xg(a+), Xm(a+) father and Xg(a-), Xm (a-) mother, no X chromosomal translocation was observed. The author concluded that by nondisjunction this child retained two maternal X chromosomes while eliminating the Y (de la Chapelle, 1972).

2. X-Y interchange. Studies of mammalian spermatocytes have revealed that homologous autosomes and the sex chromosomes form bivalents during zygotene of meiotic prophase I. By the end of zygotene, chromosomal pairing is stabilized by synaptonemal complexes extending the entire length of the autosomal bivalents and are also present within regions of the sex chromosome bivalent (Darlington, 1931; Koller and Darlington, 1934). Tres (1977 and 1979) recently demonstrated a transient but extensive side-by-side pairing of the X and Y chromosomes at early pachytene in mouse and Syrian hamster spermatocytes. By late diplotene, the association between the X and Y chromosomes was end-to-end and persisted throughout the duration of the first meiotic prophase.

In 1966, Ferguson-Smith proposed that XX males and XX true hermaphrodites were examples of X-Y interchange. Sex reversal would accordingly be the result of Y chromosomal testicular determinants translocated to an X chromosome. Support for this hypothesis is provided by the paradoxic

inheritance of Xg in three XX males and one XX true hermaphrodite (Ferguson-Smith, 1970). These intersexes were all
Xg(a-), although their fathers were Xg(a+). Reciprocal exchange of the X-linked Xg(a+) allele and Y-linked testicular
determinants would readily account for both sex reversal and
the non-X-linked inheritance of Xg, although alternative
explanations also exist.

Cytological evidence of presumptive X-Y interchange
in human XX males has been reported in a few cases (Madan and
Walker, 1974; Madan, 1976; Wachtel et al, 1976a; Bernstein
et al, 1978), but most intensive cytogenetic investigations
have failed to demonstrate abnormalities of chromosome
structure in human XX males and XX true hermaphrodites.
   3. Y-autosomal translocation. Ferguson-Smith et al
(1960) and Griboff and Lawrence (1961) favored the theory
that a Y chromosomal translocation would create testicular
development in XX individuals. Two instances of presumptive
Y-autosomal translocation in human intersexes have been reported. Dosik et al (1975) detected additional chromatin on
a No.17 autosome in an XX male and postulated that this
marker chromosome may have contained Y chromatin. Koo et al
(1977a) studied an XO phenotypic male putatively mosaic for
a marker No.22 autosome which may have carried Y chromosomal
material.

Sex determination based upon a Y-autosomal translocation has been detected in 13 species of mammals representing
five orders (Fredga, 1970). Preliminary information supports
a Y-autosomal translocation mechanism of sex determination in
three other mammalian species, the echidna (Tachyglossus
aculeatus), the platypus (Ornithorhynchus anatinus) (Fredga,
1970) and the varying lemming (Dicrostonyx torquatus) (Gileva
and Chebotar, 1979).

Males in this group of animals generally have an odd
number of chromosomes, one less than the females. This mechanism of sex determination can thus be denoted XX/XAY.
During meiosis in the male, the autosome carrying the translocated Y migrates to one pole while the non-Y-carrying
homologue and the X move together to the other pole. The
sloth (Choloepus hoffmanni) is an exceptional member in this
group. Female and male sloths alike possess a 49,XO karyotype (Corin-Frederic, 1969). Translocation of a Y to a small
autosome was described in male sloths. Meiotic preparations
from sloth testes revealed that this marker chromosome formed

one element of a sex chromosome heterotrivalent, confirming presence of Y chromatin on this chromosome. It was proposed (Fredga, 1970) that the female sloth germ line possesses two X chromosomes, producing gametes with a 25,X chromosomal constitution. Female sloth embryos would initially have a 50,XX karyotype (by fertilizaton with a 25,X sperm). Elimination of an X chromosome presumably occurs in preference to random X-inactivation, reconstituting the 49,XO karyotype in the somatic tissues of these females.

4. <u>Mutational acquisition of Y chromosomal function by autosomal or X chromosomal genes</u>. Pedigree analysis has provided evidence suggesting that a mutant gene is responsible for the occurrence of a high incidence of intersexuality in certain lines and families. Aside from a tentative Y-autosomal translocation in Sxr mice (Tres, 1978), no cytological evidence of a translocated Y chromosome has been found in the other species mentioned above. Data from human families with XX males and/or XX true hermaphrodites generally do not favor an autosomal recessive pattern of inheritance because: consanguinity among parents of these XX intersexes is rare; multiple affected siblings or incidents of intersexuality among close relatives have rarely been reported; and altered sex ratios favoring males have not been observed in these families. Indeed, in human families containing XX males there is a tendency for more <u>female</u> progeny among cousins of these intersexes (de la Chapelle, 1972).

The XX male syndrome and XX true hermaphroditism in man could be instances of a <u>de novo</u> autosomal or X-linked dominant mutation. The rare occurrence of additional affected members in a family could be due to the chance occurrence of fresh mutations. In this situation, none of the aforementioned criteria associated with an autosomal recessive inheritance pattern would be applicable (Simpson, 1976).

D. EVIDENCE FOR THE ROLE OF H-Y ANTIGEN IN PRIMARY (GONADAL) SEX DETERMINATION

While evolutionary conservation of H-Y antigen and its correlation with testicular development in normal mammals suggested that it may play a critical role in primary sex determination, evaluation of this hypothesis has been extended to the study of exceptional cases in which the chromosomal sex differs from gonadal or phenotypic sex. These special cases

help to answer whether H-Y antigen is itself of
primary importance in inducing testicular differentiation. If H-Y antigen is the testis inducer,
then it should be present whenever testicular tissue
is present. This should still be the case even
when a Y chromosome is not found (e.g., XX true
hermaphrodites). The corollary here is that testicular development should not occur in the absence
of H-Y antigen.

Exceptional Species of Rodents

The Scandinavian wood lemming (Myopus schisticolor). In
the Scandinavian wood lemming there are about four females
for every male. About half of these females produce only
female offspring whereas the other half produce equal numbers of males and females (Kalela and Oksala, 1966).

The somatic cells of those female wood lemmings which
produce only female progeny have a 32,XY karyotype. The
other females are karyotypically normal, 32,XX (Fredga et
al, 1976). Remarkably, only XX bivalents were found in the
oocytes of these XY females, suggesting that by a process
of 'double nondisjunction' the Y is replaced by a maternal
X chromosome in the germ line during early fetal gonadal
development (Fredga et al, 1976).

The existence of XY female wood lemmings has been explained by an X-linked gene that blocks Y chromosomal genes
responsible for testicular differentiation (Fredga et al,
1977). The Y chromosome is presumed normal since it was
present in the normal fathers of the XY females. Serological assays have shown that male wood lemmings have H-Y
antigen on their cell surfaces, but XX and XY females were
typed H-Y⁻ (Wachtel et al, 1976b). Thus, two types of X
chromosomes appear to be present in the wood lemming population, a normal X and an X which contains a gene or genes
which suppress the synthesis of H-Y antigen. Indeed, Herbst
et al (1978) identified two different X chromosomes. The
short arm of the normal X chromosome in the wood lemming has
four positive G-bands, the second band nearest the centromere being the widest and most darkly stained. The short
arm of the X chromosome observed in XY female wood lemmings
(the mutated X) also has four positive G-bands, but the most
prominent is the third band from the centromere. The mutated

X additionally has a narrower unstained region between the
second and third positive G-bands, giving this chromosome a
significantly smaller short arm than found with the normal X
chromosome. No simple explanation for this chromosomal re-
arrangement is apparent (Herbst et al, 1978).

The mole-vole (Ellobius lutescens). Male and female
mole-voles remarkably possess a 17,XO karyotype (Matthey,
1954). The unpaired metacentric chromosome, a No.9, may be
an original-type X chromosome (Castro-Sierra and Wolf, 1967).

The leading hypotheses explaining the development of
this exceptional karyotype center around a Y-No.9 interchange
(White, 1957) or translocation of the male-determining segment of the Y to one member of an autosomal pair (Castro-
Sierra and Wolf, 1967).

Although male mole-voles are H-Y$^+$ and the females are
H-Y- (Nagai and Ohno, 1977), linkage of H-Y antigen to either
the No.9 chromosome or any autosome is still an open question.
Biochemical techniques were employed to learn whether the
mole-vole possesses a heterogeneous population of X chromosomes (X^Y and X). Three X-linked enzymes (glucose-6-phosphate
dehydrogenase, phosphoglycerate kinase and alpha-galactosi-
dase) were studied in males and females. No sex differences
were observed in the electrophoretic mobilities of any of
these enzymes (Nagai and Ohno, 1977).

Mammalian Intersexes

Sex reversed mice. Sxr is an autosomal dominant mutation that causes XX and XO mice to develop as phenotypic,
albeit sterile males. The condition is transmitted solely
by 40,XY Sxr/- males. Serological studies were performed on
40,XX Sxr/- and 40,XY Sxr/- males, using non-Sxr female and
male siblings as controls. H-Y antigen was found on the cell
surfaces of both 40,XX Sxr/- and 40,XY Sxr/- males (Bennett
et al, 1977). Thus Sxr mice apparently possess autosomal
male-determining genes originating either by a Y-autosome
translocation or autosomal mutation.

The Y-autosome translocation model in Sxr must preserve a
Y capable of inducing testicular differentiation. Cattanach
et al (1971) proposed that Sxr originated from a Y chromatid
translocation. This event would occur during meiosis, when

the chromosomes duplicate. Translocation of the male-determining genes of one of the duplicated Y chromosomes to an
autosome would make only this Y deficient in its genetic
constitution, the other copy would still retain a full complement of genes. The original XY carrier male could thus have
transmitted an intact Y and an autosome containing a full
quotient of male determinants.

Citing the Sxr condition, Wachtel and Ohno (1979) proposed that multiple copies of testis-determining genes may
exist on the mammalian Y chromosome. A derivative Y resulting from loss of a portion of these genes could still retain
sufficient numbers to induce testicular differentiation. In
this situation, no Y-autosomal translocation need occur
during meiosis to preserve a functional Y chromosome while
establishing an autosomal locus of testis-determining genes.

The testicular feminization syndrome. Complete testicular feminization syndrome (TFS) in man is a condition in
which 46,XY individuals become phenotypic females with bilateral testes. Secondary sexual characteristics are female
(although the Mullerian ducts are suppressed) and the condition appears to be inherited either as an X-linked recessive
or a male-limited autosomal dominant mutation (Simpson,
1976).

The etiology of TFS is hormonal; a target organ insensitivity to androgens prohibits development of the male habitus.
Plasma testosterone and androstenedione levels are as high
as for normal males and may even be elevated. Intracellular
conversion of testosterone to dihydrotestosterone by 5 alpha-
reductase appears normal in these individuals (Tremblay et
al, 1972). Thus, the underlying defect in TFS seems to be
associated with the cytosol androgen receptor. The receptor
protein is either produced in abnormally low quantities or
possesses a reduced binding affinity for the androgen liquid
(Gehring and Tomkins, 1974). The significance of this defective androgen-binding protein is that the nuclei of the
target cells do not receive the androgenic message to undergo
masculinization.

This condition has been observed in the mouse (Lyon and
Hawkes, 1970) and rat (Stanley and Gumbreck, 1964). The rat
is distinctive in having low levels of testosterone in the
testicular vein (Bardin et al, 1970), suggesting a deficiency
in 17-ketosteroid reductase. Inheritance of TFS in rats and

mice is X-linked recessive (Lyon and Hawkes, 1970; Stanley and Gumbreck, 1964).

Serological studies revealed H-Y antigen in the tissues of TFS humans (Koo et al, 1977b) and mice (Bennett et al, 1975). The data are consistent with the presumptive role of H-Y antigen in primary sex determination, showing that this molecule does not require a male hormonal milieu for its occurrence on the cell surface.

Polled goats. Genetic female goats homozygous for the polled gene (60,XX P/P) are sex-reversed, possessing either testes or ovotestes. They range in appearance from nearly normal males to nearly normal females. H-Y antigen was studied in a family of polled Toggenburg goats which included an intersex offspring with bilateral testes and a sexually normal polled female twin. An Alpine-Toggenburg polled inter-sex goat with bilateral testes was also included in this study (Wachtel et al, 1978). H-Y+ phenotypes were reported in the heterozygous father and the two intersex goats. The mother was typed H-Y-, even though she was an obligatory heterozygote for the 'H-Y gene'.

Shalev (1980) investigated the expression of H-Y antigen on fibroblasts from seven Saanen goats. A polled hetero-zygote male (A) was mated to two polled heterozygote females (B,C) producing an intersex offspring in each case (D,E). An additional mating between A and a horned female (L, not studied) produced a horned male (F). H-Y antigen assays were performed on F and an unrelated polled heterozygote male (G) after they were castrated. The findings can be summarized as follows: (1) male A and both intersexes (D and E) were typed H-Y+ and (2) heterozygote female C was typed H-Y$^-$ and hetero-zygote female B may have possessed some H-Y antigen.

Several conclusions can be drawn from these two investi-gations on polled goats.

1. XX or XY polled goats possessing testicular tissue are H-Y+, a finding consistent with the contention that H-Y is the testis-determinant.

2. Horned males (60,XY +/+) are H-Y+, indicating that the wild type Y chromosome in these goats is intact or possesses a sufficient complement of H-Y genes to in-duce testicular differentiation.

3. There is reason to believe that goats of the same chromosomal sex and genotype at the polled locus may differ in their H-Y antigen phenotypes. Although the source of this variation may be technical, it is conceivable that additional factors, genetic and/or in utero might be responsible. The presence of these modifiers might explain the varying degrees of masculinization observed in the gonads and somatic tissues of these polled goats and other sex-reversed mammals.

The XX male syndrome and XX true hermaphroditism in man. Wachtel et al (1976a) found H-Y antigen on the cells of four human XX males and three human XX true hermaphrodites. Cells from the three XX true hermaphrodites absorbed significantly less H-Y antibody than did equal numbers of cells from male controls suggesting that human XX true hermaphrodites may possess less H-Y antigen on their cell surfaces than normal human males.

H-Y antigen assays were run with peripheral blood leukocytes of a human XX true hermaphrodite before and after removal of the gonads (Saenger et al, 1976). H-Y antigen was present on both occasions. A third study employed a direct H-Y antigen cytotoxicity test on peripheral blood lymphocytes of two unrelated human XX true hermaphrodites. Both individuals were H-Y+ (Ghosh et al, 1978).

H-Y antigen cytotoxicity and MHA.HA tests were performed on three XX males who shared a common ancestry. All three XX males were typed H-Y+. The mothers and fathers of these individuals were also typed H-Y+. Cells from male and female sibs of two of the XX males were unremarkable in their H-Y antigen phenotypes (de la Chapelle et al, 1978).

Serological investigations have been performed on one additional XX male (Dosik et al, 1976) and four human XX true hermaphrodites (Fraccaro et al, 1979; Winters et al, 1979; Moreira-Filho et al, 1980). In the study by Moreira-Filho et al (1980), an XX true hermaphrodite possessed H-Y antigen at a level intermediate between that of normal males and females. In that case, the mother was H-Y- and the father was H-Y+. Incidentally, a cytogenetic investigation discovered that the father is a 46,XX/46,XY mosaic; 8 of 65 metaphases derived from peripheral blood lymphocytes had a 46,XX karyotype.

The XX male syndrome and XX true hermaphroditism in the
dog. In a family of American cocker spaniels an XX male was
the offspring of an XX true hermaphrodite (Selden et al,
1978).

The XX male had a hypoplastic penis, was cryptorchid (right
inguinal testicle), and possessed a uterus. Histologic examination of the cryptorchid testicle revealed seminiferous tubules of varying shape and size. Spermatogenesis was absent;
the Sertoli cells contained vacuoles.

The external phenotype of the XX true hermaphrodite
mother was female, but at the age of 6 months an enlarged
clitoris containing an os was found protruding from her vulva.
Internally, a uterus, fallopian tubes and epididymides were
present. Bilateral ovotestes were located in the normal
ovarian position. Testicular regions of the ovotestis contained lobulated seminiferous tubules. As in the XX male,
spermatogenesis was absent and the Sertoli cells contained
vacuoles. All stages of oogenesis including development of
ova and mature graafian follicles were noted in the ovarian
regions of these ovotestes. Both XX true hermaphrodite
"mother" and XX male were typed H-Y+.

These findings suggest (a) that the XX male syndrome and
XX true hermaphroditism represent alternative manifestations
of a common masculinizing event associated with abnormal
transmission of H-Y genes, and (b) that an H-Y+ phenotype
does not preclude development of testes (or other male reproductive organs). Indeed a dog with an H-Y+ phenotype
possessed a functional female reproductive tract. The study
described below shows that this occurrence is not unique
to the dog.

A fertile female horse with an XY karyotype. Sharp et
al (1980) reported that a phenotypically female horse with
abnormally small ovaries (2 x 2 cm) and uterus, and a 64,XY
karyotype (from peripheral blood lymphocytes and fibroblasts
from skin biopsies) delivered a normal female offspring. The
mare's white blood cells contained H-Y antigen. However,
the quantity present may have been less than that present in
the corresponding cells of normal stallions. Thus, despite
the presence of a Y chromosome and H-Y antigen, this animal
was a fertile female.

SUMMARY. In all instances described, H-Y antigen was found when testes were present. Extragonadal tissues in androgen-insensitive individuals with TFS were typed H-Y$^+$, indicating that this cell surface component is hormone-independent. Thus, association of H-Y antigen and primary sex determination is reinforced. But variation in the degree of masculinization observed in certain mammalian intersexes (e.g., polled goats) is not explained by simple H-Y antigen dosage effects. Additional genetic and/or intrauterine modifiers may influence both gonadal and somatic tissue target cell sensitivity to hormones.

Acknowledgements

This work was supported in part by grants from the National Institutes of Health (CA-08748, AI-11982, GM-20138, HD-10065 and HL-05515).

This manuscript is taken from a dissertation submitted to the Graduate Group in Genetics, College of the Graduate Faculty, University of Pennsylvania, in partial fulfillment of the requirements for the degree of Doctor of Philosophy.

I thank Drs. Paul S. Moorhead, Donald F. Patterson and Stephen S. Wachtel for their helpful criticisms. I am especially grateful to Eunice D. Smith for her support in the preparation of the manuscript.

References

Adams RA (1958). Recent experiments with skin grafting in Syrian hamsters. Transpl Bull 5:24.
Andersson T (1956). Om intersexualitet hos svin. Kungl Skogs- och Lantbruksakad T 95:257.
Arey L (1965). "Developmental Anatomy: A textbook and laboratory manual of embryology." Philadelphia:Saunders.
Armendares S, Salamanca F, Cantu JM, Del Castillo V, Nava S, Dominquez De La Piedra E, Cortes-Gallegos V, Gallegos A, Cervantes C, Parra A (1975). Familial true hermaphroditism in three siblings. Humangenetik 29:99.
Asdell SA (1936). Hermaphroditism in goats. Dairy Goat J 14:3.

Asdell SA (1944). The genetic sex of intersexual goats and a probable linkage with the gene for hornlessness. Science 99:124.

Baker JR (1928). A new type of mammalian intersexuality. Br J Exp Biol 6:56.

Bardin CW, Bullock L, Schneider G, Allison JE, Stanley AJ (1970). Pseudohermaphrodite rat: end organ insensitivity to testosterone. Science 167:1136.

Basrur PK, Coubrough RI (1964). Anatomical and cytological sex of a Saanen goat. Cytogenetics 3:414.

Basrur PK, Kanagawa H (1969). Anatomic and cytogenetic studies on 19 hornless goats with sexual disorders. Ann Genet Sel Anim 1:349.

Bauer JA (1960). Genetics of skin transplantation and an estimate of the number of histocompatibility genes in inbred guinea pigs. Ann NY Acad Sci 87:78.

Bennett D, Boyse EA, Lyon MF, Mathieson BJ, Scheid M, Yanagisawa K (1975). Expression of H-Y (male) antigen in phenotypically female Tfm/Y mice. Nature 257:236.

Bennett D, Mathieson BJ, Scheid M, Yanagisawa K, Boyse EA, Wachtel SS, Cattanach B (1977). Serological evidence for H-Y antigen in Sxr, XX sex-reversed phenotypic females. Nature 265:255.

Berg K (1969). Mapping the X chromosome: discussion paper. Bull Europ Soc Hum Genet 3:29.

Berg K, Bearn AG (1968). Human serum protein polymorphisms: a selected review. Ann Rev Genet 2:311.

Bernstein R, Wagner J, Isdale J, Nurse GT, Lane AB, Jenkins T. (1978). X-Y translocation in a retarded phenotypic male. Clinical, cytogenetic, biochemical and serogenetic studies. J Med Genet 15:466.

Bernstein SE, Silvers AA, Silvers WK (1958). An attempt to demonstrate a Y-linked histocompatibility gene in the house mouse. J Natl Cancer Inst 20:577.

Billingham RE, Hildemann WH (1958). Studies on the immunological responses of hamsters to skin homografts. Proc Roy Soc Lond B 149:216.

Billingham RE, Hodge BA, Silvers WK (1962). An estimate of the number of histocompatibility loci in the rat. Proc Nat Acad Sci USA 48:138.

Billingham RE, Silvers WK (1958). Induction of tolerance of skin isografts from male donors in female mice. Science 128:780.

Billingham RE, Silvers WK (1959). Inbred animals and tissue transplantation immunity. Transpl Bull 6:399.

Billingham RE, Silvers WK (1960). Studies on tolerance of the Y chromosome antigen in mice. J Immunol 85:14.

Bishop MWH (1972). Genetically determined abnormalities of the reproductive system. J Reprod Fert Suppl 15:51.

Blank CE, Zachary RB, Bishop AM, Emery JC, Dewhurst CJ, Bond JH (1964). Chromosome mosaicism in a hermaphrodite. Br Med J 2:90.

Boveri T (1909). Über "geschlechts-chromosomen" bei nematoden. Arch Zellf 1:132.

Breeuwsma AJ (1969). Intersexualiteit bij varkens. T Diergeneesk 94:493.

Breeuwsma AJ (1970). Studies on intersexuality in pigs. Ph.D. thesis, University of Utrecht.

Brøgger A, Aagenaes Ö (1965). The human Y chromosome and the etiology of true hermaphroditism, with the report of a case with XX/XY sex chromosome mosaicism. Hereditas 53:231.

Brown TT, Burek JD, McEntee K (1976). Male pseudohermaphroditism, cryptorchism and Sertoli cell neoplasia in three miniature Schnauzers. J Am Vet Med Ass 169:821.

Bruere AN, Fielden ED, Hutchings H (1968). XX/XY mosaicism in lymphocyte cultures from a pig with freemartin characteristics. New Zealand Vet J 16:31.

Buechi HF (1963). Intersexuality in mammals. In Overzier C (ed): "Intersexuality," New York: Academic Press, p 35.

Buyse M, Fordney-Settlage D, Towner JW, Wilson MG (1975). 46,XX/47,XYY mosaicsm in a true hermaphrodite. Lancet 1:1300.

Castro-Sierra E, Wolf U (1967). Replication patterns of the unpaired chromosome No.9 of the rodent Ellobius lutescens Th. Cytogenetics 6:268.

Cattanach BM (1975). Sex reversal in the mouse and other mammals. In Balls M, Wild A (eds): "The Early Development of Mammals," Cambridge:Cambridge Univ Press, p 305.

Cattanach BM, Pollard CE, Hawkes SG (1971). Sex reversed mice: XX and XO males. Cytogenetics 10:318.

Celada F, Welshons WJ (1963). An immunogenetic analysis of the male antigen in mice utilizing animals with an exceptional chromosome constitution. Genetics 48:139.

Chai CK (1968). The effect of inbreeding in rabbits. Skin transplantation. Transplantation 6:689.

Chai CK (1973). The response of females to male grafts in inbred lines of rabbits. J Hered 64:321.

Corin-Frederic J (1969). Les formules gonosomiques dites aberrantes chez les mammifères euthériens. Example particulier du paresseux Choloepus hoffmanni Peters (Edente, Xenarthre, familles des Bradypodidae). Chromosoma 27:268.

Corner GW (1920). A case of true lateral hermaphroditism in a pig with a functional ovary. Carneg Inst Publ 274:137.

Coulombre JC, Russell ES (1954). Analysis of the pleiotropism at the W-locus in the mouse. The effects of W and W^v substitution upon postnatal development of germ cells. J Exp Zool 126:277.

Court Brown WM, Harnden DG, Jacobs PA, MacLean N, Mantle DJ (1964). Abnormalities of the sex chromosome complement in man. Med Res Counc No 305.

Cox JE (1968). A case of a fertile intersex pig. J Reprod Fert 16:321.

Crew FAE (1923). Studies in intersexuality. I. A peculiar type of developmental intersexuality in the male of domesticated mammals. Proc Roy Soc Lond B 95:90.

Darlington CD (1931). Meiosis. Biol Rev 6:221.

Davies CJ (1913). Caprine freemartins. Vet J 20:62.

de la Chapelle A (1972). Nature and origin of males with XX sex chromosomes. Amer J Human Genet 24:71.

de la Chapelle A (1981). The etiology of maleness in XX men. Hum Genet 58:105.

de la Chapelle A, Hortling H, Niemi M, Wennstrom J (1964). XX sex chromosomes in a human male. First Case. Acta Med Scand Suppl 412:25.

de la Chapelle A, Koo GC, Wachtel SS (1978). Recessive sex-determining genes in human XX male syndrome. Cell 15:837.

Dosik H, Madashur DP, Khan F, Spergel G (1975). The XX male: apparent translocation of Y chromosome material to chromosome 17. Clin Res 23:261A.

Dosik H, Wachtel SS, Khan F, Spergel G, Koo GC (1976). Evidence for the presence of Y-chromosomal genes in a phenotypic male with a 46,XX karyotype. J Amer Med Assoc 236: 2505.

Eaton ON (1945). The relation between polled and hermaphroditic characters in dairy goats. Genetics 30:51.

Eaton ON, Simmons VL (1939). Hermaphroditism in milk-goats. J Hered 30:261.

Eichwald EJ and Silmser CR (1955). Untitled communication. Transplant Bull 2:148.

Eichwald EJ, Silmser CR, Weissman I (1958). Sex-linked rejection of normal and neoplastic tissue. I. Distribution and specificity. J Nat Cancer Inst 20:563.

Eichwald EJ, Silmser CR, Wheeler N (1957). The genetics of skin grafting. Ann NY Acad Sci 64:737.

Engelstein JM (1967). Induced expression of the male iso-antigen in the skin of female mice. Proc Soc Exp Biol Med 126:907.

Epstein CJ, Smith S, Travis B (1980). Expression of H-Y antigen on preimplantation mouse embryos. Tissue Antigens 15:63.

Evans HJ, Buckton KE, Spowart G, Carothers AD (1979). Heteromorphic X chromosomes in 46,XX males: evidence for the involvement of X-Y interchange. Hum Genet 49:11.

Ferguson-Smith MA (1966). X-Y chromosomal interchange in the etiology of true hermaphroditism and of XX Klinefelter's syndrome. Lancet 2:475.

Ferguson-Smith MA (1970). Observations on X-Y homology in man. Bull Eur Soc Hum Genet 4:39.

Ferguson-Smith MA, Johnston AW, Weinberg AN (1960). The chromosome complement in true hermaphroditism. Lancet 2:126.

Fraccaro M, Tiepolo L, Zuffardi O, Chiumello G, DiNatale B, Gargantini L, Wolf U (1979). Familial XX true hermaphroditism and the H-Y antigen. Hum Genet 48:45.

Fredga K (1970). Unusual sex chromosome inheritance in mammals. Phil Trans Roy Soc Lond B 259:15.

Fredga K, Gropp A, Winking H, Frank F (1976). Fertile XX- and XY-type females in the wood lemming Myopus schisticolor. Nature Lond 251:225.

Fredga K, Gropp A, Winking H, Frank F (1977). A hypothesis explaining the exceptional sex ratio in the wood lemming Myopus schisticolor. Hereditas 85:101.

Freudenberg F (1957). Die bedeutung der intersexualität beim schwein als erbliche geschlechtsmissbildung. Mhefte Vet Med Leipsig 12:608.

Furusawa M, Kotani M, Takeuchi H (1963). Male-specific haemagglutination in mice. Nature 200:182.

Gehring U, Tomkins GM (1974). Characterization of a hormone receptor defect in the androgen insensitivity mutant. Cell 3:59.

Gerneke WH (1967). Cytogenetic investigations on normal and malformed animals with special reference to intersexes. Onderstepoort J Vet Res 34:219.

Ghosh SN, Shah PN, Gharpure HM, Athreya U (1978). H-Y antigen in human intersexuality. Clinical Genetics 14:31.

Gileva EA, Chebotar NA (1779). Fertile XO males and females in the varying lemming, Dicrostonyx torquatus pall (1979). A unique genetic system of sex determination. Heredity 42:67.

Griboff SI, Lawrence R (1961). The chromosomal etiology of congenital gonadal defects. Amer J Med 30:544

Grumbach MM, Ducharme JR (1960). The effects of androgens on fetal sexual development. Fertil Steril 11:157.

Hamerton JL, Dickson JM, Pollard CE, Grieves SA, Short RV (1969). Genetic intersexuality in goats. J Reprod Fertil Suppl 7:25

Hammond J (1912). A case of hermaphroditism in the pig. J Anat Physiol 7:307.

Hare WCD (1976). Intersexuality in the dog. Can Vet J 17:7.

Hare WCD, McFeely RA, Kelly DF (1974). Familial 78XX male pseudohermaphroditism in three dogs. J Reprod Fert 36:207.

Harnden DG, Armstrong CN (1959). Chromosomes of a true her-maphrodite. Brit Med J 2:1287.

Hauschka TS (1955). Probable Y-linkage of a histocompatibili-ty gene. Transplant Bull 2:154.

Hecht F, Antonius JI, McGuire P, Hale CG (1966). XXY cells in predominantly XX human male: evidence for cell se-lection. Pediatrics 38:982.

Herbst EW, Fredga K, Frank F, Winking H, Gropp A (1978). Cytological identification of two X-chromosome types in the wood lemming (Myopus schisticolor). Chromosoma 69:185.

Heslop BF (1968). Histocompatibility antigens in the rat: the AS2 strain in relation to the AS, BS and HS strains. Austr J Exp Biol Med Sci 46:479.

Heslop BF (1973). The male antigen in the rat. Transplanta-tion 15:31.

Hirota Y, Suzuki T, Chazono Y, Bito Y (1976). Humoral immune responses characteristic of testosterone proprionate-treated chickens. Immunology 30:341.

Hulland TJ (1964). Pregnancy in a hermaphrodite sow. Can Vet J 5:39.

Hungerford DA. Donnelly AJ, Nowell PC, Beck S (1959). The chromosome constitution of a human phenotype, intersex. Amer J Hum Genet 11:215.

Jacobs PA, Melville M, Ratcliffe S, Keay AJ, Syme J (1974). A cytogenetic survey of 11,680 newborn infants. Ann Hum Genet 37:359.

Jirásek JE (1971). "Development of the Genital System and Male Pseudohermaphroditism." Baltimore:The Johns Hopkins Press.

Johnston EF, Zeller JH, Cantwell G (1958). Sex anomalies in swine. J Hered 49:254.

Jost A (1947). Recherches sur la differenciation sexuelle de l'embryon de lapin. Archs Anat Microsc Morph Exp 36:271.

Jost A (1953). Problems of fetal endocrinology. The gonadal and hypophyseal hormones. Recent Prog Horm Res 8:379.

Jost A (1970). Hormonal factors in the sex differentiation of the mammalian foetus. Phil Trans Roy Soc Lond B 259:119.

Kalela O, Oksala T (1966). Sex ratio in the wood lemming, Myopus schisticolor (Lilljeb.) in nature and in captivity. Ann Univ Turkuensis Ser A 2:1.

Kasdan R, Nankin HR, Troen P, Wald N, Pan S, Yanaihara T (1973). Paternal transmission of maleness in XX human beings. New Engl J Med 288:539.

Koller PC, Darlington CD (1934). The genetical and mechanical properties of the sex chromosomes. I. Rattus norvegicus. J Genet 24:159.

Kondo K (1952). Studies in intersexuality in milk goats. Jap j Genet 27:131.

Koo GC, Mittl LR, Goldberg CL (1979). Expression of H-Y antigen during spermatogenesis. Immunogenetics 9:293.

Koo GC, Wachtel SS, Krupen-Brown K, Mittl LR, Breg WR, Genel M, Rosenthal IM, Borgaonkar DS, Miller DA, Tantravahi R, Schreck RR, Erlanger BF, Miller OJ (1977a). Mapping the locus of the H-Y gene on the human Y chromosome. Science 198:940.

Koo GC, Wachtel SS, Saenger P, New MI, Dosik H, Amarose AP, Dorus E, Ventruto V (1977b). H-Y antigen: expression in human subjects with the testicular feminization syndrome. Science 196:655.

Krco CJ, Goldberg EH (1976). H-Y (male) antigen: detection on eight-cell mouse embryos. Science 193:1134.

Laor M, Barnea R, Angel H, Soller M (1962). Polledness and hermaphroditism in Saanen goats. Israel J Agric Res 12:83.

Lindsten J, Bergstrand CG, Tillinger K-G, Schwarzacher H-G, Tiepolo L, Muldal S, Hokfelt B (1966). A clinical and cytogenetical study of three patients with male phenotype and apparent XX sex chromosome constitution. Acta Endocr 52:91.

Lyon MF (1974). Mechanisms and evolutionary origins of variable X-chromosome activity in mammals. Proc Roy Soc Lond B 187:243.

Lyon MF, Hawkes SG (1970). X-linked gene for testicular feminization in the mouse. Nature Lond 227:1217.

McClung CE (1902). The accessory chromosome-sex determinant? Biol Bull 3:43.

McFee AF, Knight M, Bauner MW (1966). An intersex pig with XX/XY leukocyte mosaicism. Canad J Genet Cytol 8:502.

McLaren A (1980). Oocytes in the testis. Nature 283:688.

Madan K (1976). Chromosome measurements on an XXp$^+$ male. Hum Genet 32:141.

Madan K, Walker S (1974). Possible evidence for Xp$^+$ in an XX male. Lancet 1:1223.

Matthey R (1954). Un nouveau type de chromosomes sexuels chez un mammifère (Ellobius lutescens Thomas-Rodentia-Microtinae. Experientia 10:18.

Mayou BJ, Armon P, Lindenbaum RH (1978). Pregnancy and childbirth in a true hermaphrodite following reconstructive surgery. Br J Obstet Gynecol 85:314.

Medawar P (1944). The behaviour and fate of skin autografts and skin homografts in rabbits. J Anat 78:176.

Merchant H (1975). Rat gonadal and ovarian organogenesis with and without germ cells. An ultrastructural study. Dev Biol 44:1

Minowada S, Kobayashi K, Isurugi K, Fukutani K, Ikeuchi H, Hasegawa T, Yamada K (1979). Two XX male brothers. Clin Genetics 15:399.

Miró R, Caballín MR, Marsini S, Egozcue J (1978). Mosaicism in XX males. Hum Genet 45:103.

Mittwoch U, Buehr ML (1973). Gonadal growth in embryos of sex reversed mice. Differentiation 1:219.

Moreira-Filho CA, Otto PG, Mustacchi Z, Frota-Pessoa O, Otto PA (1980). H-Y antigen expression in a case of XX true hermaphroditism. Hum Genet 55:309.

Mori Y, Mitzutani S (1968). Familial true hermaphroditism in genetic females. Japan J Urol 59:857

Mullen Y, Hildemann WH (1972). X- and Y-linked transplantation antigens in rats. Transplantation 13:521.

Nagai Y, Ohno S (1977). Testis-determining H-Y antigen in XO males of the mole-vole (Ellobius lutescens). Cell 10:729.

Narita O, Manba S, Nakanishi T, Ishizuka N (1975). Pregnancy and childbirth in a true hermaphrodite. Obstet Gynecol 45:593.

Nes HM, Andersen, K, Slagsvold P (1963). Kromosomunders kelse hos hermafroditte geiter. Saetr Med Iemsld Norski Vet Forb 7:155.

Nicolis GL, Hsu LY, Sabetghadam R, Kardon NB, Chernay NB, Mathur DP, Rose HG, Hirschhorn K, Gabrilove JL (1972). Klinefelter's syndrome in identical twins with the 46,XX chromosome constitution. Am J Med 52:482.

Pelliniemi LJ, Niemi M (1969). Fine structure of human fetal testes. I. The interstitial tissue. Z Zellforsch 99:507.

Petersen WW (1952). So-hermafrodit, der har faret fire gange. Dansk Maanedsskr Dyrlaeg 62:343.

Poláčková M (1969). Attempt at inducing male-specific antigen in female species. Folia Biol (Praha) 15:181.

Poláčková M, Vojtíšková M (1968). Inhibitory effect of early orchidectomy on the expression of the male antigen in mice. Folia Biol (Praha) 14:93.

Raynaud A, Frilley M (1947). Destruction des glandes géni-
tales, de l'embryon de souris, par une irradiation au
moyen des rayons X, à l'âge de treize jours. Annls Endocr
8:400.

Ricordeau G, Lauvergne J-J (1967). Hypothèse génétique
unique pour expliquer la presénce d'intersexués, de mâles
en excès et de mâles stériles en race caprine Saanen.
Annls Zootech 16:323.

Rosenberg HS, Clayton GW, Hsu TC (1963). Familial true
hermaphroditism. J Clin Endocr 23:203.

Sachs L, Heller E (1958). The sex-linked histocompatibility
antigens. J Natl CancerInst 20:555.

Saenger P, Levine LS, Wachtel SS, Korth-Schutz S, Doberne Y,
Koo GC, Lavengood RW, German JL, New MI (1976). Presence
of H-Y antigen and testis in 46,XX true hermaphroditism,
evidence for Y-chromosomal function. J Clin Endo Metab
43:1234.

Salkin MS (1978). Pyometra in a male pseudohermaphrodite dog.
J Amer Vet Med Ass 172:913.

Selden JR, Wachtel SS, Koo GC, Haskins ME, Patterson DF
(1978). Genetic basis of XX male syndrome and XX true
hermaphroditism: evidence in the dog. Science 201:644.

Shalev A (1980). Immunogenetic studies on H-Y antigen. Ph.D.
thesis, University of Manitoba.

Shalev A, Berczi I, Hamerton JL (1978). Detection and cross-
reaction of H-Y antigen by haemagglutination. J Immuno-
genet 5:303.

Sharp AJ, Wachtel SS, Benirschke K (1980). H-Y antigen in a
fertile XY female horse. J Reprod Fert 58:157.

Siiteri PK, Wilson JD (1974). Testosterone formation and
metabolism during male sexual differentiation in the human
embryo. J Clin Endocrinol Metab 38:113.

Silvers WK, Murphy G, Poole TW (1977). Studies on the H-Y
antigen in rats. Immunogenetics 4:85.

Silvers WK, Yang S-L (1973). Male specific antigen: homology
in mice and rats. Science 181:570.

Simpson JL (1976). "Disorders of Sexual Differentiation."
New York:Academic Press.

Sittman K (1973). Segregation of hermaphrodites in swine
litters. Can J Genet Cytol 15:229.

Snell GD (1956). A comment on Eichwald and Silmser's communication. Transpl Bull 3:29.

Soller M, Angel H (1964). Polledness and abnormal sex ratios
in Saanen goats. J Hered 55:139.

Soller M, Kempenich O (1964). Polledness and litter size in
Saanen goats. J Hered 55:301.

Somlev B, Hansen-Melander E, Melander Y, Holm L (1970). XX/XY chimerism in leucocytes of two intersex pigs. Hereditas 64:203.

Spoljar M, Drews U (1978). Identical action of Y chromosome and Sxr factor in early testicular development in the mouse. Anat Embryol 155:115

Stanley AJ, Gumbreck LG (1964). Male pseudohermaphroditism with feminizing testis in the male rat - a sex-linked recessive character. Program Endocr Soc p 40.

Therkelsen AJ (1964). Sterile male with the chromosome constitution 46XX. Cytogenetics 3:207.

Tran D, Meusy-Dessolli N, Josso N (1977). Anti-Mullerian hormone is a functional marker of foetal Sertoli cells. Nature Lond 269:411.

Tremblay RR, Foley TP, Corvol P, Park I-J, Kowarski A, Blizzard RM, Jones HW, Migeon CJ (1972). Plasma concentration of testosterone, dihydrotestosterone, testosterone-oestradiol binding globulin, and pituitary gonadotrophins in the syndrome of male pseudo-hermaphroditism with testicular feminization. Acta Endocrinol 70:331.

Tres LL (1977). Extensive pairing of the XY bivalent in mouse spermatocytes as visualized by whole-mount electron microscopy. J Cell Sci 25:1.

Tres LL (1978). Translocation of the Y-paracentromeric region to an autosomal bivalent in Sxr, XY mouse spermatocytes. J Cell Biol 79:125a.

Tres LL (1979). Side-by-side pairing of the XY bivalent in spermatocytes and the ubiquity of the H-Y locus. Archiv Andrology 2:101.

van Niekerk WA (1974). "True Hermaphroditism." New York: Harper and Row.

van Wagenen G, Simpson ME (1965). "Embryology of the Ovary and Testis. Homo sapiens and Macaca Mulatta." New Haven: Yale University Press.

Vogt DW (1968). Sex chromosome mosaicism in a swine intersex. J Hered 59:166.

Vojtíšková M, Poláčková M (1966). An experimental model of the epigenetic mechanism of autotolerance using the H-Y antigen in mice. Folia Biol Praha 12:137.

Vojtíšková M, Poláčková M (1972). Testosterone-abolished female responsiveness to syngeneic male-skin grafts. Folia Biol Praha 18:209.

Wachtel SS, Basrur P, Koo GC (1978). Recessive male-determining genes. Cell 15:279.

Wachtel SS, Koo GC, Boyse EA (1975a). Evolutionary conservation of H-Y ('male') antigen. Nature 254:270.

Wachtel SS, Koo GC, Breg WR, Thaler HT, Dillard GM, Rosenthal IM, Dosik H, Gerald PS, Saenger P, New M, Lieber E, Miller OJ (1976a). Serologic detection of a Y-linked gene in XX males and XX true hermaphrodites. New Engl J Med 295:750.

Wachtel SS, Koo GC, Ohno S, Gropp A, Dev VG, Tantravahi R, Miller DA, Miller OJ (1976b). H-Y antigen and the origin of XY female wood lemmings (Myopus schisticolor). Nature 264:638.

Wachtel SS, Koo GC, Zuckerman EE, Hämmerling U, Scheid MP, Boyse A (1974). Serological cross-reactivity between H-Y (male) antigens of mouse and man. Proc Nat Acad Sci USA 71:1215.

Wachtel SS, Ohno S (1979). The immunogenetics of sexual development. In Steinberg AG, Bearn AG, Motulsky AG, Childs B (eds): "Progress in Medical Genetics," Philadelphia: WB Saunders Co, p 109.

Wachtel SS, Ohno S, Koo GC, Boyse EA (1975b). Possible role for H-Y antigen in the primary determination of sex. Nature 257:235.

Waxman SH, Gartler SM, Kelley VC (1962). Apparent masculinization of the female fetus diagnosed as true hermaphroditism by chromosomal studies. J Pediat 60:540.

Weissman I (1973). Failure to demonstrate postnatal testicular dependent expression of the male-specific transplantation antigen in mice. Transplantation 16:122.

White MJD (1957). An interpretation of the unique sex chromosome mechanism of the rodent Ellobius lutescens. Proc Zool Foc Calcutta Mookerjee Mem Vol p 113.

Widmaier R (1957). Untersuchungen an intersexuellen ziegenlammern im hinblick auf die unfruchtbarkeit der bucke. Wiss Z Martin-Luther-Univ Halle-Wittenb 6:67.

Williamson JH (1979). Intersexuality in a family of kerry blue terriers. J Heredity 70:138.

Wilson JD, Lasnitzki I (1971). Dihydrotestosterone formation in fetal tissues of the rabbit and rat. Endocrinology 89:659.

Winters SJ, Wachtel SS, White BJ, Koo GC, Javadpour N, Loriaux DL, Sherins RJ (1979). H-Y antigen mosaicism in the gonad of a 46,XX true hermaphrodite. New Engl J Med 300:745.

Witschi E (1948). Micration of the germ cells of human embryos from the yolk sac to the primitive gonadal folds. Contrib Embryol Carnegie Inst 32:67.

Zenzes MT, Müller U, Aschmoneit I, Wolf U (1978). Studies on H-Y antigen in different cell fractions of the testis during pubesence. Hum Genet 45:297.

SECTION VII.
OTHER ANIMAL MODELS SYSTEMS AND CONSIDERATIONS

Animal Models of Inherited Metabolic Diseases, pages 421–433
© 1982 Alan R. Liss, Inc., 150 Fifth Avenue, New York, NY 10011

ANIMAL MODELS OF HUMAN ERYTHROCYTE METABOLISM

Joseph E. Smith DVM, PhD

Department of Pathology,
Kansas State University
Manhattan, Kansas   66506

Erythrocytes are unique among mammalian cells.   They lack the subcellular organelles found in most cells such as nucleus, mitochrondria, endoplasmic reticulum, and Golgi apparatus. Consequently, their metabolism is limited and any abnormality may have serious effects on function and viability.

Availability of blood has made erythrocyte disorders the most intensively studied inherited diseases. The disorders provide valuable information on gene structure, protein synthetic mechanisms, and relationship of protein structure to function.

Although the number of erythrocyte disorders found in man is higher than in other mammals for a variety of reasons, erythrocyte disorders in animals provide valuable information about erythrocyte pathophysiology. The disorders may be classified into three general categories: enzymopathies and enzyme polymorphisms, membrane defects, and hemoglobinopathies.

ENZYMOPATHIES AND ENZYME POLYMORPHISMS

Enzymopathies and enzyme polymorphorisms can be subdivided into several functional units: glycolytic pathway, hexose monophosphate pathway, glutathione detoxification system, methemoglobin reduction system, porphyrias, nucleotide metabolism, and miscellaneous enzymes.

Glycolytic enzymes

Pyruvate kinase deficiency was the first enzymopathy found to cause chronic hemolytic anemia (Tanaka et al. 1962). Subsequently, other glycolytic enzymes - glucose phosphate isomerase, hexokinase, phosphofructokinase, aldolase, triose phosphate isomerase, phosphoglycerate kinase, and diphosphoglycerate mutase - have been found to be deficient in patients with chronic hemolytic disease. In contrast, deficiencies of glyceraldehyde phosphate dehydrogenase, enolase, and lactate dehydrogenase do not appear to cause any abnormalities (Beutler 1979).

Pyruvate kinase deficiency occurs in Basenji and Beagle dogs (Searcy et al. 1979). In Basenjis the fetal pyruvate kinase persists, causing a severe hemolytic anemia (Black et al. 1978). That disorder, including the myelofibrosis resulting from the aberrant iron metabolism, can be corrected by bone-marrow transplantation (Weiden et al. 1981).

Other glycolytic enzyme deficiencies have not been found in the erythrocytes of nonhuman species. Electrophoretic variation occurs with phosphohexose isomerase in dogs (Tanaba et al. 1977), horses (Sandberg 1973), pigs (Saison & O'Reilly 1971), cats (O'Brien 1980), chinchilla (Carter et al. 1972), Lestho gerbils (Op't Hof et al. 1974), and Australian hopping mice (Baverstock et al. 1977); phosphofructokinase in cats (O'Brien 1980); and phosphoglycerate kinase in kangeroos (Cooper et al. 1971).

Hexose monophosphate pathways

Glucose-6-phosphate dehydrogenase (G6PD) is one of the most polymorphic of all human enzymes. Clinically, symptoms in man range from chronic hemolytic disease to an unusual sensitivity to "oxidant" drugs. G6PD deficiency was reported in a colony of rats and one dog, but unfortunately the rats died from respiratory disease (Werth & Muller 1967) and close relatives of the dog could not be found or produced (Smith et al. 1976). Though normally their G6PD activity, when expressed as per gram of hemoglobin, is about 14 percent of that of human erythrocytes, ovine and caprine erythrocytes do not lyse when exposed to "oxidant" drugs. Apparently G6PD in ovine and caprine erythrocytes operates at a higher percentage of its potential than does human G6PD (Smith 1981).

Electrophoretic variants for G6PD occur in pigs (Verhorst 1972), chimpanzees (Beutler & West 1978), pikas (Vergnes et al. 1974), and hybrid-hares. G6PD in hybrid hares has been used as a monotypic marker in atherosclerotic studies (Lee et al. 1981).

6-Phosphogluconate dehydrogenase deficiency might be expected to cause chronic hemolytic disease or drug sensitivity, but currently it is believed to be a nondisease condition. Although 6PGD deficiency has not been detected in nonhuman populations, electrophoretic polymorphisms occur in pigs (Saison & Giblett 1969), horses (Bender et al. 1970), cats (O'Brien 1980), rats (Carter & Parr 1969), wild rabbits (Coggan et al. 1974), and marsupial mice (Cooper & Hope 1971).

Glutathione detoxification system

Erythrocyte glutathione is decreased by deficiency of the two synthetic enzymes, γ - glutamylcysteine synthetase and glutathione synthetase, and the cysteine transport system. In man, enzyme deficiency causes chronic hemolytic disease and drug sensitivity, but in sheep it does not result in anemia or drug sensitivity (Smith 1976; Young et al. 1975).

Two other enzymes in the glutathione detoxification system, glutathione reductase and glutathione peroxidase, have been reported to cause chronic hemolytic disease, but the cause-and-effect relationship has not stood the test of time. Both enzymes can become deficient as a result of poor nutrition, but that will not result in hematologic difficulties. Glutathione reductase decreases due to suboptimal riboflavin intake, and glutathione peroxidase reflects selenium nutrition particularly in sheep and cattle. Lowered glutathione peroxidase does occur, but as a nondisease, in the Jewish population (Beutler 1979).

Methemoglobin reduction

Methemoglobinemia occurs sporadically in dogs as a

result of NADH-methemoglobin reductase deficiency (Harvey et al. 1974; Letchworth et al. 1977). Sheep (Tucker & Clarke 1980) and horses (Sandberg 1974) are polymorphic, by electrophoresis for the same enzyme, but do not suffer any adverse consequences.

Porphyrias

Congenital porphyria in cattle causes a chronic hemolytic anemia, erythrodonia, bone discoloration, and photosensitivity. The presumed defect, a deficiency of uroporphyrinogen III cosynthetase, is similar to the disease in man (Levin 1968). Similarly, a deficiency of the enzyme in all members of Sciurus niger (fox squirrels) causes erythrodonia and bone discoloration, but they do not suffer from anemia and photosensitivity (Levin & Flyger 1973).

Bovine protoporphyria results from heme synthetase deficiency in both erythroid and nonerythroid tissues. Both signs (photosensitivity without anemia) and mode of inheritance (autosomal recessive) are similar to that in man (Ruth et al. 1977).

Other porphyric diseases occur in cats (Livingston 1971) and pigs (With 1979) as an autosomal dominant disorder characterized by bone and teeth discoloration without anemia or photosensitivity. The pathogenesis of those disorders remains unknown.

Nucleotide metabolism

In man adenylate kinase deficiency, hyperactivity of adenosine deaminase, and pyrimidine nucleotidase deficiency induce inherited hemolytic anemia of variable severities. Acquired deficiency of pyrimidine nucleotidase may result from lead toxicity. When pyrimidine nucleotidase activity is inadequate, reticulocyte RNA remains uncatabolized and basophilic stippling results (Paglia & Valentine 1981). The propensity of bovine erythrocytes to develop basophilic stippling may be related to the extremely low pyrimidine nucleotidase activity (10 mU/g hemoglobin) compared with that of human erythrocytes (152 mU/g hemoglobin). (George 1980). Activity of adenosine deaminase is also lower in cattle than in human erythrocytes (Larsen et al. 1978).

Four phenotypic patterns of adenosine deaminase occur in porcine erythrocytes. These phenotypes are determined by two codominant alleles ADA^A and ADA^B and a recessive silent allele ADA^O at an autosomal locus (Widar et al. 1974). Baboons and vervet monkeys are also polymorphic (McDermid et al. 1975).

A polymorphism of purine nucleoside phosphorlyase occurs in ovine and bovine erythrocytes (Ansay 1975; Board & Smith 1977). One isozyme has high activity, another has activity close to zero, and still another in cattle (and possibly sheep) has extremely high activity.

Nucleoside transport in ovine erythrocytes is controlled by two genes: one that codes for a functional absence of a high-affinity system, and one that codes for presence of the transport system but is recessive to the other gene; the locus may be a regulator gene (Jarvis & Young 1978).

Miscellaneous enzymes

Some enzymes are not connected with any particular pathway yet are polymorphic or show unusual activity. None are associated with pathological changes.

Arginase deficiency in certain ovine erythrocytes is inherited as an autosomal recessive trait. Arginase-negative sheep have normal liver arginase activity with normal plasma amino acid and urea (Wright et al. 1977).

Sheep and goats are polymorphic with respect to erythrocyte potassium. Low-potassium sheep have the Lp blood-group antigen and high-potassium sheep have the allelic M antigen. The association of potassium types in goats is not so clear (Tucker & Clarke 1980).

Feline and canine erythrocytes lack a Na+-K+ adenosine triphosphatase and a Na+-K+ exchange pump. Consequently, their erythrocyte sodium approximates that of plasma. Cellular hydration is regulated by a calcium-dependent, sodium-extrusion system (Parker 1977).

Several enzymes in this category are polymorphic when examined by electrophoretic techniques. They provide markers for bone-marrow transplantation, genetic studies, and paternity testing.

In dogs soluble aspartic aminotransferase, indophenol oxidase, acid phosphatase, superoxide dismutase, phosphoglucomutase, and esterase D (Weiden et al. 1974, Weiden et al. 1981) are polymorphic; in cats - esterase 1 and glucose dehydrogenase 2 (O'Brien 1980); in sheep - malic enzyme and carbonic anhydrase (Tucker & Clarke 1980); in horses - malic enzyme (Guttormsen & Weitkamp 1981), catalase (Kelly et al. 1971), phosphoglucomutase (Bengtsson & Sandberg 1972), acid phosphatase (Podliachouk et al. 1972), and carbonic anhydrase (Sanberg 1970); in pigs - esterase D (Tanaka et al. 1980), catalase (Baranov 1970), and phosphoglucomutase (Ansay et al. 1971); in chinchilla (Chinchilla laniger) - carbonic anhydrase (Carter 1974); in cattle - phosphoglucomutase, (Ansay et al. 1971), carbonic anhydrase (Satore et al. 1969), acid phosphatase (Dogrul 1970), and aspartate aminotransferase (Ansay & Hanset 1972); in goats - carbonic anhydrase (Tucker & Clarke 1980); and in mice - phosphoglucomutase (Rice & O'Brien 1980), and alanine aminotransferase (Chen et al. 1973).

Acid phosphatase is polymorphic in foxes (Balbierz & Nitotajczuk 1972), southern elephant seal (Ananthakrishnan & McDermid 1971), and buffalo (Makaveev 1972); phosphoglucomutase - in inbred rabbits (McDermid et al. 1975), wild rabbits (Coggan et al. 1974), and wild rats (Koga et al. 1972); and carbonic anhydrase - in bison (Satore et al. 1969), water buffalo (Makaveev 1972), and rabbits (Bernoco 1969).

MEMBRANE DEFECTS

As an outer cover of a cell that traverses miles of vessels, the erythrocyte membrane possesses unique characteristics. It allows the erythrocytes to deform sufficiently to pass through the microcirculation and reduce bulk viscosity of blood in large vessels. Any membrane abnormality will cause premature removal of erythrocytes and may influence the release of immature erythrocytes into circulation (Chien 1975).

Membranes exist as structures and thus the components must be understood relative to surrounding components. That makes their study difficult. Membrane abnormalities usually change the erythrocyte from a biconcave disc to such abberant shapes as spherocytes, stomatocytes, elliptocytes, and acanthocytes. The biochemical basis for the changes is being determined slowly.

Spectrin (a major protein in erythrocyte membranes) is important in maintaining membrane integrity. Four mutants of Mus musculus (common house mouse) have recessively inherited deficiency of spectrin. All manifest hemolytic anemia, spherocytosis, erythrocyte budding, and unstable membranes. The clinical severity correlates closely with the degree of spectrin deficiency (Lux et al. 1979; Bernstein 1980).

Hereditary spherocytosis also occurs in some deer mice (Peromyscus maniculatus). These mice are mildly anemic and have reticulocytosis, splenomegaly and increased osmotic fragility. Unfortunately, the metabolic defect has not been determined (Huestis et al. 1956).

Hereditary stomatocytosis with chondrodysplasia occurs in Alaskan Malamute dogs as an autosomal recessive pleomorphic trait. Affected erythrocytes have a shortened life span, lower reduced glutathione, and increased sodium and water. The biochemical lesion responsible for both skeletal and erythrocyte defects has not been found (Pinkerton et al. 1974).

Membrane instability in man has been attributed to an inherited deficiency of band 4.1 (Tchernia et al. 1981), defective self-association of spectrin dimers into tetramers (Liv et al. 1981), and abnormal spectrin structure (Coetzer & Zail 1981).

HEMOGLOBINOPATHIES

Hemoglobin is probably the most studied protein and hemoglobinopathy, the most studied inherited disease. In man more than 250 different abnormal hemoglobins have been discovered and characterized. With one exception abnormal hemoglobins have not been located in nonhuman species. Radiation-induced mutants in mice have deleted a portion

∝-gene complex that results in a thalassemia-like syndrome (Martinell et al. 1981).

Several species have more than one normal hemoglobin type, some (sheep and goats) change the hemoglobin type under hypoxic conditions by derepressing inactive genes. A few species switch from a fetal hemoglobin to an adult type postnatally.

CONCLUDING REMARKS

Despite intense investigations on the erythrocyte's form and function, its enzymatic components and pathways, and its formation and demise, chronic hemolytic disease remains undiagnosed in three-quarters of the patients with with the disease even after the most exacting examination possible (Beutler 1979). Obviously, there is more to learn about this simplest of all cells. The study of nonhuman erythrocytes that are normally "deficient" when compared with human red cells and those that are genetically abnormal should provide some help toward successfully diagnosing human hemolytic anemias (Smith 1981).

ACKNOWLEDGMENTS

Supported in part by USPHS Grant HL-12972 and the Kansas Agricultural Experiment Station. I thank Dr. S. M. Dennis for his comments about the manuscript.

REFERENCES

Anantharishnan R, McDermid EM (1971). Two possible genetic variants of red cell acid phosphatase in seals. Anim Blood Grps Biochem Genet 2:113.
Ansay M (1975). Note on a third allele in the erythrocytic NP system of cattle. Anim Blood Grps Biochem Genet 6:121.
Ansay M, Hanset R (1972). Soluble glutamic oxalacetic transaminase (GOT) polymorphism in cattle. Anim Blood Grps Biochem Genet. 3:163.
Ansay M, Hanset R, Esser-Coulon J (1971). Phosphoglucomutase polymorphism in cattle. Annls Genet Sci Anim 3:413.

Balbierz, Nikotajczuk M (1972). Further immunogenetic investigation of breeding foxes. Proc 12th Eur Conf Anim Blood Grps Biochem Polymorphism (Budapest):673.

Baranov OK (1970). An immunological study of protein polymorphism in haemolysates of pigs and cattle. Biochem Genet 4:549.

Baverstock PR, Watts CHS, Cole SR (1977). Inheritance studies of glucose phosphate isomerase, transferrin and esterases in the Australian hopping mice Notomys alexis, N. cervinus, N. mitchellii and N. fuscus (Rodentia: Muridae). Anim Blood Grps Biochem Genet 8:3.

Bender K, Op't Hof J, Engel W (1970). Zur Genetik der 6-Phosphogluconate-Dehydrogenase (ec 1.1.1.44) bei Saugern Humangenetik 11:59.

Bengtsson S, Sandberg K (1972). Phosphoglucomutase polymorphism in Swedish horses. Anim Blood Grps Biochem Genet 3:115.

Bernoco D (1969). Electrophoretic variants of carbonic anhydrases in rabbit red cells. Att. Ass Genet Hzl 15:226.

Bernstein SE (1980). Inherited hemolytic disease in mice: A review and update. Lab Anim Sci 30:197.

Beutler E (1979). Red cell enzyme defects as nondiseases and as diseases. Blood 54:1.

Beutler E, West C (1978). Glucose-6-phosphate dehydrogenase variants in the chimpanzee. Biochem Med 20:364.

Black JA, Rittenberg MB, Standerfer RJ, Peterson JS (1978). Hereditary persistence of fetal erythrocyte pyruvate kinase in the Basenji dog. Prog Clin Biol Res 21:275.

Board PG, Smith JE (1977). Purine nucleoside phosphorylase polymorphism in sheep erythrocytes. Biochem Genet 15:439.

Carter ND (1974). Deficiency of a carbonic anhydrase (CAI) isoenzyme in the chinchilla. Anim Blood Grps Biochem Genet 5:53.

Carter ND, Hill MR, Weir BJ (1972). Genetic variation of phosphoglucose isomerase in some hystricomorph rodents. Biochem Genet 6:147.

Carter ND, Parr CW (1969). Phosphogluconate dehydrogenase polymorphism in British wild rats. Nature 224:1214.

Chen S-H, Donahue RP, Scott CR (1973). The genetics of glutamic-pyruvic transaminase in mice: inheritance electrophoretic phenotypes and post natal changes. Biochem Genet 10:23.

Chien S (1975). In Bishop C, Surgenor DM (eds): "The Blood Cell," 2nd ed, New York: Academic Press, p 1031.

Coetzer T, Zail SS (1981). Tryptic digestion of spectrin in variants of hereditary elliptocytosis. J Clin Invest 67:1241.

Coggan M, Baldwin J, Richardson BJ (1974). Ecological genetics of the wild rabbit in Australia. 1. Geographical distribution and biochemical characterization of 6-phosphogluconate dehydrogenase variants. Aust J Biol Sci 27:671.

Cooper DW, Hope RM (1971). 6-phosphogluconate dehydrogenase polymorphism in the marsupial mouse, Sminthopsis crassicaudata. Biochem Genet 5:65.

Cooper DW, Van der Berg JL, Sharman GB, Poole WE (1971). Phosphoglycerate kinase polymorphism in kangaroos. Nature New Biol 230:115.

Dogrul F (1970). Investigations on erythrocyte acid phosphatase in cattle. Proc 11th Eur Conf Anim Blood Grps Biochem Polymorphism (Warsaw):223.

George JW (1980). Pyrimidine specific 5' nucleotidase activity in bovine erythrocytes: Effect of phlebotomy and experimental lead poisoning. Vet Clin Path 9:43.

Guttormsen SA, Weitkamp LR (1981). Equine marker genes: Polymorphism for soluble erythrocyte malic enzyme. Anim Blood Grps Biochem Genet 12:53.

Harvey JW, Ling GV, Kaneko JJ (1974). Methemoglobin reductase deficiency in a dog. J Am Vet Med Ass 164:1030.

Huestis RR, Anderson RS, Motulsky AG (1956). Hereditary spherocytosis in peromyscus. J Hered 47:225.

Jarvis SM, Young JD (1978). Genetic control of nucleoside transport in sheep erythrocytes. Biochem Genet 16:1035.

Kelly EP, Stormont C, Suzuki Y (1971). Catalase polymorphism in the red cells of horses. Anim Blood Grps Biochem Genet 2:135.

Koga A, Harada S, Omoto K (1972). Polymorphisms of erythrocyte 6-phosphogluconate dehydrogenase and phosphoglucomutase in Rattus norvegicus in Japan. Jap J Genet 46:335.

Larsen B, Hyldgaard-Jensen J, Aagaard L (1978). Studies on adenosine deaminase (ADA) polymorphism in Danish cattle. Anim Blood Grps Biochem Genet 9:191.

Lee KT, Thomas WA, Janakidevi K, Kroms M, Reiner JM, Borg KY (1981). Mocaicism in female hybrid hares heterozygous for glucose-6-phosphate dehydrogenase (G-6-PD) 1. General properties of the hare model with special reference to atherogenesis. Eyptl Mol Path 34:191.

Letchworth GJ, Bentinck-Smith J, Bolton GR, Wootton JF, Family L (1977). Cyanosis and methemoglobinia in two dogs due to a NADH methemoglobin reductase deficiency. J Am Anim Hosp Ass 13:75.

Levin EY (1968). Uroporphyrinogen III cosynthetase in bovine erythropoietic porphyria. Science 161:907.

Levin EY, Flyger V (1973). Erythropoietic porphyria of the fox squirrel Scuirus niger. J Clin Invest 52:96.

Liv S-C, Palek J, Prchal J, Castleberry RP (1981). Altered spectrin dimer-dimer association and instability of erythrocyte membrane skeletons in hereditary pyropoikilocytosis. J Clin Invest 68:597.

Livingston JN (1971). "Characterization of Feline Porphyria: Biochemical Features and Selected Enzyme Assays. PhD Thesis, Oklahoma State University.

Lux SE, Pease B, Tomaselli MB, John KM, Bernstein SE (1979). Hemolytic anemias associated with deficient or dysfunctional spectrin. In Lux SE, Marchesi VT, Fox CF (eds): "Normal and Abnormal Red Cell Membranes," New York: AR Liss, p 463.

Makaveev T (1972). Study on the genetic polymorphism of some blood serum enzymes in water buffalo (Bos bubalus). Anim Blood Grps Biochem Genet 3 (Suppl 1):38.

Martinell J, Whitney III JB, Popp RA, Russell LB, Anderson WF (1981). Three mouse models of human thalassemia Proc Natl Acad Sci 78:5056.

McDermid EM, Agar NS, Chai CK (1975). Electrophoretic variation of red cell enzyme systems in farm animals. Anim Blood Grps Biochem Genet 6:127.

O'Brien SJ (1980). The extent and character of biochemical genetic variation in the domestic cat. J Hered 71:2.

Op't Hof J, Maurer F, Osterhoff DR (1974). Biochemical gene markers in the gerbil Tatera brantsi. 14th Int Conf Anim Blood Grps Biochem Polymorphism

Paglia DE, Valentine WN (1981). Haemolytic anaemia associated with disorders of the purine and pyrimidine salvage pathways. Clin Haemat 10:81.

Parker JC (1977). Solute and water transport in dog and cat red blood cells. In Ellory JC, Lew VL (eds): "Membrane Transport in Red Cells," London: Academic Press, p 427.

Pinkerton PH, Fletch SM, Brueckner PJ, Miller DR (1974). Hereditary stomatocytosis with hemolytic anemia in the dog. Blood 44:557.

Podliachouk L, Balbierz H, Kaminski M, Nikotojczuk M, Strzelecka A (1972). Immunogenetic study of the Mur Insulan horses. Proc 12th Eur Conf Anim Blood Grps Biochem Polymorphism (Budapest):533.

Rice MC, O'Brien SJ (1980). Genetic variance of laboratory outbred Swiss mice. Nature 283:157.

Ruth GR, Schwartz S, Stephenson B (1977). Bovine protoporphyria: The first nonhuman model of this hereditary photosensitizing disease. Science 198:199.

Saison R, Giblett ER (1969). 6-phosphogluconate dehydrogenase polymorphism in the pig. Vox Sang 76:514.

Saison R, O'Reilly M (1971). Phosphohexose isomerase variants in pigs. Vox Sang 20:274.

Sandberg K (1970). Blood group factors and erythrocytic protein polymorphism in Swedish horses. Proc 11th Eur Conf Anim Blood Grps Biochem Polymorphism (Warsaw):447.

Sandberg K (1973). Phosphohexose isomerase polymorphism in horse erythrocytes. Anim Blood Grps Biochem Genet 4:79.

Sandberg K (1974). Genetically controlled variants of NADH diaphorase from horse red cells. Anim Blood Grps Biochem Genet 5 (Suppl 1):23.

Satore G, Stormont C, Morris BG, Grunder AA (1969). Multiple electrophoretic forms of esterases in red cells of cattle and bison. Genetics 61:823.

Searcy GP, Tasker JB, Miller DR (1979). Animal model: Pyruvate kinase deficiency in dogs. Am J Path 94:689.

Smith JE (1976). Glutathione deficiency and partial gamma-glutamylcysteine synthetase in sheep. Am J Path 82:147.

Smith JE (1981). Animal models of human erythrocyte abnormalities. Clin Haemat 10:239.

Smith JE, Ryer K, Wallace L (1976). Glucose-6-phosphate dehydrogenase deficiency in a dog. Enzyme 21:379.

Tanaba Y, Omi T, Obe K (1977). Genetic variants of glucose phosphate isomerase (E.C. 5.3.1.9) in canine erythrocytes. Anim Blood Grps Biochem Genet 8:191.

Tanaka K, Kurosawa Y, Kurokawa K, Oishi T (1980). Genetic polymorphism of erythrocyte esterase-D in pigs. Anim Blood Grps Biochem Genet 11:193.

Tanaka KR, Valentine WN, Miwa S (1962). Pyruvate kinase (PK) deficiency hereditary non-spherocytic hemolytic anemia. Blood 19:267.

Tchernia G, Mohandas N, Shohet SB (1981). Deficiency of skeletal membrane protein band 4.1 in homozygous hereditary elliptocytosis. J Clin Invest 68:454.

Tucker EM, Clarke SW (1980). Comparative aspects of biochemical polymorphism in the blood of caprinae species and their hybrids. Anim Blood Grps Biochem Genet 11:163.

Vergnes H, Puget A, Govarderes C (1974). Comparative study of red-cell enzyme polymorphism in the pikas and the rabbit. Anim Blood Grps Biochem Genet 5:181.

Verhorst D (1972). Polymorphism in glucose-6-phosphate dehydrogenase in the German large white. Anim Blood Grps Biochem Genet 4:65.

Weiden PL, Hackman RC, Deeg HJ, Graham TC, Thomas ED, Storb R (1981). Long-term survival and reversal of iron overload after marrow transplantation in dogs with congenital hemolytic anemia. Blood 57:66.

Weiden P, Storb R, Kolb HJ, Graham T, Anderson J, Giblett E (1974). Genetic variation of red blood cell enzymes in the dog. Transplantation 17:115.

Werth G, Muller G (1967). Vererbbarer glucose-6-phosphat dehydrogenase mangel in den erythrocyten von ratten. Klin Wochen 45:265.

Widar J, Ansay M, Hanset R (1974). Polymorphism of adenosine deaminase in the pig: allelic variation in erythrocytes. Anim Blood Grps Biochem Genet 5:115.

With TK (1979). Porphyrias in animals. Clin Haematol 9:345.

Wright PC, Young JD, Mangan JL, Tucker E (1977). An inherited arginase deficiency in sheep erythrocytes. J Agric Sci 88:765.

Young JD, Ellory JC, Tucker EM (1975). Amino acid transport defect in glutathione-deficient sheep erythrocytes. Nature 254:156.

Animal Models of Inherited Metabolic Diseases, pages 435–447
© **1982 Alan R. Liss, Inc., 150 Fifth Avenue, New York, NY 10011**

RENAL TUBULAR DEFECTS OF SPONTANEOUS FANCONI SYNDROME
IN DOGS

Kenneth C. Bovee, DVM, M.Med.Sc.
Thaddeus Anderson, VMD
Scott Brown, VMD
Michael H. Goldschmidt BVMS, MSc
Stanton Segal, MD

School of Veterinary Medicine
University of Pennsylvania and
Children's Hospital of Pennsylvania
Philadelphia, Pennsylvania

INTRODUCTION

Spontaneous animal models of renal tubular transport
are rare. Recognized defects in the dog include those
involving uric acid in the Dalmatian (Zins 1962) and
canine cystinuria (Bovee 1974) reported in many breeds.
Other spontaneous tubular defects appear to occur in dogs.
A renal tubular disease in the Basenji breed associated
with glycosuria, polyuria, generalized debilitation and
electrolyte disturbances have been reported (Easley 1976).
Previously reported from our laboratory were abnormal
reabsorption of several solutes and reduced uptake of amino
acids and a model sugar in renal tissue from 3 dogs of
various breeds (Bovee 1978). These descriptions of renal
tubular disease seem to resemble Fanconi syndrome in man.

Fanconi syndrome in man is a constellation of abnormalities associated with renal tubular reabsorption defects
(Hunt 1966). These defects lead to excessive urinary loss
of water, glucose, phosphate, sodium, potassium, amino
acids, and bicarbonate. Clinical expression varies widely
but commonly includes polydipsia, weight loss, growth
retardation, and bone deformities. The disease is seen in
adults as well as children and renal failure is a common
sequelae.

In this paper, we describe a syndrome in 15 dogs that is similar to idiopathic Fanconi syndrome in man.

METHODS

Clinical signs in dogs include polyuria and weight loss for 2 to 12 months. Glycosuria was present in 13 of 15 dogs. Thirteen of the dogs were Basenjis; the others were a Norwegian Elkhound and Shetland Sheep dog. Four were males, and the remainder were intact females. Age ranged from 1 to 7 years.

Urine specimens were screened for sugars, amino acids, and organic acids, using paper chromatography. Renal clearance studies were performed on anesthetized dogs using a method previously described (Bovee 1979). Conventional renal clearance studies were performed for creatinine, glucose, phosphate, sodium, potassium, uric acid, and amino acids. The tubular maximum (Tm) for glucose was measured after the infusion of a 20% glucose solution sufficient to gradually raise plasma glucose concentration to 400 mg/dl. Bicarbonate reabsorption was measured in 6 dogs while arterial PCO_2 was stabilized using a positive pressure ventilation system.

A wedge renal biopsy was removed from the renal cortex. The specimen was divided into thirds. One portion was placed in a chilled buffer solution for in vitro studies, a second portion was placed in gluteraldehyde for electron microscopy, and the third portion was placed in formalin for routine histologic examination. The in vitro uptake of labeled lysine, glycine and a model amino acid, alpha-D-glucoside, a non-metabolized model sugar, was measured. The methodology of in vitro uptake measurement was previously described (Bovee 1978). The uptake of solutes in tissue slices is expressed as the distribution ratio, the ratio label in intracellular fluid to label in media.

The clearance of creatinine was used to estimate glomerular filtration rate (GFR). Conventional clearance formula were used. Results for most solutes were expressed as percentage reabsorption of filtered load. Potassium and uric acid data were expressed as the ratio of urinary excretion divided by filtered load. All clearance values represent the mean of 3 consecutive collection measurements from both kidneys.

Five clinically normal Basenji dogs were used as control animals for all clearances. These dogs were found to be the same as normal non-Basenjis in regard to these renal function measurements.

Acid-base status was determined using a pH radiometer. Radiographs of the abdomen and long bones were made to determine whether there was nephrocalcinosis or changes in bone density. Bone density was determined in one affected dog using a bone mineral analyzer. A complete necropsy was performed on 11 dogs.

The possibility of heavy metal toxicity causing nephro-toxicosis was investigated in 3 dogs; spectrographic analysis of liver and kidney tissue for heavy metals was negative. Long term chronic lead intoxication was negative in three dogs using an EDTA infusion test.

Pedigrees of affected dogs were carefully studied and compared to urine screening tests of related dogs.

RESULTS

Excessive quantities of sugars, amino acids, and organic acids were found in the urine of most dogs as determined by paper chromatography. Glucose was found in 14 of the dogs. Urine specific gravity was low in 10 dogs (range, 1.005-1.018); and normal in other dogs. Otherwise, results of analyses were normal.

Twenty-four hour urinary excretion of glucose ranges from 2-16 grams. Glucose was the only sugar found in the urine. Hemograms were normal in all dogs at the time of initial examination. Plasma electrolytes, chemistries, and enzymes were normal. Evidence of diabetes mellitus was not found.

The only abnormalities found in plasma chemical analysis were moderately increased concentrations of creatinine and blood urea nitrogen in 4 dogs. Glomerular filtration rate was reduced approximately 50% in these 4 dogs, but was normal in other affected dogs.

Table 1.

RENAL CLEARANCE OF DOGS WITH FANCONI SYNDROME
COMPARED TO NORMALS

% Reab.	Normal (N=5)	Affected	P
Glucose	99.9	90.0	<.05
Sodium	97.7	92.8	<.001
Chloride	96.0	92.0	<.05
Phosphate	90.8	64.7	<.05
Calcium	97.9	94.1	<.05
Bicarbonate	97.6	94.8	N.S.
Potassium $\frac{U_k V}{F_k}$	0.21	1.2	<.01
GFR, ml/min	35.0	22.9	

The renal clearance studies indicated the fractional reabsorption of filtered glucose was reduced in 14 dogs (Table 1). Results are shown as the mean of 3 consecutive clearance periods. Fractional reabsorption of glucose ranged from 40% to 97%. After infusion of glucose to measure glucose Tm, tubular reabsorption of glucose increased only slightly. When plasma glucose concentration increased to greater than 400 mgs/dl, fractional reabsorption of glucose was approximately 10% of filtered load.

A defect for sodium reabsorption was found in 13 of 15 dogs studied. A defect was also found for chloride. All dogs had a defect for phosphate reabsorption (Table 1). Normal dogs reabsorb approximately 90% of filtered phosphate.

Table 2
REABSORPTION OF AMINO ACIDS

Amino Acid	Percent Reabsorption	
	Dog 1	Dog 5
Cystine	50	38
Methionine	82	86
Lysine	65	100
Threonine	60	88
Glycine	73	87
Phenylalanine	92	100
Asparagine	78	100
Glutamic Acid	75	99

The renal clearance of amino acids was abnormal in all dogs studied. Two patterns of aminoaciduria were found. Most dogs had a generalized aminoaciduria; reabsorption was only 50% to 96% of filtered amino acid. This aminoaciduria included acidic, basic, and a neutral amino acid. Two dogs had aminoaciduria characteristic of canine cystinuria; defects for cystine and dibasic amino acids only. Reabsorption of amino acids in normal dogs is 97% to 100% of filtered load.

A tubular defect for potassium handling was found in 9 of 12 dogs studied. Because potassium is reabsorbed and secreted by tubular cells, results are expressed as a ratio of excreted potassium to filtered potassium. Normally, approximately 20% of filtered potassium is excreted in the urine. Potassium defect was variable, two dogs had a defect whereby approximately 60% of filtered potassium was in the urine while other dogs had excessive potassium loss with a ratio greater than 1.0 (Table 1). These results are consistent with excessive efflux from tubular cells or secretion of potassium.

A defect for uric acid transport was found in 7 of the dogs studied. Reabsorption of calcium was variable; 3 dogs had a minor reduction in calcium reabsorption.

Radiographs of kidneys were normal; bone density was normal by radiogrpahic and densitometry studies.

Acid-base status was variable. Three dogs measured periodically over a one-year period had moderate metabolic acidosis: mean pH, 7.37 ± 0.03; mean PCO_2, 23.0 ± 4.0; and mean HCO_3, 15.7 ± 2.5. Three dogs had severe metabolic acidosis associated with acute renal failure.

The renal clearance of bicarbonate was reduced in some dogs and normal in others. Preliminary results suggest a defect in the proximal tubular reabsorption of bicarbonate.

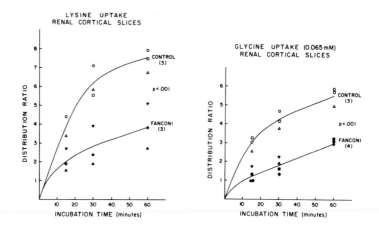

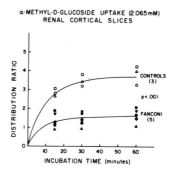

Fig. 1. The time accumulation of L-lysine, glycine, and α-methyl-D-glucoside by kidney cortex slices. Uptake is designated by the distribution ratio. ratio of counts/min/ml of intracellular fluid to counts/min/ml of medium. Different symbols are individual dogs. (Reproduced by permission Sci. 201:1129, 1978)

In vitro uptake of lysine, glycine and the model non-metabolized sugar, alpha-methyl-D-glucoside, was lower than normal, especially after 30 minute incubation (Figure 1) (p <0.001). These data demonstrate an in vitro transport defect for amino acids and a sugar in the affected renal tissue.

Six of the affected dogs died within 6 months of initial examination. The others have remained well for a period of more than 2 years; two females were bred and have produced pups. The dogs that died had rapidly progressive dehydration, profound polyuria, weight loss, anorexia and death within two weeks. Azotemia, hyperphosphatemia, and hyperkalemia developed suddenly. Hypochloremia and hyponatremia were detected in two dogs. Severe metabolic acidosis was present in these dogs (mean arterial pH, 7.15-7.29) before the onset of severe azotemia. Necropsy examination of these dogs revealed papillary necrosis with acute inflammatory cell infiltration, bacterial colonization, and mineral deposition in the renal papilla.

Histologic examination of kidneys of other affected dogs revealed tubule dilation with marked karyomegaly of the tubular cells. The nuclei are 2-3x normal size and are elongated with a vesicular nucleoplasm (Fig 2 &3). The extent of this change is variable; dogs in the early stage of the disease have moderate karyomegaly. Other changes are interstitial fibrosis with lymphocytic and plasma cell infiltration, moderate glomerulosclerosis, and protein casts in tubules. Electron microscopic examination of renal tubule cells found no abnormalities.

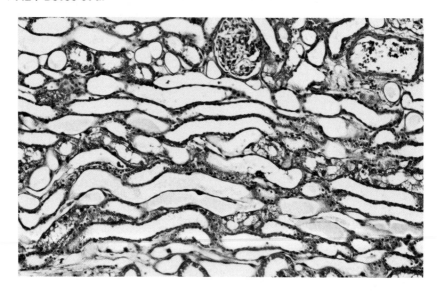

Fig. 2. Dilated tubules lined by flattened cells showing marked karyomegaly. (H.E. x 140).

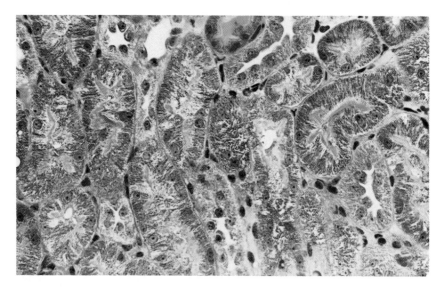

Fig. 3. Tubules showing karyomegaly from young dog. Plastic embedded section of 1 micron thickness. (H.E. x 360).

DISCUSSION

These data describe a new entity of renal tubular
disease in dogs. Results of renal clearance studies
indicate tubular defects for glucose, phosphate, sodium,
potassium, uric acid, calcium, bicarbonate, and amino acids.
The plasma concentration of these solutes remain relatively
normal despite the tubular defects. While renal failure
may result in some affected dogs, the pattern of tubular
defects is markedly different from changes in solute
handling associated with either primary acute renal
failure or chronic renal failure.

A reabsorptive defect for phosphate was found in dogs
regardless of state of renal function. During chronic
renal failure phosphate reabsorption is decreased.
Though renal failure was not a uniform finding in these
dogs, it may have played a role in phosphaturia in some
dogs. Plasma inorganic phosphate remained normal in all
dogs suggesting enhanced gastrointestinal absorption of
phosphate to balance the renal loss.

The sodium defect is of clinical importance because
it would lead to polyuria, extracellular fluid depletion,
and reduced GFR. While the polyuria in these dogs was
probably due to glycosuria and natriuresis, the most
important defect may be the natriuresis. It is likely
that the sodium loss is associated with excessive
bicarbonate loss as the transport system for these
solutes is related in dogs. A defect in bicarbonate
reabsorption could lead to acidosis seen in these dogs.
The characterization of renal tubular acidosis in this
syndrome is under further investigation.

Alpha-methyl-D-glucoside is known to have shared
transport processes with D-glucose in the renal tubule
cell (Silverman 1974, Segal 1973). The observed in vitro
defect in alpha-methyl-D-glucoside uptake in these dogs
is consistent with this concept. The inability of the
in vitro uptake method to detect the presence of a
transport defect for amino acids remains unexplained.
The magnitude of a transport abnormality may not be
involved in the defective transport system.(Bovee 1978).

Results of oral glucose tolerance tests indicate
normal gastrointestinal transport for glucose in these dogs.

The same is probably true of other solutes because normal plasma chemical values persist in the face of marked renal tubular defects.

The cause of death in these dogs appears to be chronic debilitation due to renal tubular defects including acidosis. Papillary necrosis was associated with the terminal event. The acidosis likely enhanced the debilitation of these dogs. Our findings indicate that this disease can be diagnosed early in its course and the dogs may remain clinically stable for prolonged periods. It is curious that a disease of membrane transport does not become clinically visible until adulthood or middle age.

The syndrome described in this paper may represent a genetically determined disease in the Basenji breed, since examination of pedigrees reveals several common ancestors. However, the mode of transmission remains unknown.

The unusual megalocytic nuclei in renal tubular cells of affected dogs of the Basenji breed is of unknown significance.

Fanconi syndrome in humans is characterized as idiopathic or associated with diseases such as cystinosis, Lowe's syndrome, and tyrosinemia. An acquired form occurs with multiple myeloma, amyloidosis, or drug intoxication (Wallis 1957). A mild form of this syndrome may also be associated with other metabolic diseases in humans. Inheritance of the idiopathic form is variable. Widespread derangement of transport by renal tubular cells could result from altered membrane structure or abnormal cell metabolism. The underlying mechanism of all forms of this syndrome remains unknown.

The syndrome in these dogs may be compared with adult or idiopathic Fanconi syndrome without cystinosis in man. Glycosuria, hyperphosphaturia, aminoaciduria, bicarbonaturia, and acidosis appear to be characteristics in both species. Dissimiliarities appear to be retarded bone growth, stunting and abnormal gastrointestinal absorption of calcium, seen in man but not in dogs. It is concluded that these multiple renal tubular transport defects are similar to the idiopathic Fanconi syndrome in man and represent a useful animal model for the study of transport defects.

Bovee KC, Joyce T, Blazer-Yost B, Goldschmidt, MH, Segal S (1979). Characterization of renal defects in dogs with a syndrome similar to the Fanconi syndrome in man. JAVMA 174:1094.

Bovee KC, Joyce T, Reynolds R, Segal S (1978). Spontaneous Fanconi syndrome in the dog. Metabolism 27:45.

Bovee KC , Thier SO, Rea C, et al (1974). Renal clearance of amino acids in canine cystinuria. Metabolism 23:51.

Easley JR, Breitschwerdt EB (1976). Glycosuria associated with renal tubular dysfunction in three Basenji dogs. J Am Vet Med Assoc 168:938.

Hunt DD, Sterns G, McKinley JB, et al (1966. Long term study of family with Fanconi syndrome without cystinosis. Am J Med 40:492.

Segal S, Roscenhagen M, Rea C (1973). Developmental and other characteristics of alpha methyl D-glucoside by rat kidney cortex slices. Biochim Biophys Acta 291:519.

Silverman M (1974). The chemical and steric determinants governing sugar interactions with renal tubular membranes. Biochim Biophys Acta 332:248.

Wallis LA, Engle RL (1957). The adult Fanconi syndrome. II. Review of eighteen cases, Am J Med 22:13-20.

Zins GR, Weiner IM (1968). Bi-directional urate transport limited to the proximal tubule in dogs. Am J Physiol 215:411.

DR. K. SMITH: Have you looked at the nuclei of renal tubular epithelial megalocytic cells with electron microscopy, and if so, what did you find?

DR. BOVEE: We have looked in a preliminary manner at renal tubular cells with EM and there appear to be no abnormalities in brush borders and cytoplasmic structures. We have not systematically looked at the nuclei.

DR. J. SMITH: Have you tested your animals for erythrocyte pyruvate kinase deficiency?

DR. BOVEE: That disease seems to be relatively uncommon at the present time. We have not screened our dogs for that disease, and they have no clinical signs of that disease.

DR. SEGAL: Maybe I should follow up the discussion. The question about these dogs and the Fanconi syndrome, a question that also has been raised in man, is whether this is a disorder primarily of the brush-border membrane or whether it is due to a secondary metabolic event.

You can produce Fanconi syndrome in rats and dogs by the injection of certain toxic materials, such as maleic acid, and in man, for example, in patients that have hereditary fructose intolerance, you can turn on and off the Fanconi syndrome just by the infusion of fructose. This seems to indicate that there may be a primary metabolic component in some of the patients that have Fanconi syndrome.

In order to try to get at this question we have isolated brush border membranes from these dogs, prepared membrane vesicles and studied the uptake of amino acids and glucose by these membrane vesicles. In the two dogs that we have studied there is a defect in the isolated membrane vesicle uptake of these two substrates.

At first glance one might assume that this is a primary defect in the membrane. However, we still cannot be certain because it could be that metabolic events in the cell influence the nature of the membrane itself.

DR. SCARPELLI: Dr. Segal, have you looked at the lipid composition of the proximal tubular brush border derived vesicles? I think this might be interesting and may negate the need for a "toxic" metabolite.

DR. SEGAL: I think the big problem is in acquiring these dogs and being able to sacrifice them and get their kidneys. We have tried a breeding program, which is supported by the Arthritis Institute. The biggest problem, of course, is the cost of breeding and caring for these animals to establish a colony so that they are available to us on demand to do experiments.

DR. BOVEE: We have had to use most of the dogs for the breeding program up to this time.

DR. BUSS: Have you determined whether or not arginine vasopressin or arginine vasotocin has any effect on this renal function?

DR. BOVEE: We have not studied that.

Animal Models of Inherited Metabolic Diseases, pages 449-458
© **1982 Alan R. Liss, Inc., 150 Fifth Avenue, New York, NY 10011**

HEREDITARY CANINE SPINAL MUSCULAR ATROPHY:
A CANINE MODEL OF HUMAN MOTOR NEURON DISEASE

Linda C. Cork. D.V.M.. Ph.D..
Robert J. Adams. D.V.M..
John W. Griffin. M.D..
Donald L. Price. M.D..
Division of Comparative Medicine and
Departments of Pathology and Neurology.
The Johns Hopkins University
School of Medicine. Baltimore. Maryland

INTRODUCTION

    Hereditary canine spinal muscular atrophy (HCSMA) is
a motor neuron disease originally identified in purebred
Brittany Spaniels [Cork. et al 1979]. Like the human
motor neuron diseases. a devastating group of disorders
characterized by specific dysfunction and death of motor
neurons [Price. et al in press]. HCSMA is associated with
weakness and muscle atrophy [Lorenz. et al 1979; Cork. et
al 1980]. The unifying feature of the canine and human
motor neuron diseases is the selective vulnerability of
neurons in the motor system. The spectrum of disease in
man spans all age groups ranging from infancy and
childhood (Werdnig-Hoffmann disease and Kugelberg-Welander
disease, respectively) to the adult onset form,
amyotrophic lateral sclerosis (ALS)[Andrews, Andrews 1976;
Byers, Banker 1961; Iwata, Hirano 1979]. Like the human
disorders, HCSMA also shows variation in the age of onset
and progression of clinical signs. Three phenotypes of
this dominantly inherited motor neuron disease have been
recognized: accelerated, intermediate and chronic [Lorenz,
et al 1979; Sack, et al in preparation].

CLINICAL AND LABORATORY STUDIES

    All affected dogs become weak and have progressive

denervation atrophy of limb, trunk, and bulbar muscles.
Extraocular muscles and vesicorectal sphincters are
spared. Pups with accelerated disease are weak by six
weeks of age and are tetraparetic by three to four months
of age. Brittany spaniels with intermediate disease
develop weakness between six and twelve months of age and
become tetraparetic by two to three years. In both the
accelerated and intermediate form of the disease,
electromyographic examination of affected muscles
demonstrates widespread positive sharp waves,
fibrillations, and fasciculations. Extraocular muscles
and vesico-rectal sphincters are spared. Finally, a few
dogs within the colony have chronic disease manifest by
mile weakness, abnormal electromygrams, and histologic
abnormalities on muscle biopsy.

GENETICS

        Inspection of the initial pedigree disclosed a
pattern which appeared to be consistent with a simple
Mendelian recessive trait. In particular, two
observations on the first litter suggested this mode of
inheritance: 1) phenotypically normal parents produced
affected progeny; and, 2) a backcross mating between a
clinically normal father and daughter produced affected
offspring. Since both parents were normal and have
remained so, the disease did not appear to be caused by a
simple autosomal dominant trait. This hypothesis was
tested by subsequent genetic studies. However, when
affected Brittany spaniels were mated with normal
Brittanies or Beagles, affected progeny appeared in the
F_1 generation, and their phenotypes were similar to that
of the affected parent. Furthermore, the progeny of two
affected Brittanies or of two affected F_1 Brittany/
Beagles were phenotypically similar. Both Brittanies and
Brittany/Beagles showed a marked phenotypic variation in
expression of disease, e.g., some pups developed rapidly
progressive disease, but others remained normal or had
intermediate disease. These genetic investigations
suggested that the trait was inherited as a dominant, and
that there were modifying genes which influenced the
expression of the trait or, alternatively, that the
accelerated pattern of the disease might represent
homozygosity for the dominant trait. Genetic studies in
progress should clarify the relationship between genetic

factors and the phenotypic expression of the disease
[Sack, et al in preparation].

The inbred matings which have been used to study the
mode of inheritance of motor neuron disease revealed a
second, unrelated trait within this kindred of Brittany
Spaniels. Some dogs within the colony are deficient in
the third component of complement, C_3 [Winkelstein, et
al 1981]. There was no cosegregation of the HSCMA trait
with C_3 deficiency. The C_3 deficiency appears to be
inherited as a codominant trait, and dogs heterozygous
for C_3 deficiency have decreased levels of C_3 in their
serum compared to normal dogs.

PATHOLOGY

The clinical features of HCSMA are reflected in the
character and distribution of the pathology.
Abnormalities are present in the lower motor neurons of
the spinal cord and brain stem nuclei including the
hypoglossal and the motor nucleus of the trigeminal nerve.
In contrast to ALS, dogs with HCSMA do not show evidence
of upper motor neuron signs or lesions in corticospinal
pathways.

Accelerated form

In these pups there is marked chromatolysis of motor
neurons, and the ventral horn region contains massive
numbers of neurofilament-filled swellings of the proximal
portions of axons [Cork, et al 1980; Cork in press](Figs.
1 and 2). Ultrastructurally, the chromatolytic neurons
show dispersion of ribosomes and fragmentation of the
endoplasmic retuculum. Some neurons contain increased
numbers of the neurofilaments within the perikaryon and
some dendrites are focally enlarged with accumulations of
maloriented neurofilaments and entrapped organelles
including mitochondria, endoplasmic reticulum, and other
membranous structures. The most striking pathology is in
the proximal axon or dendrites. The swollen axons are
greatly enlarged and filled with maloriented fascicles of
neurofilaments. The swellings appear to involve proximal
internodes with relative sparing of the initial segment in
the nodes of Ranvier. Distended internodal segments show

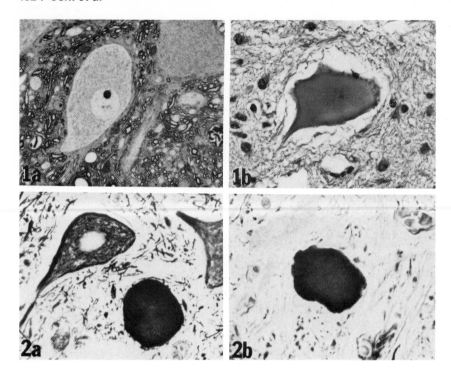

Figure 1a. Chromatolytic motor neuron from pup with
          HCSMA. Note dispersion of Nissl and eccentric
          nucleus.Tol. blue, epon X 400.
       1b. Chromatolytic motor neuron from 12-week-old
          infant with Werdnig-Hoffmann disease. Note
          small rim of Nissl at periphery. Cresyl
          violet, paraffin, X 400.
       2a. Motor neuron and axonal swelling from dog with
          HCSMA. Axonal swelling stains strongly with
          silver. Sevier-Munger, paraffin, X 400.
       2b. Axonal swelling from patient with ALS. Axonal
          swelling is strongly silver positive.
          Sevier-Munger, paraffin, X 600.

passive demyelination with displacement of the terminal
loops of the myelin sheath. Some of the most severe
swellings contain accumulations of entrapped particulate
organelles (Fig. 3). Other axons show Wallerian

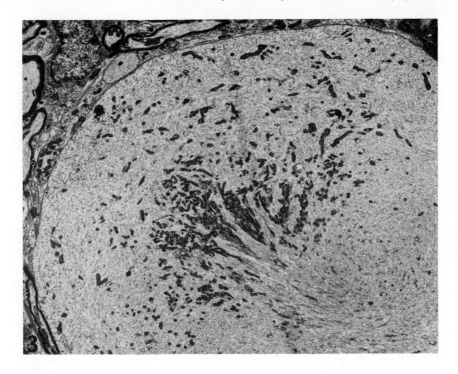

Figure 3. Electron micrograph of neurofilament- filled cell process (probably a dendrite) from pup with HCSMA. Entrapped within swirls of neurofilaments are various membranous organelles, X5000.

degeneration. Some of the neurofilament-filled axonal swellings extend into the proximal portion (5mm) of the ventral root, but they have not been identified in peripheral nerve. Glial bundles, similar to those described in Werdnig-Hoffmann disease [Chou, Fakadej 1971], have been found in the proximal ventral root.

Intermediate form

Affected dogs have a reduced number of motor neuronswithin the ventral horn. The number of neurofilament-filled axonal swellings is fewer than in the accelerated form, probably because of the slower evolution of the process and the loss of neurons. The pathologic process appears to be more slowly evolving than in the accelerated disease. Some myelin sheaths around the swollen axons are thin, and occasional intramyelinic vacuoles are present.There is some degree of Wallerian-like degeneration and axonal loss in the ventral roots during the advanced stage of the disease. As in the pups with accelerated disease, the axons within the distal portion of the root appeared smaller than normal and glial bundles were sometimes present in the proximal part of the root.

PATHOGENETIC MECHANISMS

As was noted previously, motor neurons are selectively involved in both the human and canine disease. In Werdnig-Hoffmann disease, the most striking feature is severe chromatolysis of motor neurons. Although not as frequently described in ALS, chromatolysis certainly does occur in the adult form of the disease [Price, et al in press; Inoue, Hirano 1980; Iwata, Hirano 1979; Wohlfart 1959; Wohlfart, Swank 1941]. Of particular interest in ALS is the recognition by Wolfhart [1959], Carpenter [1968], Chou [1979], and Inoue and Hirano [1980], of the presence of neurofilament-filled axonal swellings in affected individuals. These axonal swellings appeared to be most frequent in patients with a rapid clinical course, and are most common in regions of the neuraxis in which clinical disease was active in the interval before death. In his pioneering paper on the human disease, Carpenter [1968] suggested that this change might result from an abnormality in axonal transport. The presence of chromatolysis and axonal swellings strongly suggest that affected motor neurons do not suddenly die, but over time a series of complex degenerative changes evolve which are not well understood. Thus, in ALS and HCSMA we are not dealing with sudden deaths of neurons as occurs in poliomyelitis [Bodian 1949], but rather a more slowly evolving degenerative process.

Chromatolysis has usually been interpreted to be the result of changed metabolic priorities which occur during regeneration after axonal injury, e.g., the neuron is reversibly reprogrammed to manufacture materials needed for regeneration [Price, Porter 1972; Lieberman 1971; Price, et al in press]. A similar ultrastructural appearance could result from a disturbance in the synthesis/processing/transport of proteins important for maintaining the intracellular organization of the peri-karyon. One group of proteins which may be important in maintaining the structural properties of nerve cells are the cytoskeletal proteins. These proteins are synthesized in the cell body and dendrites and in these regions presumably help to maintain cell shape. In addition, because the axon and nerve terminal lack the ability to synthesize proteins, these cytoskeletal proteins must be delivered to the axon by axonal transport.

A primary role for impaired axonal transport in the pathogenesis of proximal axonal swellings and distal axonal atrophy as observed in ALS and HCSMA, has been recently demonstrated in experimental studies of β, β'-iminodipropionitrile (IDPN) intoxication. This toxin causes large neurofilament-filled swellings in proximal axons, [Chou, Hartmann 1964, 1965; Clark, et al 1980], and chronic intoxication causes reduction in the caliber of distal axons. Studies of axonal transport have demonstrated a selective impairment in slow axonal transport of cytoskeletal proteins, particularly neurofilaments [Griffin, et al 1978; Griffin, Price 1980]. These observations strongly suggest that the functional abnormality underlying the axonal swellings may be an impairment in slow axonal transport, particularly of neurofilaments.

Although the above observations suggest there may well be an abnormality in axonal transport in HCSMA, and by implication ALS, it is also possible that this type of axonal pathology (and the putative transport defect) is part of a more generalized dysfunction of motor neurons, but that the other functional abnormalities do not result in readily discernable structural pathology. Thus, it is very important to examine not only axonal transport, but other important properties of affected motor neurons, including the ability of these cells to synthesize specific enzymes like choline acetyltransferase (CAT) and acetylcholinesterase (AChE) and to evaluate the ability of these cells to synthesize and maintain specific receptors on their surface. In this context it is important to recall that young pups are profoundly weak, yet show very little in the way of loss of neurons. Why are these pups weak? Is it because of a conduction block due to passive demyelination from the axonal swellings, or perhaps the failure of synthesis of specific proteins or receptors? We do not yet know the answers to these questions, but the HCSMA model provides an opportunity to study the clinical development of motor neuron disease, temporal and spatialevolution of the pathology, and to relate these findings to investigation of axonal transport, activities of specific synthesizing enzymes, and to expression of receptors on motor neurons. Once we know the temporal and spatial profile of motor neurons in dogs with HCSMA, we will be in a much better position to understand some ofthe functional abnormalities which underly the clinical expression of human motor neuron diseases.

ACKNOWLEDGEMENTS

These studies were supported in part by USPHS Grant numbers NS 10580, NS 14784, NS 10920, N01-RR-A-2145, and NS 15721-01, and grants from the Amyotrophic Lateral Sclerosis Society of America and the H. Burnett Robinson Memorial Fund. USPHS Research Career Development Awards support Dr. Griffin (NS 004501) and Dr. Cork (NS 00488). We thank Dr. Richard Lindinberg for providing the Werdnig-Hoffmann and ALS cases. We thank Chiyin Choy and Elizabeth Sanders for their assistance in the preparation of this manuscript, and Jeanette Morris, Lula Winkler, and Harold Scott for technical assistance.

REFERENCES

Andrews JM, Andrews RL (1976). The comparative neuropathology of motor neuron diseases. In Andrews JM, Johnson RT, Brazier MA (eds): "Amyotrophic Lateral Sclerosis, UCLA Forum in Medical Science, No. 19," New York: Academic Press, p 181.
Bodian D (1949). Histiopathologic basis of clinical findings in poliomyelitis. Amer J Med 6:563.
Byers RK, Banker BQ (1961). Infantile muscular atrophy. Arch Neurol Psychiatry (Chi) 5:140.
Carpenter S (1968). Proximal axonal enlargement in motor neuron disease. Neurology 18:841.

Chou SM, Fakadej AV (1971). Ultrastructure of
chromatolytic motoneurons and anterior spinal roots
in a case of Werdnig-Hoffman disease. J Neuropathol
Exp Neurol 30:368.

Chou SM, Hartmann HA (1964). Axonal lesions and waltzing
syndrome after IDPN administration in rats. Acta
Neuropathol (Berl) 3:428.

Chou SM, Hartmann HA (1965). Electron microscopy of focal
neuro-axonal lesions produced by β,β'-
iminodipropionitrile (IDPN) in rats. Acta Neuropathol
(Berl) 4:590.

Chou SS (1979). Pathognomy of intraneuronal inclusions in
ALS. In Tsubaki T, Toyokura Y (eds): "Amyotrophic
Lateral Sclerosis," Baltimore: University Park Press,
p 135.

Clark AW, Griffin JW, Price DL (1980). The axonal
pathology in chronic IDPN intoxication. J Neuropathol Exp Neurol 39:42.

Cork LC, Griffin JW, Adams RJ, Price DL (1980). Motor
neuron disease: spinal muscular atrophy and amyotrophic
lateral sclerosis. Animal model: hereditary canine
spinal muscular atrophy. Am J Pathol 100:599.

Cork LC, Griffin JW, Munnell JF, Lorenz MD, Adams RJ,
Price DL (1979). Hereditary canine spinal muscular
atrophy. J Neuropathol Exp Neurol 38:209.

Cork LC, Price DL, Griffin JW, Choy C, Padula CA (1981).
Accelerated Hereditary Canine Spinal Muscular Atrophy
(HCSMA). J Neuropathol Exp Neurol 40:314.

Griffin JW, Hoffman PN, Clark AW, Carroll PT, Price DL
(1978). Slow axonal transport of neurofilament
proteins: impairment by β,β'-iminodipropionitrile
administration. Science 202:633.

Griffin JW, Price DL (1980). Proximal axonopathies
induced by toxic ch chemicals. In Spencer PS,
Schaumburg HH (eds): "Experimental and Clinical
Neurotoxicology," Baltimore: Williams and Wilkins,
p 161.

Inoue K, Hirano A (1980). Early pathological changes in
Amyotrophic Lateral Sclerosis: a reappraisal of the
spheroid, Bunina Body, and morphometry of the ventral
spinal root. J Neuropathol Exp Neurol 39:363.

Iwata M, Hirano A (1979). Current problems in the
pathology of Amyotrophic Lateral Sclerosis. In
Zimmerman HM (ed): "Progress in Neuropathology,
Vol. 4," New York: Raven Press, p 277.

Lorenz MD, Cork LC, Griffin JW, Adams RJ, Price DL
(1979).Hereditary spinal muscular atrophy in Brittany
Spaniels: clinical manifestations. J Am Vet Med Assoc
175:833.

Price DL, Griffin JW, Hoffman PN, Cork LC, Spencer PS (In
press). The response of motor neurons to injury and
disease. In Dyck PJ, Thomas PK, Lambert EH (eds):
"Peripheral Neuropathy, 2nd ed," Philadelphia: W.B.
Saunders.

Price DL, Porter KR (1972). The response of ventral horn
neurons to axonal transection. J Cell Biol 53:24.

Winklestein JA, Johnson JP, Ferry F, Yolken R and Cork LC:
Genetically determined deficiency of the third component
of complement in the dog. Submitted for presentation at
the IX International Complement Workshop, Key Biscayne,
Florida, November, 1981.

Wohlfart G (1959). Degenerative and regenerative changes
in the ventral horns, brainstem and cerebral cortex in
amyotrophic lateral sclerosis. Acta Univ Lundensis (new
series 2) 56:1.

Wohlfart G, Swank RL (1941). Pathology of amyotrophic
lateral sclerosis: fiber analysis of the ventral roots
and pyramidal tracts of the spinal cord. Arch Neurol
Psychiatry 46:783.

Animal Models of Inherited Metabolic Diseases, pages 459–461
© 1982 Alan R. Liss, Inc., 150 Fifth Avenue, New York, NY 10011

CHOOSING ANIMAL MODELS OF HUMAN INBORN ERRORS OF METABOLISM

L.W. Gerrity, D.V.M. and J.M. Friedman, M.D., Ph.D.

Division of Clinical Genetics
University of Texas Health Science Center
Dallas, Texas   75235

Selection of animal models for investigation of human
inborn errors of metabolism should be based on their appropriateness for a particular project. An animal with clinical
features and a pathogenetic defect similar to those of an
affected human is suitable for studies of disturbed biochemical pathways or potential treatment protocols. Extra-
polation of data from these models to humans is often valid.
Animals exhibiting a disease with similar symptomatology but
a different etiology are useful in general studies of metabolic pathways; however, they are unlikely to be relevant to
determining the abnormalities at the gene level responsible
for the human disease. Animals which appear to have a similar pathogenetic defect but differ in symptomatology from
affected humans are appropriate for studies of phylogenetic
variations in anatomical and physiological responses.

To emphasize the suitability of various animal models
for studies of different aspects of human metabolic defects
and to encourage the selection of appropriate models, a
comparability scoring system has been devised. The score
is composed of three digits separated by hyphens. Each
digit represents a different category: the first, etiology;
the second, pathogenesis; and the third, clinical features.
Within each category, there are four levels of comparability
ranging from X to 2 (Table 1). Examples of scores assigned
to various animal models of human inborn errors of heme
metabolism are listed in Table 2.

This simple scoring system provides a method for
rapidly evaluating the suitability of animal models for the

Table 1.

COMPARABILITY SCORE

X--Information about the characteristics of the
disease in the human and/or the animal is unavail-
able.

0--The characteristics of the human and the animal
disease are different.

1--The characteristics of the human and the animal
disease are similar but not exactly alike, or information is insufficient to judge if they are exactly
alike.

2--The characteristics in the human and the animal are
essentially the same.

investigation of various aspects of human inborn errors of
metabolism. The subjective nature of the system allows
evaluation of a variety of species in which the clinical
features of interest occur spontaneously or are experimentally induced. The different animals may then be judged
for appropriateness for a particular project on a relatively equal basis. Use of this system may reduce the
potential for extrapolating misleading data to human
diseases and wasting time, money, and experimental animals.

Table 2.   SCORED ANIMAL MODELS OF HUMAN INBORN ERRORS OF HEME METABOLISM

HUMAN DISEASE	McKUSICK #	ANIMAL MODEL	COMPARABILITY SCORE
Crigler-Najjar Syndrome	21880	Gunn Rat	1-2-2
Hyperbilirubinemia I (Gilbert Disease)	14350	Southdown Sheep	0-1-1
Hyperbilirubinemia II (Dubin-Johnson Syndrome)	23750	Corriedale Sheep	1-1-1
Porphyria, Congenital Erythropoietic (Gunther Disease)	26370	DSH Cat	0-1-1
		Siamese Cat	1-1-1
		Cattle	1-1-2
		Dog	X-X-1
		Fox Squirrel	1-1-1
		Swine	0-1-1
Protoporphyria, Erythropoietic	17700	Cattle	0-1-1
		Mice	0-1-1

(References are available upon request.)

Animal Models of Inherited Metabolic Diseases, pages 463–470
© 1982 Alan R. Liss, Inc., 150 Fifth Avenue, New York, NY 10011

MASKING OF MUTANT METABOLIC PHENOTYPES BY PRENATAL MATERNAL INFLUENCES.

George L. Wolff, Ph.D.

National Center for Toxicological Research, Food and Drug Administration, Jefferson, Arkansas 72079

Variable phenotypic expressivity of mutations which affect metabolic regulation increases the difficulty of identifying carriers of such mutations (Vogel & Motulsky 1979). This is especially true of mutations which do not induce gross abnormalities at an early age but alter normal function(s) in a relatively subtle quantitative manner. The absence of a visual or other easily detected marker indicating presence of the mutation is the chief problem.

Thus, a primary requirement for an animal model system to be used for gaining insight into the mechanisms involved in the variable expressivity of mutations affecting metabolic regulation is that the different phenotypes induced by the mutation used as a model be easily identified.

This requirement arises from the necessity of comparing judiciously chosen biochemical, metabolic, and physiologic parameters among the phenotypes to identify the chief differences among the phenotypic classes. These comparisons must be made not only between the overtly mutant phenotype and its variants, but also with the phenotype induced by a "normal" congenic genotype. The information obtained in these initial comparisons can then be applied to the design of efforts to identify one or more invariant molecular characteristics which distinguish all phenotypes induced by the mutation from the phenotype of the "normal" genotype. Once such invariant characteristics are identified, they can be used to identify all carriers of the mutation. The mechanisms involved in the variable expressivity can then be investigated in the whole phenotypic spectrum of carriers of the mutation.

All such comparisons must be carried out in inbred or F-1 hybrid animals so that the genetic background of the mutants and normal controls is identical; otherwise, uncontrolled genetic heterogeneity will make the comparisons unreliable.

Inbred or F-1 hybrid "viable yellow" (A^{vy}/-) mice fulfill the above requirements for a model system if the A^{vy} mutation is maintained in the population by forced heterozygosis with another allele which does not induce the agouti coat color pattern. The A^{vy} mutation induces adult-onset obesity, enhances growth of hyperplastic and neoplastic cells, and alters the qualitative regulation of hair pigment production. The latter effect results in a spectrum of coat color phenotypes varying from clear orange-yellow through different degrees of black and agouti spotting on a yellow background to completely agouti. The latter phenotypic class, "pseudoagouti", resembles the species-type coat color pattern, is free of obvious metabolic alterations such as obesity, and in all physiological characteristics examined resembles the non-A^{vy} genotype (Wolff 1971).

The A^{vy} mutation is located at the agouti locus on chromosome 2 of the house mouse, Mus musculus. Another mutation at this locus, "mottled agouti" (a^m), is also expressed in a spectrum of coat color phenotypes ranging from completely black through degrees of intermingling of yellow and agouti patches on a black background to completely agouti. This "pseudoagouti" phenotype cannot be distinguished visually from that induced by A^{vy}/- or from the species-type agouti pattern. No other effects on metabolic regulation have as yet been associated with the a^m/- genotype (Wolff 1978).

The major effects of the mutations at the agouti locus are exerted on the tissue in which the cells expressing the observed phenotypic endpoint reside (Meade et al 1979, Silvers 1979, Wolff 1970). Thus, the mutations appear not to act directly in the cell which expresses the altered endpoint. Rather, they seem to change the conditions in the tissue surrounding the cell and thus cause the cell to respond in an altered manner.

For example, the hair bulb melanocytes which synthesize the hair pigment respond to rhythmically changing, but as yet unidentified, conditions in the hair bulb by producing either phaeomelanosomes (yellow) or eumelanosomes (black or brown) (Silvers 1979). These differ ultrastructurally, phaeomelanosomes being round with a diffuse filamentous matrix and eumelanosomes being oblong with a matrix of crosslinked parallel fibrils. In the species-type coat color pattern, agouti, a yellow subterminal band in an otherwise black or brown hair results from cyclical changes in pigment production, by the same melanosomes, from eumelanin to phaeomelanin and back to eumelanin. Among $A^{vy}/-$ mice the relative amounts of phaeomelanin and eumelanin in the pelage vary widely, as do the patterns of yellow and black in the individual hairs. Yellow hairs with black bands, alternating yellow and black bands, black hairs with yellow bases, etc., are found even in the pseudoagouti phenotype (Galbraith & Wolff 1974). Such aberrant pigment patterns are not found in genetically agouti $A/-$, mice.

The "mottled yellow" $A^{vy}/-$ phenotypes constitute a continuum of individuals with different degrees of intermingling of agouti and black hair patches on a yellow background to mice which are almost completely agouti except for a few yellow areas. An early attempt to determine whether the degree of black and agouti spotting could be correlated with the degree of obesity was inconclusive (Wolff 1965). It has not been repeated because of the difficulty in separating the various degrees of spotting into discrete categories. Thus, for practical purposes, $A^{vy}/-$ mice can be grouped into three phenotypic classes: clear yellow, mottled yellow, and pseudoagouti.

As will be discussed later, the proportion of the pseudoagouti phenotype is determined to a major degree by prenatal influences of the strain and agouti locus genotype of the dam (Wolff 1978).

The obesity induced by the A^{vy} mutation appears to result from failure of the rate of lipogenesis to decrease from the juvenile to the adult level (Yen et al 1976). In contrast, this age-related decrease in lipogenesis rate does occur in obese ob/ob and db/db mice as well as in the non-A^{vy} littermates of the yellow mice (Yen et al 1976). Thus, the metabolic dysregulation induced by the A^{vy} gene, resulting in adult-onset obesity, is different from that occurring in ob/ob and db/db mice which exhibit juvenile-onset obesity and diabetes.

This different etiology of the A^{vy}/- induced syndrome, compared to the ob- and db-induced syndromes, is also indicated by the increased fat-free dry weight of A^{vy}/- mice compared to the decreased carcass size of ob/ob mice (Heston & Vlahakis 1962). Similarly, spontaneous pulmonary tumor formation is enhanced in A^{vy}/- mice (Heston & Deringer 1947) but inhibited in ob/ob mice (Heston & Vlahakis 1962). Additionally, ob/ob and db/db mice are functionally sterile, due to deficiency of pituitary gonadotropin, whereas A^{vy}/- mice are fertile.

The degree of obesity of A^{vy}/- mice is regulated by the strain genome of these mice as well as by that of the dam (Wolff & Pitot 1973). Whether this maternal effect is exerted prenatally, as in the differentiation of the pseudoagouti phenotype, or postnatally through lactational capacity is unknown. Transplantation studies using the lethal yellow (A^{y}) allele indicate that the obesity is a function of the adipose tissue rather than of the adipocytes themselves (Meade et al 1979).

The third major phenotypic endpoint known to be affected by the A^{vy} mutation is the proliferation of hyperplastic and neoplastic cells. Spontaneous neoplasms in numerous tissues appear earlier in yellow mice, either A^{vy}/- or A^{y}/-, than in their non-mutant littermates (Heston & Deringer 1947, Deringer 1970); however, the identity of the tissues in which the neoplasms appear and the absolute incidence of the lesions depend on the strain background.

Nodule-transformed cells in the mammary glands of C3H mice carrying the murine mammary tumor virus form hyperplastic alveolar nodules (HAN) earlier if the A^{vy} gene is present. The earlier appearance of mammary adenocarcinoma in these yellow mice seemed to be related to the earlier formation of HAN rather than to an increased sensitivity of A^{vy}/A cells to malignant transformation (Wolff et al 1979).

When similar numbers of allogeneic ascites cells of two different tumor cell lines were implanted subcutaneously in yellow $(A^{vy}$/a and A^{y}/a) and normal (a/a) mice of two different inbred strains, more "large" solid tumors were found in the yellow mice eight days after implantation than in the normal mice (Wolff 1970). This suggests a systemic effect of the yellow phenotype on an unknown parameter involved in regulation of the rate of division of neoplastic cells.

In another study, mammary adenocarcinomas were induced with 7,12-dimethylbenz(a)anthracene (DMBA) in yellow (A^{vy}/A) and agouti (A/a) (BALB/c x VY) F-1 hybrid female mice not carrying the mammary tumor virus. Especially at the low dose of DMBA, palpable tumors appeared earlier in the A^{vy}/A mice than in their A/a sisters (Wolff et al submitted for publication). Since no mammary adenocarcinomas were found in any control mice, yellow or agouti, the earlier appearance of the tumors in yellow mice suggests that in these mice the cells transformed by DMBA proliferated more rapidly.

In contrast to the magnitude of the metabolic dysregulations in the mottled yellow A^{vy}/- phenotypes, the pseudoagouti A^{vy}/- phenotype seems almost completely normal. That this phenotype is not completely normal, however, is indicated by the wide variation in pigment patterns found in the individual hairs which does not occur in genetically agouti A/- mice (Galbraith & Wolff 1974). However, pseudoagouti mice without yellow spots do not become obese or even noticeably heavier than their non-A^{vy} littermates (Wolff 1978). Pseudoagouti mice respond to castration like non-A^{vy} mice, i.e., their rate of weight gain is decreased, whereas mottled yellow A^{vy}/- mice exhibit no effect of castration on their rate of weight gain (Wolff 1971). The only available data, which are inadequate for a definitive statement, suggest that spontaneous hepatoma incidence in pseudoagouti A^{vy}/a males resembles that of their non-A^{vy} littermates rather than the higher incidence found among the mottled yellow A^{vy}/a males (Wolff & Pitot 1972).

The novel finding regarding the A^{vy}/-, as well as a^m/-, pseudoagouti phenotype is that its differentiation apparently depends to a considerable extent on unknown conditions in the reproductive tract of the dam which in turn are determined by her strain genome and agouti locus genotype (Wolff 1978). In a reciprocal cross between two very different inbred strains (VY/Wf and YS/ChWf) in which the dams were black (a/a) and the sires mottled yellow (A^{vy}/a), about 10% of the A^{vy}/a offspring from VY dams and about 21% of the A^{vy}/a young from YS dams were pseudo-agouti. Matings within each inbred strain confirmed this strain-specific difference in the proportion of pseudo-agouti A^{vy}/a offspring. Within each strain, A^{vy}/a dams mated by a/a sires produced extremely few pseudoagouti young; however, a/a dams mated by A^{vy}/a sires produced 10% or 17% pseudoagouti offspring depending on the strain. The parameters involved in this phenomenon are unknown. Since pseudoagouti A^{vy}/a mice produce the same proportions of mottled yellow and black or brown offspring as yellow A^{vy}/a mice, spontaneous mutation is apparently not involved.

Qualitatively, regulation of the differentiation of the a^m/a zygotes appears to be similar to that of the A^{vy}/a zygotes. In a reciprocal cross between the AM/Wf and C57BL/6JNctr strains, AM-a^m/a^m dams produced no pseudoagouti offspring; however, C57BL/6J dams produced about 30% pseudoagouti a^m/a young. When C57BL/6J dams were mated by AM-A^{vy}/a^m sires, about 5% of the A^{vy}/a offspring and about 30% of the a^m/a young were pseudoagouti (Wolff 1978). Thus, it seems that A^{vy}/a zygotes are more resistant to the conditions favoring differentiation of the pseudoagouti phenotype than are the a^m/a zygotes.

It should be pointed out that the agouti locus begins acting very early in the life of the zygote. Among putative homozygous A^y/A^y embryos, retardation of cell division in vitro as early as the second cleavage division has been reported (Pedersen & Spindle 1976). In vivo, A^y/A^y embryos die about the time of implantation (Eaton & Green 1962). Thus, the agouti locus acts throughout the life of the organism and appears to affect cellular metabolism at a very fundamental level of regulation.

In using these agouti locus mutations in model systems for studying factors influencing variable expressivity of mutations which affect metabolic regulation, comparison of selected parameters between the non-mutant and pseudoagouti phenotypes provides the best prospect for identifying molecular differences most closely related to the primary effect of the polypeptide specified by the mutation. Once such differences are identified, parameters of interest can be compared among the variable mottled phenotypes and the mechanisms of their variation investigated.

ACKNOWLEDGEMENTS

The expert typing of this manuscript by Ms. Ruth York is much appreciated.

REFERENCES

Deringer MK (1970). Influence of the lethal yellow (A^y) gene on development of reticular neoplasms. J Natl Cancer Inst 45:1205.

Eaton GJ, Green MM (1962). Implantation and lethality of the yellow mouse. Genetica 33:106.

Galbraith DB, Wolff GL (1974). Aberrant regulation of the agouti pigment pattern in the viable yellow mouse. J Hered 65:137.

Heston WE, Vlahakis G (1962). Genetic obesity and neoplasia. J Natl Cancer Inst 29:197.

Heston WE, Deringer, MK (1947). Relationship between the yellow (A^y) gene of the mouse and susceptibility to spontaneous pulmonary tumors. J Natl Cancer Inst 7:263.

Meade CJ, Ashwell M, Sowter C (1979). Is genetically transmitted obesity due to an adipose tissue defect? Proc Roy Soc London B 205:395.

Pedersen RA, Spindle AI (1976). Genetic effects on mammalian development during and after implantation. CIBA Found Symp 40:133.

Silvers WK (1979). "The Coat Colors of Mice. A Model for Mammalian Gene Action and Interaction." New York: Springer, p 23.

Vogel F, Motulsky AG (1979). "Human Genetics. Problems and Approaches." New York: Springer, p 84.

Wolff GL, Kodell RL, Cameron AM, Medina D (Submitted for publication). Accelerated appearance of chemically induced mammary carcinomas in obese yellow (A^{vy}/A) (BALB/c x VY) F-1 hybrid mice.

Wolff GL, Medina D, Umholtz RL (1979). Manifestation of hyperplastic alveolar nodules and mammary tumors in "viable yellow" and non-yellow mice. J Natl Cancer Inst 63:781.

Wolff GL (1978). Influence of maternal phenotype on metabolic differentiation of agouti locus mutants in the mouse. Genetics 88:529.

Wolff GL, Pitot HC (1973). Influence of background genome on enzymatic characteristics of yellow $(A^y/-, A^{vy}/-$ mice. Genetics 73:109.

Wolff GL, Pitot HC (1972). Variation of hepatic malic enzyme capacity with hepatoma susceptibility in mice of different genotypes. Cancer Res 32:1861.

Wolff GL (1970). Stimulation of growth of transplantable tumors by genes which promote spontaneous tumor development. Cancer Res 30:1731.

Wolff GL (1971). Genetic modification of homeostatic regulation in the mouse. Am Nat 105:241.

Wolff GL (1965). Body composition and coat color correlation in different phenotypes of "viable yellow" mice. Science 147:1145.

Yen TT, Allan JA, Yu P, Acton JM, Greenberg MM (1976). Triacylglycerol contents and in vivo lipogenesis of ob/ob, db/db, and A^{vy}/a mice. Biochim Biophys Acta 441:213.

SECTION VIII.
COMPENDIUM OF INHERITED METABOLIC DISEASES IN ANIMALS

Animal Models of Inherited Metabolic Diseases, pages 473-501
© **1982 Alan R. Liss, Inc., 150 Fifth Avenue, New York, NY 10011**

COMPENDIUM OF INHERITED METABOLIC DISEASES IN ANIMALS

George Migaki
Registry of Comparative Pathology
Armed Forces Institute of Pathology
Washington, D.C. 20306

During the past decade there have been reports of significant new information on biochemical defects as related
to inherited metabolic diseases in animals. Since reports
of these diseases appear in a wide variety of journals and
textbooks, an attempt has been made to collect and assemble
this material and then to present it in tabular form with
suitable references. Included are only those diseases of
animals in which the clinical and pathological findings are
attributed to an inborn error of metabolism; experimentally
induced metabolic diseases, e.g. phenylketonuria, etc., are
not included in this report unless genetic factors form an
important permissive or conditioning prerequisite. For each
disease one key reference has been selected. Genetic defects
in metabolism generally result from 1) deficiency of a specific enzyme, 2) disorders of transport or 3) disorders of
synthesis. Although there are many useful methods of group-
ing these diseases, we have selected the scheme outlined by
Stanbury, Wyngaarden and Fredrickson, 1978.

Excellent general sources of information on inherited
metabolic diseases in animals are the following: Andrews,
Ward and Altman, 1979; Bustad, Hegreberg and Padgett, 1975;
Capen, Jones, Hackel and Migaki, 1972-81; Cornelius, 1969;
Hegreberg and Leathers, 1981; Jones, 1969; Kaneko, 1980;
Leader and Leader, 1971; Leipold, 1980; Mitruka, Rawnsley
and Vadehra, 1976; and Patterson, 1974. For references on
specific inherited metabolic diseases in animals, the following are recommended: Bannerman et al, 1973 (anemias); Hunt
et al, 1976 (diabetes mellitus); Smith, 1981 (errors in
erythrocyte metabolism); Kitchen and Boyer, 1974 (hemoglobin-

opathies); Dodds et al, 1981 (hemorrhagic defects); Altman
and Katz, 1979 (inbred and genetically defined strains of
laboratory animals); Jolly and Blakemore, 1973 (lysosomal
diseases); Harris, 1979 (muscular dystrophies); Gershwin and
Merchant, 1981 (immune defects); and Bulfield, 1977
(nutrition-related diseases).

This compendium was prepared at the suggestion of the
planning committee of this symposium and with their
encouragement. Special thanks go to Drs. Gerald Hegreberg
and Donald Patterson for supplying valuable references; to
Drs. Leslie Bullock, Charles Capen, Robert Desnick, Jean
Dodds, Carl Jones, Lance Perryman, Dante Scarpelli, Joseph
Smith, and Robert Wissler for their helpful suggestions; to
Charlotte Kenton of the National Library of Medicine for her
computer search of the literature; to Merryanna Swartz for
assistance in the literature search; and to Charmaine Goetz
and Susan Stolze for technical assistance.

CARBOHYDRATE METABOLISM

Disorder	Primary Defect	Animal	Inherit*	Reference**
Diabetes mellitus	Insulin action def.	Mouse	AR	Kahn et al, 1973
Diabetes mellitus	Insulin action def.	Cat	NM	Gembardt and Loppnow, 1974
Diabetes mellitus	Insulin action def.	Rat	NM	Nakhooda et al, 1977
Diabetes mellitus	Insulin action def.	Hamster	AR	Butler, 1967
Diabetes mellitus	Insulin action def.	Sand rat	NM	Schmidt-Nielsen et al, 1964
Diabetes mellitus	Insulin action def.	G. pig	NM	Munger and Lang, 1973
Diabetes mellitus	Insulin action def.	Mystromys	AR	Stuhlman et al, 1972
Diabetes mellitus	Insulin action def.	Monkey	NM	Howard, 1974
Diabetes mellitus	Insulin action def.	Carp	NM	Yokote, 1970
Diabetes mellitus	Insulin action def.	Dog	AR	Kraner et al, 1980
Galactokinase deficiency	Galactokinase	Kangaroo	NM	Stephens et al, 1974
Galactosemia	Galactose-1-phosphate uridyl transferase	Kangaroo	NM	Richardson et al, 1979
Galactosemia	Galactose-1-phosphate uridyl transferase	Rat	NM	Solov'eva et al, 1975
Glycogenosis II	α-1,4-glucosidase	Cat	NM	Sandstrom et al, 1969
Glycogenosis II	α-1,4-glucosidase	Sheep	NM	Manktelow and Hartley, 1975
Glycogenosis II	α-1,4-glucosidase	Dog	NM	Mostafa, 1970
Glycogenosis II	α-1,4-glucosidase	Cattle	NM	Cook et al, 1980
Glycogenosis II	α-1,4-glucosidase	Quail	NM	Murakami et al, 1980
Glycogenosis III	Amylo-1,6-glucosidase	Dog	AR	Ceh et al, 1976
Glycogenosis VIII	Phosphorylase b kinase	Mouse	XL	Lyon et al, 1967
Glycogenosis VIII	Phosphorylase b kinase	Rat	AR	Clark et al, 1980

*Mode of inheritance: AR=Autosomal recessive; AD=Autosomal dominant; XR=X-Linked recessive; XD=X-Linked dominant; NM=Not mentioned.
**Complete listing of authors in reference list.

Disease	Defect	Species		Reference
Lipoamide dehydrogenase deficiency	Lipoamide dehydrogenase	Pigeon	NM	Zemplenyi et al, 1975
Mannosidosis	α-mannosidase	Cattle	AR	Hocking et al, 1972
Mannosidosis	α-mannosidase	Cat	NM	Burditt et al, 1980
Mannosidosis	β-mannosidase	Goat	AR	Jones and Dawson, 1981
Neuronal glycoproteinosis	Unknown	Dog	NM	Holland et al, 1970
Pituitary dwarfism	Growth hormone deficiency	Mouse	AR	Eicher and Beamer, 1976
Pituitary dwarfism	Growth hormone deficiency	Dog	AR	Willeberg et al, 1975
Pituitary dwarfism	Growth hormone and prolactin deficiency	Mouse	NM	Sinha et al, 1975
AMINO ACID METABOLISM				
Albinism	Tyrosinase-positive	Goldfish	NM	Abramowitz et al, 1977
Albinism	Tyrosinase-positive	Mouse	NM	Pomerantz and Li, 1974
Albinism	Tyrosinase-positve	Hamster	NM	Pomerantz and Li, 1974
Albinism	Tyrosinase-positive	Frog	AR	Smith-Gill et al, 1972
Albinism	Tyrosinase-positive and negative	Chicken	AR	Brumbaugh and Lee, 1976
Albinism	Tyrosinase-negative	Mouse	NM	Coleman, 1962
Alcaptonuria	Homogentisic acid oxidase	Orangutan	AR	Keeling et al, 1973
Arginase deficiency in erythrocytes	Arginase	Monkey	AR	Shih et al, 1972
Chediak-Higashi syndrome	Unknown	Cattle	AR	Padgett et al, 1964
Chediak-Higashi syndrome	Unknown	Mink	AR	Padgett et al, 1964

Disease	Defect	Species	Inheritance	Reference
Chediak-Higashi syndrome	Unknown	Mouse	AR	Lutzner, 1967
Chediak-Higashi syndrome	Unknown	Cat	AR	Kramer et al, 1977
Chediak-Higashi syndrome	Unknown	Whale	NM	Taylor and Farrell, 1973
Cystathioninuria pyridoxine responsive	Unknown	Rat	NM	Sturman et al, 1970
Familial goiter	Thyroglobulin synthesis	Sheep	AR	Falconer et al, 1970
Familial goiter	Thyroglobulin synthesis	Goat	AR	de Vijlder et al, 1978
Familial goiter	Thyroglobulin synthesis	Cattle	AR	Van Jaarsveld et al, 1972
Gyrate atrophy of choroid & retina	Ornithine-δ-aminotransferase	Cat	NM	Valle et al, 1981
Histidinemia	Histidase	Mouse	AR	Kacser et al, 1973
Hyperammonemia (citrullinemia)	Arginosuccinate synthetase	Dog	NM	Strombeck et al, 1975
Hyperammonemia II	Ornithine transcarbamylase	Mouse	XD	Qureshi et al, 1979
Hyperprolinemia I	Proline oxidase	Mouse	AR	Blake, 1972
Hyperprolinemia II	Proline dehydrogenase	Mouse	AR	Blake et al, 1976
Riboflavinuria	Protein binding	Chicken	AR	Ramanathan et al, 1980
Tyrosinemia II	Tyrosine aminotransferase	Mink	AR	Goldsmith et al, 1981

LIPID METABOLISM

Disease	Defect	Species	Inheritance	Reference
Cholesterosis	Unknown	Parakeet	NM	Leav et al, 1968
Gangliosidosis GM1	β-galactosidase	Cattle	AR	Donnelly et al, 1973

Disease	Enzyme defect	Species	Inheritance	Reference
Gangliosidosis GM1	β-galactosidase	Cat	AR	Baker et al, 1971
Gangliosidosis GM1	β-galactosidase	Dog	AR	Read et al, 1976
Gangliosidosis GM1	Hexosaminidase A and B	Cat	AR	Cork et al, 1977
Gangliosidosis GM2	Hexosaminidase A	Dog	AR	Bernheimer and Karbe, 1970
Gangliosidosis GM2	Hexosaminidase A	Pig	AR	Kosanke et al, 1978
Gaucher's disease	Glucocerebrosidase	Sheep	NM	Laws and Saal, 1968
Gaucher's disease	β-glucosidase	Dog	NM	Van De Water et al, 1979
Gaucher's disease	β-xylosidase	Mouse	NM	Stephens et al, 1979
Globoid cell leuko-dystrophy	Galactocerebroside β-galactosidase	Dog	AR	Fletcher et al, 1966
Globoid cell leuko-dystrophy	Galactocerebroside β-galactosidase	Cat	XL	Johnson KH, 1970
Globoid cell leuko-dystrophy	Galactocerebroside β-galactosidase	Mouse	AR	Kobayashi et al, 1980
Globoid cell leuko-dystrophy	Galactocerebroside β-galactosidase	Sheep	NM	Pritchard et al, 1980
Hypercholesterolemia	Unknown	Rat	NM	Müller et al, 1979
Hypercholesterolemia	LDL receptor activity	Rabbit	NM	Kita et al, 1981
Hypercholesterolemia	Unknown	Pigeon	NM	Patton et al, 1974
Hyperlipidemia	Unknown	Chicken	NM	Ho et al, 1974
Hyperlipoproteinemia type IIb	Unknown	Rabbit	NM	Pescador, 1980
Hyperlipoproteinemia type III	Unknown	Dog	NM	Rogers et al, 1975
Hyperlipoproteinemia type IV	Unknown	Rat	AR	Koletsky, 1975

Disease	Defect	Species	Inheritance	Reference
Lysozyme deficiency	Lysozyme	Rabbit	AR	Prieur et al, 1974
Metachromatic leukodystrophy	Arylsulfatase A	Mink	AR	Christensen et al, 1965
Neuraminidase deficiency	Neuraminidase	Mouse	NM	Potier et al, 1979
Neuronal ceroid-lipofuscinosis	Unknown	Dog	AR	Patel et al, 1974
Neuronal ceroid-lipofuscinosis	Unknown	Cat	NM	Green and Little, 1974
Neuronal ceroid-lipofuscinosis	Unknown	Sheep	AR	Jolly et al, 1980
Niemann-Pick disease type A	Sphingomyelinase	Cat	AR	Wenger et al, 1980
Niemann-Pick disease type A	Sphingomyelinase	Dog	AR	Bundza et al, 1979
Niemann-Pick disease type C	Sphingomyelinase	Mouse	AR	Adachi et al, 1976
Sudanophilic leukodystrophy	Unknown	Mouse	XR	Torii et al, 1971
Tissue cholesterol storage	Unknown	Mouse	AR	Pentchev et al, 1980
STEROID METABOLISM				
Intersexuality	Unknown	Dog	NM	Selden et al, 1978
Lipoidal adrenal cortical hyperplasia	Unknown	Rabbit	AR	Fox and Crary, 1978
Male pseudo-hermaphroditism II	17-β-hydroxysteroid dehydrogenase	Rat	XR	Schneider and Bardin, 1970
Testicular feminization	Androgen receptor	Mouse	XR	Wieland and Fox, 1979

Testicular feminization	Androgen receptor	Rat	XL	Bardin et al, 1973

PURINE AND PYRIMIDINE METABOLISM

Xanthinuria	Xanthine oxidase	Dog	NM	Delbarre et al, 1969

METAL METABOLISM

Copper storage	Biliary excretion of copper	Dog	AR	Ludwig et al, 1980
Hemochromatosis	Increased iron absorption	Hyrax	NM	Rehg et al, 1980
Hemochromatosis	Increased iron absorption	Bird	NM	Lowenstine and Petrak, 1980
Menkes' kinky hair syndrome	Intestinal copper absorption	Mouse	XR	Prins and Van den Hamer, 1980

PORPHYRIN AND HEME METABOLISM

Crigler-Najjar syndrome	Glucuronyl transferase	Gunn Rat	AR	Johnson et al, 1959
Dubin-Johnson syndrome	Bilirubin excretion	Sheep	AR	Cornelius et al, 1965
Erythropoietic porphyria	Uroporphyrinogen-III cosynthetase	Cattle	AR	Batlle et al, 1979
Erythropoietic porphyria	Uroporphyrinogen-III cosynthetase	Squirrel	NM	Levin and Flyger, 1971
Erythropoietic porphyria	Unknown	Pig	AD	Jorgensen and With, 1963
Erythropoietic and hepatic porphyria	Unknown	Cat	AD	Glenn et al, 1968
Gilbert's syndrome	Bilirubin uptake	Sheep	AR	Cornelius and Gronwall, 1968
Protoporphyria	Ferrochelatase	Cattle	AR	Ruth et al, 1977

CONNECTIVE TISSUE, MUSCLE AND BONE

Disease	Defect	Species	Inheritance	Reference
Amyloidosis	Unknown	Cat	NM	Clark and Seawright, 1969
Amyloidosis	Unknown	Bird	NM	Covan, 1968
Amyloidosis	Unknown	Duck	NM	Rigdon, 1961
Amyloidosis	Unknown	Mouse	NM	Glenner et al, 1971
Amyloidosis	Unknown	Mink	NM	Schwartz et al, 1971
Ehlers-Danlos syndrome	Procollagen peptidase	Cattle	AR	Lapière et al, 1971
Ehlers-Danlos syndrome	Procollagen peptidase	Sheep	AR	Fjølstad and Helle, 1974
Ehlers-Danlos syndrome	Procollagen peptidase	Cat	NM	Counts et al, 1980
Ehlers-Danlos syndrome	Unknown	Dog	AD	Hegreberg et al, 1970
Ehlers-Danlos syndrome	Unknown	Mink	AD	Hegreberg et al, 1970
Ehlers-Danlos syndrome	Unknown	Cat	AD	Patterson and Minor, 1977
Ehlers-Danlos syndrome	Lysyl oxidase	Mouse	XL	Rowe et al, 1977
Hurler's syndrome (MPS I H)	α-L-iduronidase	Cat	AR	Haskins et al, 1979
Maroteaux-Lamy syndrome (MPS VI)	Arylsulfatase B	Cat	AR	Jezyk et al, 1977
MPS VII	β-glucuronidase	Mouse	AD	Yatziv et al, 1978
Mucopolysaccharidosis	Unknown	Cattle	NM	Hurst et al, 1975
Muscular dystrophy	Unknown	Chicken	AR	Julian and Asmundson, 1963
Muscular dystrophy	Unknown	Turkey	AR	Harper and Parker, 1967
Muscular dystrophy	Unknown	Dog	AR	Kramer et al, 1976
Muscular dystrophy	Unknown	Hamster	AR	Bajusz et al, 1966

Disease	Defect	Species	Inheritance	Reference
Muscular dystrophy	Unknown	Sheep	NM	McGavin and Baynes, 1969
Muscular dystrophy	Unknown	Mink	AR	Hegreberg et al, 1974
Muscular dystrophy	Unknown	Mouse	AR	Michelson et al, 1955
Osteogenesis imperfecta	Synthesis of bone matrix	Cattle	AR	Jensen et al, 1976
Osteogenesis imperfecta	Synthesis of bone matrix	Sheep	NM	Holmes et al, 1964
Osteogenesis imperfecta	Synthesis of bone matrix	Mouse	AR	Guénet et al, 1982
Osteopetrosis	Bone resorption	Cattle	AR	Leipold et al, 1970
Osteopetrosis	Bone resorption	Rat	AR	Cotton and Gaines, 1974
Osteopetrosis	Bone resorption	Rabbit	AR	Pearce and Brown, 1948
Osteopetrosis	Bone resorption	Mouse	AR	Raisz et al, 1977
Rickets (vitamin D resistant)	Renal 1-α-hydroxylase	Pig	AR	Wilke et al, 1979
BLOOD AND BLOOD-FORMING TISSUES				
Cyclic neutropenia	Stem cell defect	Dog	AR	Lund et al, 1967
γ-glutanylcysteine synthetase deficiency	γ-glutanylcysteine synthetase	Sheep	AR	Smith et al, 1973
Hereditary spherocytosis	Spectrin	Mouse	AR	Lux et al, 1979
Hereditary spherocytosis	Unknown	Mouse	AR	Huestis et al, 1956
Hemolytic anemia with stomatocytosis	Unknown	Dog	AR	Fletch and Pinkerton, 1973
Hemolytic anemia III	Glucose-6-phosphate dehydrogenase	Rat	NM	Werth and Müller, 1967
Hemolytic anemia III	Glucose-6-phosphate dehydrogenase	Mouse	A	Hutton, 1971

Disease	Substance/Enzyme	Species	Inheritance	Reference
Hemolytic anemia IV	Glucosephosphate isomerase	Mouse	A	Padua et al, 1978
Hemolytic anemia VI	Phosphofructokinase	Rat	NM	Chassin et al, 1978
Hemolytic anemia VIII	Pyruvate kinase	Dog	AR	Searcy et al, 1971
Methemoglobinemia	NADH-methemoglobin reductase	Dog	NM	Harvey et al, 1974
Microcytic anemia	Iron uptake	Mouse	AR	Edwards and Hoke, 1975
Sickling phenomena	Unknown	Deer	NM	Taylor and Easley, 1974
α-thalassemia	α-globin synthesis	Mouse	NM	Martinell et al, 1981
TRANSPORT				
Acrodermatitis enteropathica	Zinc (intestine)	Cattle	AR	Flagstad, 1976
Cysteine transport system	Erythrocyte	Sheep	AR	Young et al, 1975
Cystinuria	Cystine, lysine, arginine, ornithine (kidney)	Dog	XR	Bovée et al, 1974
Cystinuria	Cystine, lysine, arginine, ornithine (kidney)	Wolf	NM	Bovée and Bush, 1980
Cystinuria	S-sulphocysteine (kidney)	Blotched genet	NM	Elliot et al, 1968
Cystinuria	Cystine stones (kidney)	Mink	NM	Oldfield et al, 1956
Disaccharidase deficiency	Lactose, sucrose, trehalose, cellobiose (intestine)	Sea lion	NM	Kretchmer and Sunshine, 1967
Disaccharidase deficiency	Lactose (intestine)	Monkey	NM	Hart et al, 1980

Fanconi syndrome	Transport (kidney)	Dog	NM	Bovée et al, 1978
Hypertaurinuria	Taurine (kidney)	Mouse	NM	Chesney et al, 1976
Hyperuricemia	Uric acid	Chicken	NM	Zmuda and Quebbemann, 1975
Hypophosphatemic rickets	Phosphate (kidney)	Mouse	XD	Eicher et al, 1976
Iron malabsorption	Iron (intestine)	Mouse	XR	Bédard et al, 1971
Manganese deficiency	Manganese	Mouse	NM	Cotzias et al, 1972
Nephrogenic diabetes insipidus	ADH-response (kidney)	Mouse	NM	Kutscher et al, 1975
Nephrogenic diabetes insipidus	ADH-response (kidney)	Chicken	AR	Dunson et al, 1972
Renal glycosuria	Unknown	Mouse	AD	Butler, 1972
Renal glycosuria	Glucose (kidney)	Dog	NM	Easley and Breitschwerdt, 1976
Zinc deficiency	Zinc (intestine)	Mouse	AR	Piletz and Ganschow, 1978

CIRCULATING ENZYMES AND PLASMA PROTEINS

Acatalasemia	Catalase	Mouse	NM	Feinstein, 1970
Acatalasemia	Catalase	Dog	AR	Feinstein et al, 1968
Acatalasemia	Catalase	Duck	NM	Feinstein et al, 1968
Afibrinogenemia	Fibrinogen (Factor I)	Goat	AD	Breukink et al, 1972
Afibrinogenemia	Fibrinogen (Factor I)	Dog	AD	Kammermann et al, 1971
α_1-antitrypsin deficiency	α_1-antitrypsin	Turkey	NM	Meirom et al, 1974
C1 deficiency	C1	Chicken	--	Hammer et al, 1981
C2 deficiency	C2	G. Pig	AD	Bitter-Suerman et al, 1981
C3 deficiency	C3	Dog	AR	Winkelstein et al, 1981
C4 deficiency	C4	G. Pig	AR	Ellman et al, 1970
C4 deficiency	C4	Rat	AR	Arroyave et al, 1977
C5 deficiency	C5	Mouse	AR	Petit, 1980

Disease	Defect	Species	Inheritance	Reference
C6 deficiency	C6	Hamster	--	Hammer et al, 1981
C6 deficiency	C6	Rabbit	AD	Rother et al, 1966
Dysgammaglobulinemia	Unknown	Chicken	MM	Benedict et al, 1978
Factor VII deficiency	Factor VII	Dog	AR	Mustard et al, 1962
Factor X deficiency	Factor X	Dog	AD	Dodds, 1973
Hageman trait	Factor XII	Cat	AR	Kier et al, 1980
Hemophilia A	Factor VIII	Dog	XR	Dodds, 1981
Hemophilia A	Factor VIII	Cat	XR	Cotter et al, 1978
Hemophilia B	Factor IX	Dog	XR	Mustard et al, 1960
Hemophilia B	Factor IX	Cat	XR	Dodds, 1978
Hemophilia A and B	Factor VIII and IX	Dog	XL	Brinkhous et al, 1973
Hypoprothrombinemia	Factor II	Dog	AD	Dodds, 1979
Immunodeficiency, T-cell	Unknown	Mouse	AR	Crewther and Warner, 1972
PTA deficiency	Factor XI	Dog	AD	Dodds and Kull, 1971
PTA deficiency	Factor XI	Cattle	A	Kociba et al, 1969
Severe combined immunodeficiency	Unknown	Horse	AR	McGuire et al, 1975
Severe combined immunodeficiency	Unknown	Mouse	AR	Azar et al, 1980
Thrombasthenia	Platelet membrane glycoprotein III	Dog	AD	Dodds, 1967
Thrombopathia	Unknown	Dog	AD	Johnstone and Lotz, 1979
Thrombopathia	Unknown	Mouse	AR	Novak et al, 1981
Thrombopathia	Platelet serotonin deficiency	Rat	AD	Tschopp and Zucker, 1972
von Willebrand's disease	von Willebrand's factor protein	Pig	AR	Bowie et al, 1973
von Willebrand's disease	von Willebrand's factor protein	Dog	AD	Dodds, 1970

von Willebrand's disease	von Willebrand's factor protein	Rabbit	A	Benson and Dodds, 1977
X-linked agamma-globulinemia	Unknown	Horse	NN	Banks et al, 1976
X-linked agamma-globulinemia	Unknown	Mouse	XR	Scher et al, 1975

REFERENCES

Abramowitz J, Turner WA Jr, Chavin W, Taylor JD (1977). Tyro-
sinase positive oculocutaneous albinism in the goldfish,
Carassius auratus L., an ultrastructural and biochemical
study of the eye. Cell Tiss Res 182:409.
Adachi M, Volk BW, Schneck L (1976). Niemann-Pick disease
type C animal model: Mouse Niemann-Pick disease. Am J Pathol
85:229.
Altman PL, Katz DD (1979). "Inbred and Genetically Defined
Strains of Laboratory Animals." Part 1 House and Rat.
Bethesda: Federation of American Societies for Experimental
Biology.
Altman PL, Katz DD (1979). "Inbred and Genetically Defined
Strains of Laboratory Animals." Part 2 Hamsters, Guinea Pig,
Rabbit, and Chicken. Bethesda: Federation of American
Societies for Experimental Biology.
Andrews EJ, Ward BC, Altman NH (1979). "Spontaneous Animal
Models of Human Disease." Vols I and II New York: Academic
Press.
Arroyave CM, Levy RN, Johnson JS (1977). Genetic deficiency of
the fourth component of complement (C4) in Wistar rats.
Immunology 33:453.
Azar HA, Hansen CT, Costa J (1980). N:NIH(S) 11-nu/nu mice
with combined immunodeficiency: A new model for human tumor
heterotransplanation. J Nat Cancer Inst 65:421.
Bajusz E, Homburger F, Baker JR, Opie LH (1966). The heart
muscle in muscular dystrophy with special reference to
involvement of the cardiovascular system in the hereditary
myopathy in the hamster. Ann NY Acad Sci 138:213.
Baker HJ, Lindsey JR, McKhann GM, Farrell DF (1971). Neuronal
GM1 gangliosidosis in a Siamese cat with β-galactosidase
deficiency. Science 174:838.
Banks KL, McGuire TC, Jerrells TR (1976). Absence of B lymphocytes in a horse with primary agammaglobulinemia. Clin
Immunol Immunopath 5:282.
Bannerman RM, Edwards JA, Pinkerton PH (1973). Hereditary
disorders of the red cell in animals. Prog Hematol 8:131.
Bardin CW, Bullock LP, Sherins RJ, Mowszowicz I, Blackburn WR
(1973). Part II Androgen metabolism and mechanism of action
in male pseudohermaphroditism: A study of testicular feminization. Recent Prog Horm Res 29:65.
Batlle AM del C, Wider de Xifra EA, Stella AM, Bustos N, With
TK (1979). Studies on porphyrin biosynthesis and the enzymes
involved in bovine congenital erythropoietic porphyria. Clin
Sci 57:63.

Bédard YC, Pinkerton PH, Simon GT (1971). Ultrastructure of the duodenal mucosa of mice with a hereditary defect in iron absorption. J Pathol 104:45.

Benedict AA, Chanh TC, Tam LQ, Pollard LW, Kubo RT, Abplanalp HA (1978). Inherited immunodeficiency in chickens. In Gershwin ME, Cooper EL (eds.): "Animal Models of Comparative and Developmental Aspects of Immunity and Disease." New York: Pergamon Press, p 99.

Benson RE, Dodds WJ (1977). Autosomal factor VIII deficiency in rabbits: Size variations of rabbit factor VIII. Thromb Haemost 38:380.

Bernheimer H, Karbe E (1970). Morphologische und neurochemische Untersuchungen von 2 Formen der amaurotischen Idiotie des Hundes: Nachweis einer GM_2-Gangliosidose. Acta Neuropathol (Berl) 16:243.

Bitter-Suerman D, Hoffman T, Burger R, Hadding U (1981). Linkage of total deficiency of the second component (C2) of the complement system and of genetic C2-polymorphism to the major histocompatibility complex of the guinea pig. J Immunol 127:608.

Blake RL (1972). Animal model for hyperprolinaemia: Deficiency of mouse proline oxidase activity. Biochem J 129:987.

Blake RL, Hall JG, Russell ES (1976). Mitochondrial proline dehydrogenase deficiency in hyperprolinemic PRO/Re mice: Genetic and enzymatic analyses. Biochem Genet 14:739.

Bovée KC, Bush M (1980). Cystinuria in the maned wolf. In Montali RJ, Migaki G (eds): "The Comparative Pathology of Zoo Animals," Washington: Smithsonian Institution Press, p 121.

Bovée KC, Joyce T, Reynolds R, Segal S (1978). The Fanconi syndrome in Basenji dogs: A new model for renal transport defects. Science 201:1129.

Bovée KC, Thier SO, Rea C, Segal S (1974). Renal clearance of amino acids in canine cystinuria. Metabolism 23:51.

Bowie EJW, Owen CA Jr, Zollman PE, Thompson JH Jr, Fass DN (1973). Tests of hemostasis in swine: Normal values and values in pigs affected with von Willebrand's disease. Am J Vet Res 34:1405.

Breukink HJ, Hart HC, Arkel C, Veldon NA, Watering CC (1972). Congenital afibrinogenemia in goats. Zentralbl Veterinaermed Reihe A 19:661.

Brinkhous KM, Davis PD, Graham JB, Dodds WJ (1973). Expression and linkage of genes for X-linked hemophilias A and B in the dog. Blood 41:577.

Brumbaugh JA, Lee KW (1976). Types of genetic mechanisms controlling melanogenesis in the fowl. Pigm Cell 3:165.

Bulfield G (1977). Nutrition and animal models of inherited metabolic disease. Proc Nutr Soc 36:61.

Bundza A, Lowden JA, Charlton KM (1979). Niemann-Pick disease in a poodle dog. Vet Pathol 16:530.

Burditt LJ, Chotai K, Hirani S, Nugent PG, Winchester BG, Blakemore WF (1980). Biochemical studies on a case of feline mannosidosis. Biochem J 189:467.

Bustad LK, Hegreberg GA, Padgett GA (1975). "Naturally Occurring Animal Models of Human Disease: A Bibliography." Washington: National Academy of Sciences.

Butler L (1967). The inheritance of diabetes in the Chinese hamster. Diabetologia 3:124.

Butler L (1972). The inheritance of glucosuria in the KK and A^y mouse. Can J Genet Cytol 14:265.

Capen CC, Jones TC, Hackel DB, Migaki G (1972-1981). "Handbook: Animal Models of Human Disease." First to Tenth Fascicles. Washington: Armed Forces Institute of Pathology.

Ceh L, Hauge JG, Svenkerud R, Strande A (1976). Glycogenosis type III in the dog. Acta Vet Scand 17:210.

Chassin SL, Kruckeberg WC, Brewer GJ (1978). Thermal inactivation differences of phosphofructokinase in erythrocytes from genetically selected high and low DPG rat strains. Biochem Biophys Res Commun 83:1306.

Chesney RW, Scriver CR, Mohyuddin F (1976). Localization of the membrane defect in transepithelial transport of taurine by parallel studies in vivo and in vitro in hypertaurinuric mice. J Clin Invest 57:183.

Christensen E, Palludan B (1965). Late infantile familial metachromatic leucodystrophy in minks. Acta Neuropathol (Berl) 4:640.

Clark DG, Topping DL, Illman RJ, Trimble RP, Malthus RS (1980). A glycogen storage disease (gsd/gsd) rat: Studies on lipid metabolism, lipogenesis, plasma metabolites, and bile acid secretion. Metabolism 29:415.

Clark L, Seawright AA (1969). Generalised amyloidosis in seven cats. Pathol Vet 6:117.

Coleman DL (1962). Effect of genic substitution on the incorporation of tyrosine into the melanin of mouse skin. Arch Biochem Biophys 96:562.

Cook RD, Dorling PR, Gawthorne JM, Howell JMcC (1980). Generralized glycogenosis type II in cattle. Neuropathol Appl Neurobiol 6:79.

Cork LC, Munnell JF, Lorenz MD, Murphy JV, Baker HJ, Rattazzi MC (1977) GM_2 ganglioside lysosomal storage disease in cats with β-hexosaminidase deficiency. Science 196:1014.

Cornelius CE (1969). Animal models--a neglected medical resource. N Engl J Med 281:934.

Cornelius CE, Arias IM, Osburn BI (1965). Hepatic pigmentation with photosensitivity: A syndrome in Corriedale sheep resembling Dubin-Johnson syndrome in man. J Am Vet Med Assoc 146:709.

Cornelius CE, Gronwall RR (1968). Congenital photosensitivity and hyperbilirubinemia in Southdown sheep in the United States. Am J Vet Res 29:291.

Cotter SM, Brenner RM, Dodds WJ (1978). Hemophilia A in three unrelated cats. J Am Vet Med Assoc 172:166.

Cotton WR, Gaines JF (1974). Unerupted dentition secondary to congenital osteopetrosis in the Osborne-Mendel rat. Proc Soc Exp Biol Med 146:554.

Cotzias GC, Tang LC, Miller ST, Sladic-Simic D, Hurley LS (1972). A mutation influencing the transportation of manganese, L-dopa and L-tryptophan. Science 176:410.

Counts DF, Byers PH, Holbrook KA, Hegreberg GA (1980). Dermatosparaxis in a Himalayan cat: I. Biochemical studies of dermal collagen. J Invest Dermatol 74:96.

Cowan DF (1968). Avian amyloidosis. Pathol Vet 5:51.

Crewther P, Warner NL (1972). Serum immunoglobulins and antibodies in congenitally athymic (nude) mice. Aust J Exp Biol Med Sci 50:625.

Delbarre F, Holtzer A, Anscher C (1969). Xanthine urinary lithiasis and xanthinuria in a dachshund. CR Acad Sci (Paris) 269:1449.

de Vijlder JJM, van Voorthuizen WF, van Dijk JE, Rijnberk A, Tegelaers WHH (1978). Hereditary congenital goiter with thyroglobulin deficiency in a breed of goats. Endocrinology 102:1214.

Dodds WJ (1967). Familial canine thrombocytopathy. Thromb Diath Haemorrh (Suppl) 26:241.

Dodds WJ (1970). Canine von Willebrand's disease. J Lab Clin Med 76:713.

Dodds WJ (1973). Canine factor X (Stuart-Prower factor) deficiency. J Lab Clin Med 82:560.

Dodds WJ (1978). Inherited bleeding disorders. Canine Pract 5:49.

Dodds WJ (1979). Introduction to hemorrhagic disorders. In Andrews EJ, Ward BC, Altman NH (eds): "Spontaneous Animal Models of Human Disease," Vol I, New York: Academic Press, p 266.

Dodds WJ (1981). Second international registry of animal models of thrombosis and hemorrhagic diseases. ILAR News 24:R3.

Dodds WJ, Kull JE (1971). Canine factor XI (plasma thromboplastin antecedent) deficiency. J Lab Clin Med 78:746.

Dodds WJ, Moynihan AC, Fisher TM, Trauner DB (1981). The frequencies of inherited blood and eye diseases as determined by genetic screening programs. J Am An Hosp Assoc 17:697.

Donnelly WJC, Sheahan BJ, Rogers TA (1973). GM₁ gangliosidosis in Friesian calves. J Pathol 111:173.

Dunson WA, Buss EG, Sawyer WH, Sokol HW (1972). Hereditary polydipsia and polyuria in chickens. Am J Physiol 222:1167.

Easley JR, Breitschwerdt EB (1976). Glycosuria associated with renal tubular dysfunction in three Basenji dogs. J Am Vet Med Assoc 168:938.

Edwards JA, Hoke JE (1975a). Red cell iron uptake in hereditary microcytic anemia. Blood 46:381.

Eicher EM, Beamer WG (1976). Inherited ateliotic dwarfism in mice. J Hered 67:87.

Eicher EM, Southard JL, Scriver CR, Glorieux FH (1976). Hypophosphatemia: Mouse model for human familial hypophosphatemic (vitamin D-resistant) rickets. Proc Natl Acad Sci 73:4667.

Elliot JS, Ribeiro ME, Eusebio E (1968). Cystinuria in the blotched genet. Invest Urol 5:568.

Ellman L, Green I, Frank M (1970). Genetically controlled total deficiency of the fourth component of the complement in the guinea pig. Science 170:74.

Falconer IR, Roitt IM, Seamark RF, Torrigiani G (1970). Studies of the congenitally goitrous sheep. Biochem J 117:417.

Feinstein RN (1970). Acatalasemia in the mouse and other species. Biochem Genet 4:135.

Feinstein RN, Faulhaber JT, Howard JB (1968). Acatalasemia and hypocatalasemia in the dog and the duck. Proc Soc Exp Biol Med 127:1051.

Fjølstad M, Helle O (1974). A hereditary dysplasia of collagen tissues in sheep. J Pathol 112:183.

Flagstad T (1976). Lethal trait A 46 in cattle: Intestinal zinc absorption. Nord Vet Med 28:160.

Fletch SM, Pinkerton PH (1973). Inherited hemolytic anemia with stomatocytosis in the Alaskan Malamute dog. Am J Pathol 71:477.

Fletcher TF, Kurtz HJ, Low DG (1966). Globoid cell leukodystrophy (Krabbe type) in the dog. J Am Vet Med Assoc 149:165.

Fox RR, Crary DD (1978). Genetics and pathology of hereditary adrenal hyperplasia in the rabbit: A model for congenital lipoid adrenal hyperplasia. J Hered 69:251.

Gembardt C, Loppnow H (1974). Zur Pathogenese des spontanen Diabetes mellitus der Katze. Vet Pathol 11:461.

Gershwin ME, Merchant B (eds) (1981). "Immune Defects of Laboratory Animals." New York: Plenum, vol 1 and 2.

Glenn BL, Glenn HG, Omtvedt IT (1968). Congenital porphyria in the domestic cat (Felis catus): Preliminary investigation on inheritance pattern. Am J Vet Res 29:1653.

Glenner GG, Page D, Iserky C, Harada M, Cuatrecasas P, Eanes ED, De Lellis RA, Bladen HA, Keiser HR (1971). Murine amyloid fibril protein: Isolation, purification and characterization. J Histochem Cytochem 19:16.

Goldsmith LA, Thorpe JM, Marsh RF (1981). Tyrosine aminotransferase deficiency in mink (Mustela vison): A model for human tyrosinemia II. Biochem Genet 19:687.

Green PD, Little PB (1974). Neuronal ceroid lipofuscin storage in Siamese cats. Canad J Comp Med 38:207.

Guénet JL, Stanescu R, Maroteaux P, Stanescu V (1982). Fragilitas ossium (fro): A new autosomal recessive mutation in the mouse. In Desnick RJ, Scarpelli DG, (eds.): "Animal Models of Inherited Metabolic Disease," New York: Alan R. Liss.

Hammer CH, Gaither T, Frank MM (1981). Complement deficiencies of laboratory animals. In Gershwin ME, Merchant B (eds): "Immune Defects of Laboratory Animals." New York: Plenum, vol 2, p 207.

Harper JA, Parker JE (1967). Hereditary muscular dystrophy in the domestic turkey. J Hered 58:189.

Harris JB (1979). "Muscular Dystrophy and Other Inherited Diseases of Skeletal Muscle in Animals." Vol 317 New York: The New York Academy of Sciences.

Hart NA, Reeves J, Dalgard DW, Adamson RH (1980). Lactose malabsorption in two sibling rhesus monkeys (Macaca mulatta) J Med Primatol 9:309.

Harvey JW, Ling GV, Kaneko JJ (1974). Methemoglobin reductase deficiency in a dog. J Am Vet Med Assoc 164:1030.

Haskins ME, Jezyk PF, Desnick RJ, McDonough SK, Patterson DF (1979). α-L-iduronidase deficiency in a cat: A model of mucopolysaccharidosis I. Pediatr Res 13:1294.

Hegreberg G, Leathers C (1981). "Bibliography of Naturally Occurring Animal Models of Human Disease." Pullman: College of Veterinary Medicine, Washington State University.

Hegreberg GA, Hamilton MJ, Camacho Z, Gorham JR (1974). Biochemical changes of a muscular dystrophy of mink. Clin Biochem 7:313.

Hegreberg GA, Padgett GA, Ott RL, Henson JB (1970). A heritable connective tissue disease of dogs and mink resembling the Ehlers-Danlos syndrome of man. I. Skin tensile strength properties. J Invest Dermatol 54:377.

Ho K-J, Lawrence WD, Lewis LA, Liu LB, Taylor CB (1974). Hereditary hyperlipidemia in nonlaying chickens. Arch Pathol 98:161.

Hocking JD, Jolly RD, Batt RD (1972). Deficiency of α-mannosidase in Angus cattle: An inherited lysosomal storage disease. Biochem J 128:69.

Holland JM, Davis WC, Prieur DJ, Collins GH (1970). Lafora's disease in the dog: A comparative study. Am J Pathol 58:509.

Holmes JR, Baker JR, Davies ET (1964). Osteogenesis imperfecta in lambs. Vet Rec 76:980.

Howard CF Jr (1974). Correlations of serum triglyceride and prebetalipoprotein levels to the severity of spontaneous diabetes in Macaca nigra. J Clin Endocrin Met 38:856.

Huestis RR, Anderson RS, Motulsky AG (1956). Hereditary spherocytosis in peromyscus. J Hered 47:225.

Hunt CE, Lindsey JR, Walkley SU (1976). Animal models of diabetes and obesity, including the PBB/Ld mouse. Fed Proc 35:1206.

Hurst RE, Cezayirli RC, Lorincz AE (1975). Nature of the glycosaminoglycanuria (mucopolysacchariduria) in brachycephalic "snorter" dwarf cattle. J Comp Pathol 85:481.

Hutton JJ (1971). Genetic regulation of glucose-6-phosphate dehydrogenase activity in the inbred mouse. Biochem Genet 5:315.

Jensen PT, Rasmussen PG, Basse A (1976). Congenital osteogenesis imperfecta in Charollais cattle. Nord Vet Med 28:304.

Jezyk PF, Haskins ME, Patterson DF, Mellman WJ, Greenstein M (1977). Mucopolysaccharidosis in a cat with arylsulfatase B deficiency: A model of Maroteaux-Lamy syndrome. Science 198:834.

Johnson KH (1970). Globoid leukodystrophy in the cat. J Am Vet Med Assoc 157:2057.

Johnson L, Sarmiento F, Blanc WA, Day R (1959). Kernicterus in rats with inherited deficiency in glucuronyl transferase. Am J Dis Child 97:591.

Johnstone IB, Lotz F (1979). An inherited platelet function defect in basset hounds. Can Vet J 20:211.

Jolly RD, Blakemore WF (1973). Inherited lysosomal storage diseases. An essay in comparative medicine. Vet Rec 92:391.

Jolly RD, Janmaat A, West DM, Morrison I (1980). Ovine ceroid-lipofuscinosis: A model of Batten's disease. Neuropathol Appl Neurobiol 6:195.

Jones MZ, Dawson G (1981). Caprine beta-mannosidosis. Inherited deficiency of beta-D-mannosidase. J Biol Chem 256:5185.

Jones TC (1969). Mammalian and avian models of disease in man. Fed Proc 28:162.

Jorgensen SK, With TK (1963). Porphyria in domestic animals:

Danish observations in pigs and cattle and comparison with human porphyria. Ann NY Acad Sci 104:701.

Julian LM, Asmundson VS (1963). Muscular dystrophy of the chicken. In Bourne GH, Golarz MA (eds): "Muscular Dystrophy in Man and Animals," Basel: S Karger, p 457.

Kacser H, Bulfield G, Wallace ME (1973). Histidinaemic mutant in the mouse. Nature 244:77.

Kahn CR, Neville DM Jr, Roth J (1973). Insulin-receptor inter-action in the obese-hyperglycemic mouse. J Biol Chem 248:244.

Kammermann B, Gmür J, Stünzi H (1971). Afibrinogenämie beim Hund. Zentralbl Veterinaermed Reihe A 18:192.

Kaneko JJ (1980). "Clinical Biochemistry of Domestic Animals." New York: Academic Press.

Keeling ME, McClure HM, Kibler RF (1973). Alkaptonuria in an orangutan (Pongo pygmaeus). Am J Phys Anthropol 38:435.

Kier AB, Bresnahan JF, White FJ, Wagner JE (1980). The inher-itance pattern of factor XII (Hageman) deficiency in domestic cats. Can J Comp Med 44:309.

Kita T, Brown MS, Watanabe Y, Goldstein JL (1981). Deficiency of low density lipoprotein receptors in liver and adrenal gland of the WHHL rabbit, an animal model of familial hyper-cholesterolemia. Proc Natl Acad Sci USA 78:2268.

Kitchen H, Boyer S (1974). "Hemoglobin: Comparative Molecular Biology Models for the Study of Disease." Vol 241 New York: The New York Academy of Sciences.

Kobayashi T, Yamanaka T, Jacobs JM, Teixeira F, Suzuki K (1980). The Twitcher mouse: An enzymatically authentic model of human globoid cell leukodystrophy (Krabbe disease). Brain Res 202:479.

Kociba GJ, Ratnoff OD, Loeb WF, Wall RL, Heider LE (1969). Bovine plasma thromboplastin antecedent (factor XI) defi-ciency. J Lab Clin Med 74:37.

Koletsky S (1975). Pathologic findings and laboratory data in a new strain of obese hypertensive rats. Am J Pathol 80:129.

Kosanke SD, Pierce KR, Bay WW (1978). Clinical and biochemical abnormalities in porcine GM_2-gangliosidosis. Vet Pathol 15:685.

Kramer JW, Davis WC, Prieur DJ (1977). The Chediak-Higashi syndrome of cats. Lab Invest 36:554.

Kramer JW, Hegreberg GA, Bryan GM, Meyers K, Ott RL (1976). A muscle disorder of Labrador Retrievers characterized by deficiency of type II muscle fibers. J Am Vet Med Assoc 169:817.

Kramer JW, Nottingham S, Robinette J, Lenz G, Sylvester S, Dessouky MI (1980). Inherited, early onset, insulin-requiring diabetes mellitus of keeshond dogs. Diabetes

29:558.

Kretchmer N, Sunshine P (1967). Intestinal disaccharidase deficiency in the sea lion. Gastroenterology 53:123.

Kutscher CL, Miller M, Schmalbach NL (1975). Renal deficiency associated with diabetes insipidus in the SWR/J mouse. Physiol Behav 14:815.

Lapière CM, Lenaers A, Kohn LD (1971). Procollagen peptidase: An enzyme excising the coordination peptides of procollagen. Proc Nat Acad Sci USA 68:3054.

Laws L, Saal JR (1968). Lipidosis of the hepatic reticulo-endothelial cells in a sheep. Aust Vet J 44:416.

Leader RW, Leader I (1971). "Dictionary of Comparative Pathology and Experimental Biology." Philadelphia: Saunders, p 223.

Leav I, Crocker AC, Petrak ML, Jones TC (1968). A naturally occurring lipidosis in shell parakeets, Melopsittacus undulatus. Lab Invest 18:433.

Leipold HW (1980). Congential defects of zoo and wild mammals: A review. In Montali RJ, Migaki G (eds): "The Comparative Pathology of Zoo Animals," Washington: Smithsonian Institution Press, p 457.

Leipold HW, Doige CE, Kaye MM, Cribb PH (1970). Congenital osteopetrosis in Aberdeen Angus calves. Can Vet J 11:181.

Levin EY, Flyger V (1971). Uroporphyrinogen III cosynthetase activity in the fox squirrel (Sciurus niger). Science 174:59.

Lowenstine LJ, Petrak ML (1980). Iron pigment in the livers of birds. In Montali RJ, Migaki G (eds): "The Comparative Pathology of Zoo Animals," Washington: Smithsonian Institution Press, p 127.

Ludwig J, Owen CA Jr, Barham SS, McCall JT, Hardy RM (1980). The liver in the inherited copper disease of Bedlington terriers. Lab Invest 43:82.

Lund JE, Padgett GA, Ott RL (1967). Cyclic neutropenia in grey collie dogs. Blood 29:452.

Lutzner MA, Lowrie CT, Jordan HW (1967). Giant granules in leukocytes of the beige mouse. J Hered 58:299.

Lux SE, Pease B, Tomaselli MB, John KM, Bernstein SE (1979). Hemolytic anemias associated with deficient or dysfunctional spectrin. In Lux SE, Marchesi VT, Fox CF (eds): "Normal and Abnormal Red Cell Membranes," New York: AR Liss, p 463.

Lyon JB, Porter J, Robertson M (1967). Phosphorylase b kinase inheritance in mice. Science 155:1550.

Manktelow BW, Hartley WJ (1975). Generalized glycogen storage disease in sheep. J Comp Pathol 85:139.

Martinell J, Whitney JB III, Popp RA, Russell LB, Anderson WF (1981). Three mouse models of human thalassemia. Proc Natl Acad Sci USA 78:5056.

McGavin MD, Baynes ID (1969). A congenital progressive ovine muscular dystrophy. Pathol Vet 6:513.

McGuire TC, Banks KL, Poppie MJ (1975). Combined immunodeficiency in horses: Characterization of the lymphocyte defect. Clin Immunol Immunopathol 3:555.

Meirom R, Trainin Z, Barnea A, Neumann F, Klopfer U, Nobel TA, Dison MS, Plesser O (1974). Hypoproteinemia and α globulin deficiency in round heart disease of turkeys. Vet Rec 94:262.

Michelson AM, Russell ES, Harman PJ (1955). Dystrophia muscularis: A hereditary primary myopathy in the house mouse. Proc Natl Acad Sci USA 41:1079.

Mitruka BM, Rawnsley HM, Vadehra DV (1976). "Animals for Medical Research. Models for the Study of Human Disease." New York: John Wiley and Sons.

Mostafa IE (1970). A case of glycogenic cardiomegaly in a dog. Acta Vet Scand 11:197.

Müller KR, Li JR, Dinh DM, Subbiah MTR (1979). The characteristics and metabolism of a genetically hypercholesterolemic strain of rats (RICO). Biochim Biophys Acta 574:334.

Munger BL, Lang CM (1973). Spontaneous diabetes mellitus in guinea pigs. Lab Invest 6:685.

Murakami H, Takagi A, Nanaka S, Ishiura S, Sugita H (1980). Glycogenesis II in Japanese quails. Jikken Dobutsu 29:475.

Mustard JF, Rowsell HC, Robinson GA, Hoeksema TD, Downie HG (1960). Canine hemophilia B (Christmas disease). Br J Haematol 6:259.

Mustard JF, Secord D, Hoeksema TD, Downie HG, Rowsell HC (1962). Canine factor VII deficiency. Br J Haematol 8:43.

Nakhooda AF, Like AA, Chappel CI, Murray FT, Marliss EB (1977). The spontaneously diabetic Wistar rat: Metabolic and morphologic studies. Diabetes 26:100.

Novak EK, Hui SW, Swank RT (1981). The mouse pale ear pigment mutant as a possible animal model for human platelet storage pool deficiency. Blood 57:38.

Oldfield JE, Allen PH, Adair J (1956). Identification of cystine calculi in mink. Proc Soc Exp Biol Med 91:560.

Padgett GA, Leader RW, Gorham JR, O'Mary CC (1964). The familial occurrence of the Chediak-Higashi syndrome in mink and cattle. Genetics 49:505.

Padua RA, Bulfield G, Peters J (1978). Biochemical genetics of a new glucosephosphate isomerase allele (Gpi-1c) from wild mice. Biochem Genet 16:127.

Patel V, Koppang N, Patel B, Zeman W (1974). p-Phenylene-diamine-mediated peroxidase deficiency in English setters with neuronal ceroid-lipofuscinosis. Lab Invest 30:366.

Patterson DF (1974). Comparative medical genetics: Studies in domestic animals. Birth Defects 10:263.

Patterson DF, Minor RR (1977). Hereditary fragility and hyper-extensibility of the skin of cats. A defect in collagen fibrillogenesis. Lab Invest 37:170.

Patton NM, Brown RV, Middleton CC (1974). Familial cholesterolemia in pigeons. Atherosclerosis 19:307.

Pearce L, Brown WH (1948). Hereditary osteopetrosis of the rabbit. I. General features and course of disease; genetic aspects. J Exp Med 88:579.

Pentchev PG, Gal AE, Boothe AD, Fouks J, Omodeo-Sale F, Brady RO (1980). A lysosomal storage disorder in mice characterized by the accumulation of several sphingolipids. Birth Defects 16:225.

Pescador R (1980). The spontaneously hyperlipoproteinaemic rabbit. Life Sci 26:805.

Petit J-C (1980). Resistance to listeriosis in mice that are deficient in the fifth component of complement. Inf Immun 27:61.

Piletz JE, Ganschow RE (1978). Zinc deficiency in murine milk underlies expression of the lethal milk (lm) mutation. Science 199:182.

Pomerantz SH, Li JP-C (1974). Tyrosinase in the skin of albino hamsters and mice. Nature 252:241.

Potier M, Lu Shun Yan D, Womack JE (1979). Neuraminidase deficiency in the mouse. FEBS Lett 108:345.

Prieur DJ, Olson HM, Young DM (1974). Lysozyme deficiency - An inherited disorder of rabbits. Am J Pathol 77:283.

Prins HW, Van den Hamer CJA (1980). Abnormal copper-thionein synthesis and impaired copper utilization in mutated Brindled mice: Model for Menkes' disease. J Nutr 110:151.

Pritchard DH, Napthine DV, Sinclair AJ (1980). Globoid cell leucodystrophy in Polled Dorset sheep. Vet Pathol 17:399.

Qureshi IA, Letarte J, Ouellet R (1979). Ornithine transcarb-amylase deficiency in mutant mice I. Studies on the characterization of enzyme defect and suitability as animal model of human disease. Pediatr Res 13:807.

Raisz LG, Simmons HA, Gworek SC, Eilon G (1977). Studies on congenital osteopetrosis in microphthalmic mice using organ cultures: Impairment of bone resorption in response to physiologic stimulators. J Exp Med 145:857.

Ramanathan L, Guyer RB, Buss EG, Clagett CO, Listwak S (1980). Avian riboflavinuria-XI. Immunological quantitation of cross-reacting liver proteins from normal, heterozygous, and mutant hens. Biochem Genet 18:1131.

Read DH, Harrington DD, Keenan TW, Hinsman EJ (1976). Neuronal-visceral GM$_1$ gangliosidosis in a dog with β-galactosidase deficiency. Science 194:442.

Rehg JE, Burek JD, Strandberg JD, Montali RJ (1980). Hemochromatosis in the rock hyrax. In Montali RJ, Migaki G (eds): "The Comparative Pathology of Zoo Animals," Washington: Smithsonian Institution Press, p 113.

Richardson BJ, Inglis B, Poole WE, Rolfe B (1979). Galactose-1 phosphate uridyl transferase deficiency in the western grey kangaroo (Macropus fuliginosus; Marsupialia): A model system for gene therapy studies. Aust J Exp Biol Med Sci 57:43.

Rigdon RH (1961). Amyloidosis: Spontaneous occurrence in white Pekin ducks. Am J Pathol 39:369.

Rogers WA, Donovan EF, Kociba GJ (1975). Idiopathic hyperlipoproteinemia in dogs. J Am Vet Med Assoc 166:1087.

Rother K, Rother U, Müller-Eberhard HJ, Nilsson UR (1966). Deficiency of the sixth component of complement in rabbits with an inherited complement defect. J Exp Med 124:773.

Rowe DW, McGoodwin EB, Martin GR, Grahn D (1977). Decreased lysyl oxidase activity in the aneurysm-prone, mottled mouse. J Biol Chem 252:939.

Ruth GR, Schwartz S, Stephenson B (1977). Bovine protoporphyria: The first nonhuman model of this hereditary photosensitizing disease. Science 198:199.

Sandstrom B, Westman J, Öckerman PA (1969). Glycogenosis of the central nervous system in the cat. Acta Neuropath 14:194.

Scher I, Ahmed A, Strong DM, Steinberg, AD, Paul WE (1975). X-linked B-lymphocyte immune defect in CBA/HN mice. J Exp Med 141:788.

Schmidt-Nielsen K, Haines HB, Hackel DB (1964). Diabetes mellitus in the sand rat induced by standard laboratory diets. Science 143:689.

Schneider G, Bardin CW (1970). Defective testicular testosterone synthesis by the pseudohermaphrodite rat: An abnormality of 17 beta-hydroxysteroid dehydrogenase. Endocrinology 87:864.

Schwartz P, Wolfe KB, Beuttas JT (1971). Spontaneous amyloidosis in mink. J Comp Pathol 81:437.

Searcy GP, Miller DR, Tasker JB (1971). Congenital hemolytic anemia in the Basenji dog due to erythrocyte pyruvate kinase deficiency. Can J Comp Med 35:67.

Selden JR, Watchel SS, Koo GC, Haskins ME, Patterson DF (1978). Genetic basis of XX male syndrome and XX true hermaphroditism: Evidence in the dog. Science 201:644.

Sinha YN, Salocks CB, Vanderlaan WP (1975). Pituitary and serum concentrations of prolactin and GH in Snell Dwarf mice. Proc Soc Exp Biol Med 150:207.

Shih VE, Jones TC, Levy HL, Madigan PM (1972). Arginase deficiency in Macaca fascicularis. I. Arginase activity and arginine concentration in erythrocytes and in liver. Pediatr Res 6:548.

Smith JE (1981). Animal models of human erythrocyte metabolic abnormalities. Clin Haematol 10:239.

Smith JE, Lee MS, Mia AS (1973). Decreased γ-glutamylcysteine synthetase: The probable cause of glutathione deficiency in sheep erythrocytes. J Lab Clin Med 82:713.

Smith-Gill SJ, Richards CM, Nace GW (1972). Genetic and metabolic bases of two "albino" phenotypes in the leopard frog, Rana pipiens. J Exp Zool 180:157.

Solov'eva NA, Morozkova TS, Salganik RI (1975). Production of rat substrain with features of the hereditary galactosemia and studies of their biochemical characteristics. Genetika 11:63.

Stanbury JB, Wyngaarden JB, Fredrickson DS (1978). "The Metabolic Basis of Inherited Disease." New York: McGraw-Hill.

Stephens MC, Bernatsky A, Legler G, Kanfer JN (1979). The Gaucher mouse: Additional biochemical alterations. J Neurochem 32:969.

Stephens T, Irvine S, Mutton P, Gupta JD, Harley JD (1974). Deficiency of two enzymes of galactose metabolism in kangaroos. Nature 248:524.

Strombeck DR, Meyer DJ, Freeland RA (1975). Hyperammonemia due to a urea cycle enzyme deficiency in two dogs. J Am Vet Med Assoc 166:1109.

Stuhlman RA, Packer JT, Doyle RE (1972). Spontaneous diabetes mellitus in Mystromys albicaudatus: Repeated glucose values from 620 animals. Diabetes 21:715.

Sturman JA, Cohen PA, Gaull GE (1970). Metabolism of L-^{35}S-methionine in vitamin B_6 deficiency: Observations on cystathioninuria. Biochem Med 3:510.

Taylor RF, Farrell RK (1973). Light and electron microscopy of peripheral blood neutrophils in a killer whale affected with Chediak-Higashi syndrome. Fed Proc 32:822.

Taylor WJ, Easley CW (1974). Sickling phenomena of deer. Ann NY Acad Sci 241:594.

Torii J, Adachi M, Volk BW (1971). Histochemical and ultrastructural studies of inherited leukodystrophy in mice. J Neuropathol Exp Neurol 30:278.

Tschopp TB, Zucker MB (1972). Hereditary defect in platelet function in rats. Blood 40:217.

Valle DL, Boison AP, Jezyk P, Aguirre G (1981). Gyrate atrophy of the choroid and retina in a cat. Invest Ophthalmol Vis Sci 20:251.

Van De Water NS, Jolly RD, Farrow BRH (1979). Canine Gaucher disease--the enzymic defect. Aust J Exp Biol Med Sci 57:551.

Van Jaarsveld P, van der Walt B, Theron CN (1972). Afrikander cattle congenital goiter: Purification and partial identification of the complex iodoprotein pattern. Endocrinology 91:470.

Wenger DA, Sattler M, Kudoh T, Snyder SP, Kingston RS (1980). Niemann-Pick disease: A genetic model in Siamese cats. Science 208:1471.

Werth G, Müller G (1967). Vererbbarer Glucose-6-Phosphat-dehydrogenasemangel in den Erythrocyten von Ratten. Klin Wschr 45:265.

Wieland SJ, Fox TO (1979). Putative androgen receptors distinguished in wild-type and testicular-feminized (Tfm) mice. Cell 17:781.

Wilke R, Harmeyer J, von Grabe C, Hehrmann R, Hesch RD (1979). Regulatory hyperparathyroidism in a pig breed with vitamin D dependency rickets. Acta Endocrinol 92:295.

Willeberg P, Kastrup KW, Andersen E (1975). Pituitary dwarfism in German Shepherd dogs: Studies on somatomedin activity. Nord Vet Med 27:448.

Winkelstein JA, Cork LC, Griffin DE, Griffin JW, Adams RJ, Price DL (1981). Genetically determined deficiency of the third component of complement in the dog. Science 212:1169.

Yatziv S, Erickson RP, Sandman R, Robertson WVB (1978). Glycosaminoglycan accumulation with partial deficiency of β-glucuronidase in the C3H strain of mice. Biochem Genet 16:1079.

Yokote M (1970). Sekoke disease, spontaneous diabetes in carp, Cyprinus carpio, found in fish farms. I. Pathological study. Bull Freshwater Fish Res Lab 20:39.

Young JD, Ellory JC, Tucker EM (1975). Amino acid transport defect in glutathione-deficient sheep erythrocytes. Nature 254:156.

Zemplenyi T, Blankenhorn DH, Rosenstein AJ (1975). Inherited depression of arterial lipoamide dehydrogenase activity associated with susceptibility to atherosclerosis in pigeons. Circ Res 36:640.

Zmuda MJ, Quebbemann AJ (1975). Localization of renal tubular uric acid transport defect in gouty chickens. Am J Physiol 229:820.

Acknowledgements

Supported in part by Public Health Service Grant no. RR00301-16 from the Division of Research Resources, National Institutes of Health, US Department of Health and Human Services, under the auspices of Universities Associated for

Research and Education in Pathology, Inc.

SECTION IX.
SUMMATION

Animal Models of Inherited Metabolic Diseases, pages 505–514
© **1982 Alan R. Liss, Inc., 150 Fifth Avenue, New York, NY 10011**

SUMMATION

Donald F. Patterson

Section of Veterinary Medical Genetics and
Department of Human Genetics, Schools of
Veterinary Medicine and Medicine, University
of Pennsylvania, Philadelphia, PA 19104

This symposium has brought together a group of
scientists, not to address a discrete scientific question,
but for the more general purpose of fostering the recognition and study of animal models of inherited metabolic
disease. This we have attempted to do by combining papers
which review some established and developing areas of basic
genetics and metabolism with others that illustrate how
inherited metabolic defects in animals can be detected and
used to understand pathogenesis and approaches to therapy.
Our hope is that by informing and stimulating each other
and those who will read the proceedings of this symposium,
this area of research will become more widely recognized,
better organized, and more active.

In attempting to produce a summation of our meeting,
it very early became clear to me that it would be both
redundant and presumptuous to try to improve upon our very
thoughtful and lucid speakers by simply rephrasing what
they have said. Nor am I enthusiastic about preaching
again the value of animal models. That message comes
through very clearly in the excellent examples contained
in this symposium. Instead, I have chosen an approach that
I hope will convey in a concise way what I believe are
important points made by our speakers, at the same time
providing a light note on which to end our serious
discussions.

I. GENETIC BASIS OF DISEASE

Gene Structure, Organization and Expression - A.W. Nienhuis

Well, we thought that we finally had figured it out!
We knew what the structure of genes was about.
"It's simply a piece of the old DNA,
Transcribed and translated the usual way;
The way that Jacob and Monod always said.
It's simple," we said, "when it gets through your head."
But there's two kinds of Karyotes- there's Eu- and
  there's Pro-
And what's true for E coli just isn't so,
When it comes to the genes of a mouse or a man.
Mother Nature, it seems, has used more than one plan.
Dr. Nienhuis informs us it's much more exotic
When dealing with animals Eukaryotic.
Their chromosomes aren't just ribbons of genes,
One coming right after the other, it seems.
Eu-genes are in pieces - they're really quite split.
A Eu-gene's got introns in the middle of it.
And this complication just leads us to more:
RNA now needs cutting and splicing before
It can serve as a template, appropriate to
The making of proteins. That's <u>one</u> thing we knew.

Biochemical Variation and Comparative Gene Mapping
  S. J. O'Brien

Geneticists with a Darwinian zeal
Expected to find just one common allele
At a locus in animals abroad in the land.
They thought most mutations could not be so bland
As to stay, in the presence of natural selection;
But then, they were lacking the means of detection.
'Til refinement of protein electrophoresis
Provided a new and provocative thesis:
Genes for enzymes and most other proteins occur
In a number of forms that we often refer
To as polymorphistic, which happens because
Some mutants are good as the old allele was.

Whether neutral or selectionist theories prevail,
We now, so to speak, have the cat by the tail;
For with biochemically-clear variation
And use of somatic cell hybridization,
The genes can receive chromosomal assignments
Or be mapped to a chromosome arm, with refinements.
And what is the value of this, you may ask?
Evolution dissected, is one useful task.
O'Brien has told us it now would appear:
Whenever two loci in cats are quite near,
The same thing most likely is true in the pup,
And in man - they are not broken up!
Which gives us more reason for confidence that
Genetic disorders we find in a cat,
Or a dog, or a mouse, or a cow, or a goat,
Relate to the human - they're not so remote.

Hemoglobinopathies - from Phenotype to Genotype
    W. F. Anderson

We'd like to explain what pathology means,
In terms of what's wrong with the structure of genes;
Know if a control or a structural locus
Constitutes the exact pathological focus.
Dr. Anderson's talk has made it quite clear
That the answers to some of these questions are near.
At least with respect to the globins, we know
why some mutant's erythrocyte levels are low.
With the help of the enzymes that slice DNA,
And cloning techniques, we now have a way
To study the actual sequence of bases;
To know when those purines are not in their places.
In humans who have a resistant anemia
That goes by the general name, thalassemia,
Globin genes can be missing, we don't know where they went-
Perhaps an unequal crossover event
Has caused their deletion - whatever - they're gone.
In others they're present, but never turned on.
The latter are viewed with much more expectation
As keys to the problem of gene regulation.
What's needed are animal models of these
So look, animal hematologists, <u>please</u>!

II. DETECTION AND USE OF ANIMAL MODELS OF DISEASE

Recognition by Biochemical Methods - P. F. Jezyk

Having garnered some basics of genes and disease,
We moved to detection with relative ease.
Dr. Jezyk informed us of methods for screening
And showed us the defects his lab has been gleaning.
The screening of animals, canines and felines,
Selected because they had clinical signs
Suspicious of les maladies metabolique
Has been très revealing and un peu symbolique.
It's shown that they're out there, those errors inborn,
In all the variety Garrod had warned.
They'll be found in all species, if only we look,
Sufficient to fill a new Stanbury book.

Some Animal Models of Lysosomal Storage Diseases
  R. D. Jolly

To further confirm this delightful conclusion
Regarding the animal model profusion,
Dr. Jolly reviewed just what we know now
Of defects lysosomal, in especially the cow,
Where mannosidosis, a common defect,
In the Angus, no doubt, is a founder effect.

Identification of Hemostatic Defects - W. J. Dodds

Then on to the defects we call "hemostatic,"
Not "clotting," a term that is idiomatic.
Dr. Dodds in her country-wide studies of bleeding
In dogs of every conceivable breeding,
Has shown that the frequency of defects is higher
In some breeds because of a popular sire,
Who carried the Von Willebrand gene mutation
And spread it across an unwary nation!

Use of Animals for Evaluation of Therapy for
  Genetic Disease - R. J. Desnick

So what, there's a model! How can we ease
The ravages of that genetic disease?
Through the <u>use</u> of the model, when will we learn
How to treat <u>it</u>, and even beyond that, discern
How to put in a good gene to replace the bad?
Dr. Desnick has told us some thoughts that he's had:
Gene splicers are busy contriving to snip
Out a good gene which then they will carefully slip
In a host cell in which it will then integrate
With the genome and hopefully then replicate
With the cell, thus giving a guaranteed lifetime supply of
The enzyme the patient in question is shy of.
But that's in the future. For now we'll be pleased
Just to get in the enzyme and have it released
At the lysosome site of the storage, if that
Happens to be where the problem is at.
Another approach that was recently hit on
Involves enzyme manipulation.
In feline Maroteaux-Lamy,
The deficiency of ASB*
Results from a failure of dimerization
That's apparently corrected by medication:
Cysteamine and DTT**
Improve enzyme activity.
That appears to be the first time
For a CAT-abolic enzyme.

 *Arylsulfatase B
**Dithiothreitol

III. STRUCTURAL PROTEINS, ENZYMES AND RECEPTORS

Animal Models of Collagen Disease - G. A. Hegreberg

By affecting the structure of tissue connective,
We know gene mutations can make skin defective.
The enzymes and structural proteins it's got
Determine if skin will be stretchy or taut.
Dr. Hegreberg recently informed us that now
In the cat, and the sheep, and the dog and the cow,
We recognize various blocks in the plan
For the making of collagen, just as in man.
But the valuable, versatile model, I think
Is Ehlers-Danlos-like syndrome that's found in the mink.
There's cause for rejoicing by the short and the tall;
With this kind of mink, one size fits all!

Mucopolysaccharidoses - M. E. Haskins

Folks with mucopolysaccharidosis
Store glycosaminoglycan
We know in most types what the cause is,
There's at least seven types found in man.
Until recently, none were discovered
In beasts of the lab or the field,
But now screening tests have uncovered
Three models, Dr. Haskins revealed.
Two types were discovered in felines,
Type six and later type one.
In both cases clinicians could see signs
Involving the eyes and the bone.
But the sign that will most reassure 'ya,
It's almost a sine qua non,
Is mucopolysacchariduria
(That's abnormal in cats that are grown).

Immunodeficiency Disease in Animals - L. E. Perryman

As knowledge about the immune system grows,
And we learn of its parts in detail,
It's apparent how much immunology owes
To the animal models that fail
To produce a response when it's needed, and thence
Reveal a new link in the chain
Of the body's complex immunologic defense
Against antigens bugs can contain.
Dr. Perryman told us of models defined
In mice and Arabian foals.
In the latter, the defect's severe and combined,
Affecting both lymphocyte roles.
The T and B functions are both quite imperfect;
At present we're able to say
That it might be a purine kind of a defect,
But we know that it's not ADA.*

*Adenosine deaminase deficiency

Histocompatibility, Disease and Aging - E. Yunis

"The crown of life, our play's last act,"
Cicero on old age was opining.
What he didn't know, but now is a fact:
Its then your T-cells are declining.
Too many tick-tocks of the old thymic clock;
It runs down like a watch on the shelf.
Then suppressor T-cells aren't sufficient to block
B-cell clones that arise against self.
This theory's supported, Dr. Yunis explained,
By studies in mice and in man.
The data suggests that the program's ingrained;
It's a genetic kind of a plan.
It seems to depend on your HLA type.
If you have a desire to die late,
And your wish is, in time, to become overripe,
It is better not to B-8.

Inherited Defects in Receptor Function - G. D. Aurbach

A hormone may be high, and yet be ignored
By the target cells that it was meant for.
Dr. Aurbach revealed this is quite in accord
With defects that involve a receptor.
But its not quite that simple - there's more than one kind
Of hormone resistance for peptides.
Which is clear when we find its not just that they bind;
There's things that go on in cell insides.
If adenyl cyclase and a protein called G
Have relations much less than idyllic,
It's been found there's a very good chance there won't be
Enough AMP that is cyclic.
In the human condition that Albright
Appropriately called PHP,*
Parathyroid hormone is all right
Gut, kidney, and bone disagree.
Blood calcium's low and phosphorus high,
Parathormone just isn't effective.
We didn't before, but now we know why:
It's been found the G-protein's defective.

*Pseudohypoparathyroidism

H-Y Antigen and Intersexuality in Animals - J. R. Selden

When the gonad forms as a testis,
Its hormones will masculinize.
And this will insure that the rest is
Of suitable male shape and size.
But still there's a question we must face -
For years we have wondered just why
The testicle forms in the first place;
Now we think that it may be H-Y.
If H-Y's the testicular inducer,
And it's not something else from the Y,
An intersex may give the clue, sir,
Make the theory more easy to buy.
The intersex dogs Dr. Selden
Has studied lack chromosome Y,
Yet they've got ovotestes not seldom,
And they have, yes they do have, H-Y.

IV. PROFFERED PAPERS

The gangliosidoses, GM1, GM2,
Have been studied by Baker and Company, who
Reported some findings they've made in the cat
Where pathology closely resembling that
Found in children is basically due to the way
The enzymes deficient, Beta Gal and Hex-A,
Aren't breaking the substrates they're used for down right,
Thus causing in some way the meganeurite,
Which in turn has effects on neuronal geometries;
At least that is one of their current hypotheses.

The syndrome Fanconi first saw in the Swiss
Is now known in Basenjis (Bovée told us this).
In dogs, and presumably patients, there's lack
Of a way for the kidney to quickly get back
The solutes it filters, like glucose and phosphate
Amino acids, potassium, sodium and urate.

Filagrin seemingly acts to assemble
The keratin fibers of skin.
Er mice who are very deficient, resemble
A pupa, anomalous in
The ways Dr. Brown has just told us about.
While others, with just a bit more,
Survive, but he finds that their hair still falls out.
They're heterozygous Er.

Tfm's a mutation that's found in the rat
As well as the mouse and the cow.
Dr. Bullock was bothering telling you that
Because they are models of how
Cytoplasmic receptors for androgens can
Be deficient, and thereby can render
A person who's genotypically man,
Phenotypically, feminine gender.

Dr. Cork, in her Brittany Spaniel report,
Of the defect HCSMA,*
Showed neurons that seemingly fail to transport
Neurofilaments the usual way.

*Hereditary Canine Spinal Muscular Atrophy

They're not flowing to axons the way they should do,
Neurofilaments tend to meander,
Producing pathology similar to
Werdnig-Hoffman and Kugelberg-Welander.

When referring to Caprines,
One should say what that means.
What you're talking is, basically, goat,
Except in the one case
They lack mannosidase.
Then, there's something distinguished to note.
Now the search should occur,
Dr. Jones would concur,
For a human that models the goat.

Dr. Whitney's nice tale
About mice that are pale,
Because alpha globin's depleted,
Has shown their anemia
Is like thalassemia,
In which alpha chain genes are deleted.

I'm sure Chediak and Higashi must think,
"It's nice that our syndrome is now
Recognized, besides man, in the cat and the mink,
The mouse, killer whale and the cow.
But why are the leukocyte granules immense?
And why is hair color so pale?
Why does the body's own normal defense
Against microbes so commonly fail?
And what can it be, the common pathway
That ties all these defects together?"
No doubt, Chediak and Higashi would say,
"We've been wondering about it forever."
Chediak, I am sure, would be happy today,
And Higashi would doubtless agree.
Dr. Roder's results on the killer pathway
In Beige mice are exciting to see.
At the end of the tunnel, a light has been seen.
We've got a new foot in the door.
At last we may fathom that old C-H gene;
That's what animal models are for!

Index

acid phosphatase, 221, 223
acrodermatitis enteropathica, 280
adenosine deaminase, 161, 162, 273, 275,
    286-89, 294-95, 306, 309, 424-25
adenosine diphosphate, 118-19
adenylate cyclase, 353, 360, 362, 368
aging, 327-43, 349
agouti locus, 464-65, 467-68
allotransplantation, 48-50
α-globin, 135-37, 139
α-L-iduronidase, 186, 190-91, 201
α-mannosidase, 146, 148, 150, 152, 160
    162-63, 172, 176, 221, 223
α-mannosidosis, 169, 172-73, 176
amino acids, 94-103, 110, 135
amyotrophic lateral sclerosis, 449, 451,
    454-55
androgen, 369-76
    insensitivity, 369-71, 373-76
    receptor, 370, 372, 374-76, 379
    resistance, 353, 357
anemia, 11
Angus cattle, 145-50
animal disease
    enzymatic defects, 39-43
    and human disease, 32-33
animal models, 1-3, 5-6
    in collagen disease, 229-39, 243-44
    comparability of, 459
    in erythrocyte metabolism, 421-28
    in gangliosidosis, 203-9, 211
    in immunodeficiency diseases,
        275-86, 296, 306-7
    in inherited metabolic disease, 473-87
    in lysosomal storage disease, 27-32
    scoring system for, 459-60
    screening for IEM, 93-110, 114-16
    sexual determination, 381-408
    suitability of, 459
    see also specific animals
arginase, 425
arylsulfatase B, 42-43, 178, 184-86, 223
autoimmunity, 329, 331-32, 336, 340

β-globin, 134-35, 137
β-glucoronidase, 38-39, 45-46, 47, 49

β-hexosaminidase, 214-19
β-mannosidase, 166, 171-72
β-mannosidosis, 165-73
B lymphocyte, 271
    and aging, 330
    deficiency in animals, 280-84
    disorders in man, 272-74
    -T lymphocyte deficiency in animals,
        284-86
bleeding disorders, 117-26, 128-32
blood/brain barrier, 207-9, 214
body sex, 382-83
brachymorphic cartilage matrix deficien-
    cy, 245-48
brain, 374
breeding colonies, 29, 32, 43-44, 52

cancer, 67
carbohydrate, 94, 107-9
cartilage biosynthesis, 245-48
cat
    gangliosidosis in, 203-9, 211, 213-19
    and IEM, 67,85, 89-90, 93-110,
        114-16
    mucopolysaccharidosis in, 178-91
    syntenic map, 71-78, 85
cattle
    dermatosparaxis in, 238, 243
    immune disorders in, 279-80
    mannosidosis in, 145-50, 152, 153,
        163
central nervous system, 374
    in gangliosidosis, 216-17
    in mucopolysaccharidosis, 181, 187
ceroid-lipofuscin, 153-54
ceroid-lipofuscinosis, 150-56, 160-61, 163
Chediak-Higashi syndrome, 315-22
chickens, 282-83
chloroquine, 155-56, 161
chondrodystrophic dwarfism, 245
chromosome abnormalities, 389-401, 406
chromosome 17, 221-23
collagen
    animal models for disease of, 229-39,
        243-44
    composition of, 230

PROGRESS IN CLINICAL AND BIOLOGICAL RESEARCH

Vol 1: **Erythrocyte Structure and Function,** George J. Brewer, *Editor*

Vol 2: **Preventability of Perinatal Injury,** Karlis Adamsons and Howard A. Fox, *Editors*

Vol 3: **Infections of the Fetus and the Newborn Infant,** Saul Krugman and Anne A. Gershon, *Editors*

Vol 4: **Conflicts in Childhood Cancer: An Evaluation of Current Management,** Lucius F. Sinks and John O. Godden, *Editors*

Vol 5: **Trace Components of Plasma: Isolation and Clinical Significance,** G.A. Jamieson and T.J. Greenwalt, *Editors*

Vol 6: **Prostatic Disease,** H. Marberger, H. Haschek, H.K.A. Schirmer, J.A.C. Colston, and E. Witkin, *Editors*

Vol 7: **Blood Pressure, Edema and Proteinuria in Pregnancy,** Emanuel A. Friedman, *Editor*

Vol 8: **Cell Surface Receptors,** Garth L. Nicolson, Michael A. Raftery, Martin Rodbell, and C. Fred Fox, *Editors*

Vol 9: **Membranes and Neoplasia: New Approaches and Strategies,** Vincent T. Marchesi, *Editor*

Vol 10: **Diabetes and Other Endocrine Disorders During Pregnancy and in the Newborn,** Maria I. New and Robert H. Fiser, *Editors*

Vol 11: **Clinical Uses of Frozen-Thawed Red Blood Cells,** John A. Griep, *Editor*

Vol 12: **Breast Cancer,** Albert C.W. Montague, Geary L. Stonesifer, Jr., and Edward F. Lewison, *Editors*

Vol 13: **The Granulocyte: Function and Clinical Utilization,** Tibor J. Greenwalt and G.A. Jamieson, *Editors*

Vol 14: **Zinc Metabolism: Current Aspects in Health and Disease,** George J. Brewer and Ananda S. Prasad, *Editors*

Vol 15: **Cellular Neurobiology,** Zach Hall, Regis Kelly, and C. Fred Fox, *Editors*

Vol 16: **HLA and Malignancy,** Gerald P. Murphy, *Editor*

Vol 17: **Cell Shape and Surface Architecture,** Jean Paul Revel, Ulf Henning, and C. Fred Fox, *Editors*

Vol 18: **Tay-Sachs Disease: Screening and Prevention,** Michael M. Kaback, *Editor*

Vol 19: **Blood Substitutes and Plasma Expanders,** G.A. Jamieson and T.J. Greenwalt, *Editors*

Vol 20: **Erythrocyte Membranes: Recent Clinical and Experimental Advances,** Walter C. Kruckeberg, John W. Eaton, and George J. Brewer, *Editors*

Vol 21: **The Red Cell,** George J. Brewer, *Editor*

Vol 22: **Molecular Aspects of Membrane Transport,** Dale Oxender and C. Fred Fox, *Editors*

Vol 23: **Cell Surface Carbohydrates and Biological Recognition,** Vincent T. Marchesi, Victor Ginsburg, Phillips W. Robbins, and C. Fred Fox, *Editors*

Desnick, R., Patterson, D.,
Scarpelli, D.

Animal Models of Inherited
Metabolic Diseases Vol. 94

Name   Date

G. J. Brewer M.D.